S0-CQR-310

Neuromuscular Dentistry The Next Millennium

David M. Hickman, Editor

Anthology Volume V
ICCMO
The International College
of Cranio-Mandibular Orthopedics

MyoData
P.O. Box 89698
Tucson, AZ 85752
(800) 533-5121

Neuromuscular Dentistry—The Next Millennium

ISBN 0-9675046-0-0

The International College of Cranio-Mandibular Orthopedics, Seattle, Washington

Copyright © 1999 by The International College of Cranio-Mandibular Orthopedics

All rights reserved. No part of this publication may be reproduced or transmitted by any means, electronic, mechanical, or otherwise, including photocopying and recording, or by any information storage or retrieval system, without permission—in writing—from the publisher.

Design: Jamrose Design Associates
Typography and Prepress Production: Full Circle Type, Inc.
Printing: Herrmann Printing & Litho, Inc.

Table of Contents

Clinical

Politics and Philosophy

Editor's Comments

As we press on into a new millennium, one must consider the past and the lessons that we have learned to walk into this new era. To a great extent, the trials and tribulations of the past have created the character represented within those individuals who comprise a very unique organization, The International College of Cranio-Mandibular Orthopedics. As a group of health care professionals we have been forced to stand upon our knowledge of anatomy and physiology, and upon our ability to measure physiologic occurrences.

The ability to measure, envisioned by Barnard Jankelson, has given those who utilize biomedical instrumentation the ability to survive and thrive against a naïve, negative environment created by the academic community, as well as attempts from individual interest groups and financial pressures from the insurance industry to silence the truth.

At times these attacks have come from the uninformed, but often they have come from a subversive few who refuse to consider science and its applications, which are the foundation principles of neuromuscular dentistry. Often this has resulted for personal gain or lack of intellectual insight. One must continue to be mindful of the forces that would prevent all efforts to bring science and its clinical application to dentistry. As a close friend once told me, always remember that "In the Valley of the Blind the one-eyed man is King." Let us walk into this next millennium with both eyes wide open.

Remember those who have fought against this lack of vision—the Jankelsons, Garry, Cooper and many others. Soon it will be time to pass the torch and it is critical that those who press on to fight future battles be armed with a proper defense, but more importantly to create an impenetrable offence. As has already been proven, science is our only true offence.

I trust that this text will enable you to begin building your foundation, and allow you to face the opposition armed with the offensive tools to stand against whatever force may come against you. As Dr. Barney Jankelson would say "show me the facts and not your opinion." Inevitably, the art and science of neuromuscular dentistry will change, however, let us remember to base these future changes upon science and never be accused of having the inflexibility or lack of intellectual vision which often and typically has thwarted any scientific progress, ultimately resulting in *stagnation.*

David M. Hickman
Editor

Introduction to the ICCMO Anthology V

The International College of Cranio-Mandibular Orthopedics (ICCMO) was founded in 1979. The inspiration for the formation of the college was the research and teachings of Dr. Bernard Jankelson. While his contemporaries theorized about the essential role of muscle function in occlusion, Dr. Jankelson ("Dr. J"), with extraordinary perseverance and insight, proved the premise. It was under his guidance and impetus that bioelectronic instruments were created to "measure" what others only "observed".

The college was formed as an international educational forum for doctors who shared a common interest in the alleviation of pain and suffering in patients suffering from facial, head and neck pain specifically related to craniomandibular or temporomandibular disorders and in the creation of a neuromuscular based dental occlusion. ICCMO members recognize the essential role of objective measurement of the physics and physiology of the craniomandibular system.

The past twenty years have witnessed tremendous growth in numbers of members and countries of activity within North and South America, Europe and Asia and most importantly in the interrelations between members throughout the world. Scientists and health care providers from various disciplines are brought together annually at the Bernard Jankelson Memorial Lecture Forum of the American Section of the College and at the Biennial International Congresses. International meetings have successfully been held in Honolulu, Hawaii; Florence, Italy; Kyoto and Osaka, Japan; Banff, Canada and in Toulouse, France. These exciting meetings provide the opportunity for growth of interpersonal and intercultural relationships in both scientific and social areas. Together with international exchanges related to clinical practice and research, friendships have continued to grow and prosper. This is the essence of ICCMO.

This fifth anthology text represents a further maturation of the College's educational activities. The book has become the International College's vehicle for the presentation of the work of our members and invited teachers from around the world. Originally designed to publish the tests of oral presentations made at ICCMO meetings, this volume contains articles written specifically for this text. The scientific paper papers deal with basic science research on biology and biophysics and clinically applicable information. They represent the broad spectrum of activities of our members in both academic and private practice settings.

This book is designed to provide a broad base of knowledge about the interrelationships between systems in the head and neck in function and dysfunction. ICCMO is committed to the proposition that objective measurement is essential for proper diagnosis and effective therapy. Several articles are included that deal with the use and efficacy of objective measurement modalities. Through objective measurement and the creation of a healthy relationship between dental occlusion, temporomandibular joint and neuromuscular systems in the head and neck, dentistry is able to take a giant step into the new millennium with a firm footing in science.

States of perfect health and disease, optimum function and total dysfunction rarely exist in man. Rather, variable and varying intermediate states exist. In the case of musculoskeletal disorders, including temporomandibular disorders, this continuum exists. Diagnosis is often made by determining the quality of function, not in absolute black and white terms, but rather in relative terms. Treatment is designed to effect an improvement in form and function, not perfect health. Objective measurement provides the treating doctor with the ability to establish the direction of therapy with realistic treatment goals, and the capacity to measure treatment outcome along the way. This is evidence-based care. It is far more precise and effective than care based solely on subjective observations and opinions of success and failure by patients and doctors.

On behalf of the College, I wish to extend thanks to those who have contributed articles to this book. I would like to give special recognition to Dr. David Hickman, our editor, for selecting and editing the manuscripts and for the preparation of this book with our publisher. The College also recognizes the assistant editors, Dr. Rosie Rojas and Dr. Michael Mazzacco, for their efforts in reviewing and editing manuscripts and the assistance of Hallie Truswell, the College's Executive Secretary in the preparation and worldwide distribution of this book.

Barry C. Cooper, DDS
International President

Acknowledgements

At times developing and writing a text can be can be a very painful process. It requires an enormous effort by both the authors and the editors. These individuals have carried us to the threshold of "The Next Millineuum" and they are to be commended. The authors have gone far beyond the "call of duty" and I would like to thank each for their efforts: Drs. Carlo Bergamini, Maurizio Bergamini, Greg Bixby, Pietro Bracco, Barry Cooper, Andrea Deregibus, James Garry, Robert Graves, David Hickman, Robert Jankelson, Takayoshi Kawazoe, Michael Mazzocco, Allen Moses, Stefano Prayer-Galletti, Masahiro Tanaka, Mitsuhiro Tatsuta, Martyn Thomas, Norman Thomas, Richard Thomas, Larry Tilley, Bryan Weaver, and Gary Wolford.

To my associate editors, colleagues and friends, Drs. Michael Mazzocco and Rosemary Rojas, I thank you for your insight, vision and aid in completing this text.

To Hallie Truswell, exectutive secretary for the International College of Craniomandibular Orthopedics, a very special thank you for efforts which went well beyond your responsibilities.

David M. Hickman
Editor

Contributors

Carlo Bergamini, M.D., M.S.
Department of Immunology and Clinical Allergology
University of Florence, General Hospital
Florence, Italy

Maurizio Bergamini, M.D.,D.D.S., Ph.D., MICCMO
Professor and Chairman of Clinical
Odontostomathology
University of Florence Dental School
Florence, Italy

Greg Bixby, D.D.S., MICCMO
Private Dental Practice
Salida, Colorado, U.S.

Pietro Bracco, M.D., D.D.S., D.O.S., MICCMO, F.I.C.D.
Director of Orthodontics, School of Dentistry
University of Torino,
Torino, Italy

Barry C. Cooper, D.D.S., MICCMO
International President, ICCMO
Clinical Associate Professor
Department of Oral Biology and Pathology
School of Dental Medicine
S.U.N.Y., Stony Brook, NY
Private Practice
Lawrence and Manhattan, NY, U.S.

Andrea Deregibus, M.D., D.D.S., Ph.D., FICCMO
Professor, School of Dentistry
University of Torino
Torino, Italy

James F. Garry, D.D.S., MICCMO
Immediate Past International President, ICCMO
Private Practice
Fullerton, CA, U.S.

Robert Graves, D.D.S.
Professor and Chairman
Oral and Maxillofacial Surgery
School of Dentisry
West Virginia University
Morgantown, WV, U.S.

David M. Hickman, D.D.S., MICCMO
International Vice President, ICCMO
Director, Orofacial Pain Clinic
Professor, School of Dentistry
West Virginia University
Morgantown, WV, U.S.

Robert R. Jankelson, D.D.S., MICCMO
Chelan, WA, U.S.

Takayoshi Kawazoe D.D.S., Ph.D., MICCMO
Chairman and Professor
Department of Fixed Prosthodontics
Osaka Dental University
Osaka, Japan

Michael W. Mazzocco, D.M.D., Ph.D., MICCMO
Clinical Assistant Professor, School of Dentistry
West Virginia University
Morgantown, WV, U.S.

Allen J. Moses, D.D.S., MICCMO
International President Elect, ICCMO
Teaching Staff, Michael Reese Hospital
Advisor to FDA
Private Practice
Chicago, IL, U.S.

Stefano Prayer-Galletti, M.D., D.D.S., M.S., MICCMO
Assistant Professor of Clinical Odontostomathology
University of Florence Dental School
Florence, Italy.

Mitsuhiro Tatsuta, D.D.S., Ph.D.
Lecturer, Department of Fixed Prosthodontics
Osaka Dental University
Osaka, Japan

Masahiro Tanaka D.D.S., Ph.D.
Associate Professor, Department of Fixed
Prosthodontics
Osaka Dental University

Martyn R. Thomas, B.D.S., B.Sc., MICCMO
Part Time Instructor, Faculty of Medicine and
Oral Health Sciences
University of Alberta
Private Dental Practice
Edmonton, AB, Canada

Norman R. Thomas, B.D.S., Ph.D., F.R.C.D., M.C.V., MICCMO
Chancellor, ICCMO
Professor Emeritus, Faculty of Medicine and Oral Health Sciences
University of Alberta
Edmonton, AB, Canada

Richard Thomas, D.D.S., C.W.R.U.
Part Time Instructor, Faculty of Medicine and Oral Health Sciences
University of Alberta
Edmonton, AB, Canada
Private Dental Practice

Larry L. Tilley, D.M.D., MICCMO
Assistant Clinical Professor
School of Dentistry
Medical College of Georgia
Private Practice
Calhoun, GA, U.S.

Bryan Weaver, D.D.S., M.D.
Assistant Professor, Oral and Maxillofacial Surgery
School of Dentistry
West Virginia University
Morgantown, WV, U.S.

D. Gary Wolford, D.D.S.
Former Division Head of Oral and Maxillofacial Surgery
Henry Ford Hospital
Private Practice
St. Clair Shores, MI, U.S.

OVERVIEW

The Politics and Science of Neuromuscular Dentistry 1965–1999

Robert Jankelson

One Man Versus the Establishment—1965–1987

Introduction

When asked by the editor of the Anthology to contribute a chapter on the past, present and future of neuromuscular dentistry, I willingly agreed. After several months of research and 100 pages of manuscript, I conceded that a chapter was impossible to adequately capture both the science and politics which inextricably intertwine the history of neuromuscular dentistry. The science of neuromuscular dentistry is well chronicled in hundreds of scientific articles and textbooks, including past Anthologies.

I have chosen to explore two eras that define the politics that have impacted the science and progress of neuromuscular dentistry. The early years, from 1967 to 1977, gave insights and appreciation for the intellect and courage of one man, Bernard Jankelson ("Dr. J"), as he single handedly challenged the dental occlusionist establishment and their cherished dogmas. At any time during these ten years, if he had wavered in character or conviction, the science and technology we take for granted today would not be available. Dr. J's fight to bring a new technology and a new paradigm to treatment of the dental occlusion unleashed an epic confrontation with all the intrigues described by Becker. *"At this point the gloves come off. Already a lightning rod for the wrath of the Olympian peers, the would be Prometheus writhes under attacks on his or her honesty, scientific competence and personal habits. The pigeons of Zeus cover the new ideas with their droppings and conduct rigged experiments to disprove them. In extreme cases, government agencies staffed and advised by the establishment begin legal harassment."*[1]

The second political era explores the politics following Dr. J's death in 1987 and encompasses epic battles in the American Dental Association and U.S. Food and Drug Administration. By 1986 the scientific foundation for *neuromuscular* concepts and techniques was firmly rooted in the scientific literature. The technology was recognized as safe and effective for the purposes intended by the American Dental Association Council on Scientific Affairs. The clinical techniques were precise, predictable and successful. Yet, the neuromuscular clinicians, their philosophy and their instrumentation continued to be attacked by gnathological gurus whose status and livelihood depended upon the defense of the scientifically indefensible, by third party carriers intent on denial of payment, by IME's whose livelihood depended upon denial of patient claims, and by psycho-social academicians whose research funding depended upon adherence to a particular TMD paradigm.

The story of neuromuscular dentistry is not unique in the history of science and medicine. The iconoclast is labeled a pariah. His ideas, hypotheses and technologies are cast to the outer fringes of the scientific credibility. Only the preponderance of evidence and the iconoclast's conviction support him as his family, character and state of mind are impugned by the establishment priesthood. Thus is the story of Dr. J, neuromuscular concepts and neuromuscular technology.

The Neuromuscular Paradigm

Kuhn, in The Structure of Scientific Revolutions, stated: *"Led by a new paradigm, scientists adopt new instruments and look in new places. Even more important, during revolutions scientists see new and different things when looking with familiar instruments in places they have looked before."*

Many great scientific discoveries began with self doubt. As late as 1960 Bernard Jankelson wrote: *"The dentist should do everything possible to see that centric relation and centric occlusion do coincide, since instability can trigger hypertonic contraction of muscles ..."*[2] Few disciples of neuromuscular dentistry would attribute this statement to the father of neuromuscular dentistry, Dr. Bernard Jankelson. How persistent the attachment to dogma when we do not have the ability to see the truth hidden in space or submolecular spaces. Almost every scientific breakthrough has been preceded by a technologic breakthrough that allows us to see the previously unseen. Galileo's telescope opened the universe to new observation and cosmic theories. The light microscope, followed by the electron microscope, revealed previously hidden secrets of the cell, leading to previously unimaginable medical breakthroughs. Angle recognized the importance of muscle forces on occlusal form and function as early as 1906.[3] However, an occlusal paradigm that integrated the neuromusculature into a diagnostic and therapeutic protocol awaited the technological breakthrough that could predictably restore muscle to a more physiologic state prior to occlusal diagnosis.

The genesis of neuromuscular dentistry began with the collaboration of Bernard Jankelson and Dr. H.H. Dixon, a renowned muscle physiologist, working together at the University of Oregon School of Medicine in the early 1960s. In 1967 Dixon concluded, *"Experimental work with the myograph and chemical analysis indicates that fatigued muscle restores its energy with light, free motion at a rate below 60 contractions per minute. Fatigue spasm can be reduced by electrical stimulation. The device used should deliver a fraction of a milliampere, at around 100 volts, in a biphasic wave, at a rate of 40 to 60 impulses per minute."*[4]

The technology to change muscle metabolism and resting states was the breakthrough that broke the clinical dependency upon an elusive and unproven CO/CR occlusal reference. The electrical parameters established by Dixon, the serendipity of anatomic proximity of the V and VII cranial nerves to the coronoid notch and a clinical paradigm of muscle relaxation as a precursor to occlusal diagnosis and treatment culminated in Dr. J's development of the first prototype Myo-monitor in 1967.

"Transcutaneous electrical neural stimulation has the essential ability not only to relax the musculature, but also to initiate controlled isotonic muscle contraction to propel the mandible from rest position on an isotonic trajectory through the interocclusal space to a neuromuscularly oriented occlusal position in space."[5] The Myo-monitor provided a clinical tool to facilitate masticatory muscle relaxation and to generate an isotonic path of closure that was central to the neuromuscular paradigm. As so often occurs in science, the technology, i.e., the Myo-monitor, was necessary to define the new neuromuscular paradigm.

"In the past, character flaws couldn't wholly prevent the recognition of scientific truths. Both sides of a

controversy would fight with equal vehemence, and the one with better evidence would usually win sooner or later. In the past four decades, however, changes in the structure of scientific institutions have produced a situation so heavily weighted in favor of the establishment that it impedes progress in health care and prevents truly new ideas from getting a fair hearing in almost all circumstances. The present system in effect is a dogmatic religion with a self perpetuating priesthood dedicated only to preserving the current orthodoxies."[1]

The resistance to Jankelson's neuromuscular theory and the Myo-monitor was swift and predictable. Many a genius has been destroyed by people of lesser talent defending the status quo. It was inevitable that the genius and elegance of Bernard Jankelson's model for neuromuscular occlusion be challenged by a threatened establishment.

The Gnathologic Paradigm

Since 1986 TMD has been the arena for those opposing neuromuscular concepts and instrumentation. However, the early "Myo-monitor wars" were fought on the occlusal battlefield. Resistance to Barney Jankelson's neuromuscular theory came from the entrenched gnathologic school of occlusion. Gnathology had its origins in the mechanical concepts of Bonwill dating from 1850.[6] This theory postulated that during function, teeth slid against each other in a characteristic mechanical pattern. Centric relation was originally defined as *"the mandibular position when the heads of the condyles are in their most retruded positions from which the jaw can make free lateral movements."*[7] Lacking more physiologic parameters, gnathology also mandated that it is necessary to use a border reference position of the jaw as described by Posselt.[8]

Reproducibility became the operative mantra for seeking a "terminal hinge" position, however unphysiologic that position may be. Even reproducibility was an illusion.[9,10] Lacking objective physical data the gnathologic literature degenerated into semantic obfuscation as each new definition of centric relation failed to meet scientific and clinical scrutiny. In 1959, Shore listed twenty-six different definitions of centric relation.[11] After 130 years of gnathologic tradition, Dawson was describing occlusal bite registration in terms more appropriate to a Victorian novel than to scientific discourse: *"Now with gentle manipulation, the open jaw is lightly 'romanced' into the terminal hinge position."*[12] Twenty-five years later the "romancing" continues, but hard, objective evidence that CR results in the desired therapeutic effect is notably lacking. With seven different definitions of centric relation in the Prosthetic Glossary, only the definitions change to accommodate the anachronisms of a nineteenth century mechanical theory of occlusion.[13]

The apparent inadequacy of the operator explained every clinical failure. The gnathologic gurus admonished and promised more predictable results if only the clinician could be more precise, *"If the operator (or researcher) does not capture the true terminal hinge relationship, the value of a correct relationship cannot be fully appreciated. Furthermore, most experienced operators have confidence that their centric relation recordings are correct, but the study showed that experience cannot compensate for inadequate methods of manipulation or recording. Most of the methods used to manipulate the mandible into its terminal hinge axis do not work."* The author continues, *"It is also clear that recording it correctly is a demanding skill that must be carefully learned and precisely executed."*[14] Sadly, 25 years later the proponents of gnathology perpetrate the same unscientific premises. Even the most unapologetic of gnathologists concede the elusiveness of CR, yet rationalize the continuing semantic obfuscation. *"Unfortunately, the definition of centric relation keeps changing in the literature. However the changes simply relate to improvements in jaw manipulation techniques and new knowledge regarding the anatomic and physiologic position of the condyle."*[15] This is equivalent to an astronomer redefining the definition of light years with the discovery of each new star.

One Man Versus the Establishment

While electrostimulation was a familiar modality in the everyday practice of physical medicine, neurology and cardiology, such modalities were deemed inappropriate by a dental establishment searching for the perfect articulator. Early practitioners utilizing the Myo-monitor were frequently derided as *"jaw jerkers"* or *"jaw shockers."* Those of us pioneering the early use of the Myo-monitor were amazed at the dramatic patient response to the *myocentric occlusal treatment position.* A common patient response to the myocentric occlusion was *"that's where I told all those other dentists my bite should be!"* Prosthetic occlusal adjustments suddenly were reduced by 80%. No more post-insertion syndrome. Anecdotal, but the clinical evidence that the Myo-monitor was a clinical breakthrough in treatment of occlusal and TMD problems quickly mounted.[16-21]

When cherished dogma are threatened by new ideas, evidence and technology, *"The pigeons of Zeus cover the new ideas with their droppings and conduct rigged experiments to disprove them. Manuscripts submitted to scientific journals are reviewed for validity in the same way as grant requests. And who is better qualified to judge an article than those same eminent experts with their laurels to guard. Publication is accepted as evidence that an experiment has some basic value."*[1]

The Myo-monitor war of 1970–1975 found the occlusal establishment, with all the resources of their refereed journals, aligned against a singular foe, Barney Jankelson and "his" Myo-monitor.

I remember well these years when my father, a meticulous researcher and writer, had paper after paper rejected by the reviewers, only to discover an anti-Myomonitor article of questionable scientific merit in these same journals. The conclusions were always the same, the Myo-monitor centric position is always anterior to centric relation[22-24] and the Myo-monitor only stimulates muscle directly, not via neural mediation as suggested by Jankelson.[25-26] Any assault on the sanctity of centric relation upon which reputations were built was to be stopped at the castle wall. The refereed journal was the platform to repulse the invasion of original thinking. The pigeons of Zeus were circling the challenger to centric relation.

Methodology in these studies often included the use of clutches, gothic arch devices and wax bite registration materials, and protocols assured to produce the researcher's desired outcome. The finding that the Myo-monitor position was always anterior to centric relation was enough to condemn the Myo-monitor to the outer perimeters of scientific credibility. Practitioners using this device were assigned "fringe" status by the establishment. Accepting centric relation (take your choice of 26 definitions) as the occlusal gold standard was, and still is, an intellectual arrogance unsupported by scientific evidence. Yet, the CR icon stood unquestioned and off base to critical scrutiny by these men of science.

The establishment literature quickly "proved" that the observed muscle contraction was only direct muscle stimulation, not contraction neurally mediated via the V and VII motor nerves.[25,26] If this were proven it would invalidate Jankelson's theory of a Myo-monitor mediated *isotonic* closure to a *myocentric* position.

Meanwhile several studies, most conducted at Japanese Universities, supporting Jankelson's premise of neural mediation were published.[16,17,19] Jankelson's intensity duration curve studies supporting the Japanese studies, after several years of delay at the referee level, were finally published in 1975.[18] Later, Jankelson's neural mediation theory was definitively confirmed by Williamson. Patients were given succinylcholine as a muscle paralyzer at time of intubation for orthognathic surgery. Succinylcholine antagonizes acetylcholine at the myo-neural end plate preventing neurally mediated muscle contraction. The only way a muscle can contract under such conditions is by direct depolarization of the muscle itself. There was no muscle contraction with the Myo-monitor stimulus. This was definitive evidence that Myo-monitor induced muscle stimulation is neurally transmitted.[27]

By 1986 the weight of evidence began to quiet all but the most strident anti-Myomonitor foes. The period from 1977 to 1987 was marked by rapid improvement in the neuromuscular instrumentation. Neuromuscular instrumentation and techniques were routinely used in dental practices around the world.

Dr. J endured personal and professional vilification during the early years of the Myo-monitor and introduction of the neuromuscular philosophy. Strength of character and scientific validity were his only defense. After development and introduction of the J-2 Myo-monitor in 1969, he now tackled the challenge of developing objective measurement instrumentation to document masticatory function.

Dr. J's Dream—Objective Measurement of Occlusal Function

In 1973 Lerman observed that *"It cannot be overemphasized that since symptoms are muscle based, occlusal therapy of the MSD should be muscle oriented. Unfortunately, present clinical techniques which establish either terminal hinge or centric placement do not consistently accomplish this. With current techniques, an entire physiologic dimension is largely missing from analysis of the occlusion, namely the occlusion's compatibility with the muscles."*[28]

Funding the project himself, Dr. J assembled a R & D group of former Boeing engineers and biomedical engineers in 1970 to develop biomedical instrumentation to track jaw movement in three dimensions. Four years later, in 1974, the first K5 Mandibular Kinesiograph was introduced. The system sensed the spatial location of a small magnet attached to the labial of the lower incisor teeth allowing the clinician to diagnose and treat occlusal dysfunction with objective physiologic data.

Technology to monitor masticatory muscle activity at rest and in function in a clinical environment was necessary to elevate diagnosis and treatment of occlusion from art to science. Surface electromyography (EMG) is the technique by which the action potentials from muscle fibers are recorded and displayed. Surface EMG had been used in research institutions for many years to study masticatory muscle function. However, the first EMG designed specifically to monitor masticatory muscle in the dental office was introduced by Myotronics Inc. (EM-1*) in 1979. Real time EMG was integrated into the three dimensional computerized jaw tracking system in 1987, allowing the clinician to objectively correlate muscle activity and jaw position.

At the time of Dr. J's death in 1987 most of his dreams had been fulfilled. A new occlusal paradigm was gaining wide acceptance. The Myo-monitor was being used successfully by thousands of dentists around the world. He had pioneered and developed the first three dimensional jaw tracking system. He had collaborated with colleagues in Japan to develop the first clinical EMG to specifically monitor masticatory muscle activity. His contribution to the science of dentistry was a product of his professional passion and conviction. Shortly after Dr. J's death his disciples would need the same courage and conviction.

II. Posthumous Politics

ADA Politics 1988–1994

In 1986 the American Dental Association Council on Scientific Affairs granted the *Seal of Recognition* to Myotronic's neuromuscular instrumentation. The pigeons of Zeus could not abide the messengers of objective data. It threatened old dogma, it made IME rejections difficult, and as Becker described *"In general, projects that propose a search for evidence in support of new ideas aren't funded. Most review committees approve nothing that would challenge the findings their members made when they were struggling young researchers who created the current theories, whereas projects that pander to these elder egos receive lavish support."*[1]

It was now time to slay the messenger. The political battlefield shifted from occlusion to *TMD*. In 1988 a small group identified with the gnathologic occlusal paradigm joined a small group from the American Association of Orofacial Pain (AAOP), then the American Association of Craniomandibular Disorders (AACD), to exert political pressures upon the ADA to rescind the Scientific Council Seal of Recognition for neuromuscular measurement devices. Dr. Norman Mohl was retained by the ADA to review the scientific safety and efficacy of these devices as aids in diagnosis and treatment of TMD. The draft Report concluded that *"Except for devices that have been developed for electromyographic biofeedback, none of the other devices intended for treatment of TMD have the scientific evidence required for their recommendations."*

These devices included jaw tracking, surface electromyography, thermography, sonography, Doppler ultrasound, muscle stimulators. It appeared that the anti-instrumentation Luddites were strategically placed politically within the American Dental Association. Disciples of the neuromuscular paradigm were armed only with facts and conviction.

The 1989 ADA Mohl Draft Status Report rejecting the safety and efficacy of transcutaneous electrical neural stimulation (TENS), jaw tracking, and electromyography, and electrosonography became the manifesto of the anti-instrumentation Luddites. Ultimately it could not hold back the tide of scientific evidence that exposed the Mohl Report as a adhominem political diatribe, not a reasoned *scientific* document. Myotronics submitted a voluminous review of the scientific literature supporting the efficacy of surface EMG, jaw tracking and low frequency TENS for diagnosis and treatment of TMD to the ADA Council on Scientific Affairs. After unprecedented scientific scrutiny these devices were ultimately awarded the ADA Council on Scientific Affairs Seal of Acceptance.

"Manuscripts submitted to scientific journals are reviewed for validity in the same way as grant requests. And who is better qualified to judge an article than those same eminent experts with their laurels to guard?"[1]

Despite being marked **Draft Only, Not to be Referenced** and despite its rejection by the Council on Scientific Affairs the Mohl Draft Status Report appeared in over twenty refereed journals in the next six years. Many years after its rejection by the ADA Council on Scientific Affairs, the pigeon droppings from the original Draft Report trace a scatologic trail through the mainstream dental literature.[29-36]

Rigging of the FDA

"In extreme cases, government agencies staffed and advised by the establishment begin legal harassment..."[1]

Failing to achieve their political agenda through the American Dental Association, the anti-instrumentation Luddites resorted to improper and illegal distortion of the regulatory process, culminating in "rigging" of the October 1994 FDA Dental Advisory Panel convened to classify *muscle monitoring devices*. An Orwellian nightmare for the manufacturers of neuromuscular instrumentation began in 1991 when an anti-instrumentation cabal subverted certain FDA employees to bring the full wrath of the FDA regulatory process upon them. The 1994 FDA Dental Advisory Panel was designed to be the death knell of neuromuscular instrumentation and ideas.

Dickinson's FDA Review[36] in an article entitled "'Perverted' FDA: officials under criminal probe" chronicals the Machiavellian script for the panel: *"Without revealing that Myotronics' products, and similar ones made by another firm, BioResearch, were the only ones to be dealt with by the panel on a very loosely defined agenda ('muscle monitor devices,' a term that could cover over 30 other types of products as well), the FDA then appointed a notorious opponent of Myotronics' products and AADR member, State University of New York at Buffalo professor Norman Mohl as the panel's expert advisor."*

Not only did FDA conceal until the morning of the hearing its choice of old foe Bertolami to chair the hearing, but the FDA (or one of its "special government employees" on the panel) allegedly leaked Myotronics' presentation in advance to a witness who testified against the company's products.

"Myotronics and BioResearch got another shock when they saw the witness list: three well known political opponents of their technology, who had earlier fought unsuccessfully to get the American Dental

Association to rescind its approval seals for the firms' products."[37]

For two years the investigative trail of the FDA Special Investigator, the U.S. House Commerce Oversight Committee and the U.S. Department of Health and Human Services Inspector General exposed Machiavellian machinations by an anti-instrumentation group subverting FDA employees to destroy the manufacturers of neuromuscular instrumentation.

The "rigged" Panel recommended a Class III category for low frequency TENS, jaw tracking, surface electromyography and electrosonography. The class III category is reserved for implantable life threatening devices such as cardiac pacemakers, etc., and the Panel recommendation would effectively put the manufacturers of neuromuscular dental devices out of business. The principals orchestrating misuse of the FDA Dental Advisory Panel had apparent victory within their grasp. Within months the manufacturers of these devices would be forced out of business. The pigeons of Zeus had killed the messenger. The neuromuscular clinician would no longer have technology to objectively measure masticatory function or relax masticatory muscle. The neuromuscular paradigm, dependent upon its objective measurement devices, would die on the altar of FDA regulatory prohibition.

Dr. Barry Cooper and myself represented the neuromuscular position at the October 14, 1994, Advisory Panel Meeting. It is impossible to convey the shock, dismay and disappointment of that day. The pigeons of Zeus were circling vultures picking the final meat from the bones of Dr. J's neuromuscular dentistry carcass. However, the pigeons would soon be in a stew of their own making.

The next three years was a David versus Goliath battle to re-instate the legitimacy of neuromuscular instrumentation and to expose the egregious misuse of the governmental regulatory process by a small group of anti-instrumentation foes. With only conviction and facts on their side, a few neuromuscular disciples took on the AAOP academic establishment and the governmental FDA Goliath. Few could have predicted the outcome. Few will ever appreciate the price paid by the neuromuscular advocates.

The battle and its outcome was chronicled in the *Medical Devices and Diagnostic Industry* (MDDI) *Reports: "An investigation was begun by the FDA Office of the Chief Mediator in conjunction with the FDA Omsbudsman's Office in response to a 33-page letter of complaint filed in January 1995 by the Washington D.C. law firm of Hyman, Phelps & McNamara on behalf of Myotronics and BioResearch. In July 1995 Myotronics President Roland Jankelson testified at a hearing before Rep. Barton's House Commerce Oversight Subcommittee on allegations of FDA retaliation that the FDA's Office of Internal Affairs planned to conduct its own inquiry."*[38]

The House oversight Committee found Roland Jankelson's testimony so compelling, the credibility of then FDA Commissioner David Kessler's testimony to the Committee regarding the Myotronics' issues so lacking and the evidence of FDA coverup so powerful that the criminal investigation was transferred to the Inspector General, Department of Health and Human Services. The two year investigation concluded *"In 1994 the Dental Products Advisory Panel of the Center for Devices and Radiologic Health (CDRH) assessing a Myotronics Inc. dental measuring device was indeed rigged."*[39] The probe resulted in discipline and dismissal of certain FDA employees, including the author of the 1988 ADA Draft Status Report.[40]

Dr. James Garry, past President of ICCMO, Dr. Barry Cooper, President ICCMO, Dr. Larry Tilley, President of the TMD Alliance, my brother Roland Jankelson who possessed all the courage and tenacity of our father, and countless others gave their time and energies to overcome seemingly insurmountable adversaries. Yet, time after time the disciples of Dr. J have prevailed and the pigeons of Zeus retreat, only to reappear. Their venues change, but their agendas remain the same. The neuromuscular devices have the ADA Seal of Acceptance. The neuromuscular devices, after reconvening the Dental Advisory Panel, now have the lowest priority classification, which they should have been granted in 1994, and are recognized as safe and effective by the FDA.

In the face of overwhelming evidence of misbehavior and regulatory abuse by FDA employees, eight years after Norman Mohl submitted his anti-instrumentation Draft Status Report to the ADA, the FDA informed Mohl that his FDA consultantship would not be renewed. Further, the FDA accepted the voluntary resignation of Charles Bertolami, Chairman of the discredited 1994 Dental Products Panel. Other FDA employees were disciplined. The FDA admonished the 1994 Panel Secretary Carolyn Tylenda by inserting a confession of inappropriate conduct into her record. She had previously left the Agency. The FDA verbally admonished General and Restorative Device reviewer Dr. Gregory Singleton. Singleton left the Agency on August 1, 1997. An article in the Gray Sheet, an industry trade journal, reported that "Singleton was dismissed from the Agency in a quick and discreet manner, FDA says ..."

III. Future Politics

Biomechanical Versus the Psycho-social Paradigm

The pigeons of Zeus first littered the occlusal landscape with the scat of 100 year old dogma and personal agendas. When the weight of scientific evidence made flight impossible over the fields of occlusion the surrogate "TMD" landscape became littered with the scatologic refuse of their agendas. Losing the ADA and FDA battles the pigeons have now migrated to the land of psychosocial nirvana. A land where the clinician never has to worry about occlusal function or the tedium of precisely adjusting an occlusal appliance. This is the land of tricyclics, prozac and other pharmacologic wonders. A land where biomechanics and proprioception become non-operative.

"Our review of the literature revealed no substantiated theory of TMJ injury in cases of whiplash and no experimental evidence of forces that cause TMJ injury."[41]

Not surprisingly, the author is identified as a full-time independent medical examiner. The scatologic trail in this new land is easy to follow. The modus operandi varies not from the infamous Mohl Draft Status Report of 1988. The splat of pigeon droppings in the form of well placed *literature reviews* published in mainstream professional journals can now be heard in *psychosocial* land.

For the past 60 years, dating from the work of anatomist pioneer Harry Sicher and physiologist Hans Selye, clinicians and academics such as Shore and Bell have approached the problem as a primary *physical (biomechanical)* etiologic condition, albeit with concomitant secondary *psychosocial* overlays. This has been the reigning clinical paradigm for 60 years. The clinical and scientific evidence for such a model is consistent with anatomic and physiologic models of function/dysfunction. It has served our patients well.

It is only recently that a small group from the Academy of Orofacial Pain have denied occlusal causality for TMD. In its place they have attempted to posture TMD as a psychosocial disease caused by emotional stressors. The 1996 National Institute of Dental Research Consensus Conference clearly defined the *biomechanical* versus the *psychosocial* paradigm schism. This is the next field to be fertilized by the pigeons of Zeus.

The masticatory system with its unique mechanism of bilateral diarthrodial joints, precise tooth intercuspation and highly developed proprioception of the trigeminal system suggests a *biomechanical* pathogenic model that is generic to other musculoskeletal structures. Treatment to physiologically reposition the mandible to the cranium has been the foundation of TMD treatment for sixty years. The dental literature is replete with studies supporting the scientific and clinical basis for such treatment.

When *biomechanical* and *psychosocial* stressors impose demands that exceed the accommodative capacity of the organism, dysfunction and symptoms of TMD occur. The pathogenic model for TMD should logically embrace both the *biomechanical* and the *psychosocial* models.

The present effort by a small academic group to impose a strictly *psychosocial* model for TMD is more related to political agendas, allocation of grants for TMD research, IME consulting fees and pretense for denial of insurance re-imbursement, rather than sound scientific methodology.[42,43] In 1970 Dr. J was armed only with conviction and the facts. Thirty years later that is still the only defense of his neuromuscular disciples. The ADA and FDA victories attest to the strength of this conviction and fact.

The neuromuscular dentist will be well served by technologic advances in the next few years. Computer interface modules, faster hardware, easier to use software, EMG spectral analysis to give new insights into muscle fatigue states will make clinical procedures even better. However, as long as there are "pigeons of Zeus covering new ideas with their droppings" and anti-instrumentation Luddites with adhominem diatrabe there will be more political battles and more victories to win for "Dr. J" and our patients.

References

1. Becker RO, Seldon D: *The Body Electric.* New York: William Morrow, 1985.
2. Jankelson B: A technique for obtaining optimum functional relationship for the natural dentition. *Dent Clin N Am March,* 1960;132.
3. Angle E: *Malocclusion of the Teeth, 7th Ed.* Philadelphia: SS White; 1907;612
4. Dixon HH, Dickel HA: Tension headaches. *J Northwest Med* 1967;66:817-820.
5. Jankelson B: Neuromuscular aspects of occlusion: effects of occlusal position. *Dent Clin N Am* 1779;23(2):158.
6. Washburn HB: History and evaluation of the study of occlusion. *Dent Cosmos* 1925;67:223.
7. Report, National Society of Denture Prosthetists. *J Am Dent Assoc* 1930;17:1122.
8. Posselt U: Studies on the mobility of the human mandible. *J Prosthet Dent* 1957:7:787-789.
9. Dawson PE: *Evaluation, Diagnosis and Treatment of Occlusal Problems.* St. Louis: C.V. Mosby; 1974;52.
10. Jankelson B: Neuromuscular aspects of occlusion. *Dent Clin N Am* 1979;23(2):157-168.
11. Shore NA: *Temporomandibular Joint Dysfunction and Occlusal Equilibration, 2nd Ed.* Philadelphia: J.B. Lippincott; 1959;89-90.
12. Dawson, 56.
13. The Glossary of Prosthetic Terms, 6th Ed. *J. Prosthet Dent* 1994;71:59.

14. Dawson, 54.

15. McNeill C: Science and Practice of Occlusion. In: McNeill C, ed. *Fundamental treatment goals.* Quintessence Books; 1997;311.

16. Fuji H, Mitani H: Reflex responses of the masseter and temporal muscles in man. *J Dent Res* 1973;152(5):1046-1050.

17. Choi B: On the mandibular position regulated by the Myo-monitor stimulation. *J Japanese Prosthet Dent* 1973;17:73-96.

18. Jankelson B, Sparks S, Crane P: Neural conduction of the Myo-monitor stimulus: a quantitative analysis. *J Prosthet Dent* 1975;34(3):245-253.

19. Fuji H: Evoked EMG of masseter and temporalis muscles in man. *J Oral Rehab* 1977;4:291-303.

20. Jankelson B, et al.: Kinesiometric instrumentation: a new technology. *J Am Dent Assoc* 1975;90:834-840.

21. Wessberg GA, Dinham R: The Myo-monitor and the myo-facial pain dysfunction syndrome. *J Hawaii Dent Assoc* 1977;10(2):10-13.

22. Noble WH: Antero-posterior position of the Myo-monitor centric. *J Prosthet Dent* 1975;33(4):398-402.

23. Remien JC, Ash M: Myo-monitor centric and evaluation. *J Prosthet Dent* 1974;31(2):137-145.

24. Azarbal M: Comparison of Myo-monitor centric position to centric relation and centric occlusion. *J Prosthet Dent* 1977;38(3):331-337.

25. DeBoever J, McCall WD: *Physiologic aspects of masticatory muscle stimulation: the Myo-monitor.* Quintessence Int 1972;5:57-58.

26. Bessette RW, Quinlivan JT: Electromyographic evaluation of the Myo-monitor. *J Prosthet Dent* 1973;30(1):19-24.

27. Williamson EH: Myo-monitor rest position in the presence and absence of stress. *Facial Ortho and Temporomand Arthro Vol III* 1986;2:14-17.

28. Lerman MD: Unifying concept of the TMJ pain-dysfunction syndrome. *J Am Dent Assoc* 1973;86:468.

29. Mohl ND, Lund JP, Widmer CG, McCall WD: Devices for the diagnosis and treatment of temporomandibular disorders. Part II. Electromyography and sonography. *J Prosthet Dent* 1990;63(3):332-335.

30. Mohl ND, McCall WD, Lund JP, Plesh O: Devices for the diagnosis and treatment of temporomandibular disorders. Part I: Introduction, scientific evidence and jaw tracking. *J Prosthet Dent* 1990;63(2):198-201.

31. Mohl ND, Ohrbach RK, Crow CC, Gross AJ: Devices for the diagnosis and treatment of temporomandibular disorders. Part III: Thermography, ultrasound, electrical stimulation and electromyographic feedback. *J Prosthet Dent* 1990;63(4):472-477.

32. Lund JP, Widmer CG: An evaluation of the use of surface electromyography in the diagnosis, documentation and treatment of dental patients. *J Craniomandib Dis* 1989;3(3):125-137.

33. Lund JP, Lavigne G, Feine JS: The use of electronic devices in the diagnosis and treatment of temporomandibular disorders. *J Canadian Dent Assoc* 1989;55(9):749-750.

34. Mohl ND: Temporomandibular disorders: The role of occlusion, TMJ imaging and electronic devices. *J Am Coll Dent* 1991:158(3):4-10.

35. Mohl ND, Crow H: Role of electronic devices in diagnosis of temporomandibular disorders. *J NY Dent Soc* 1993;59(10):57-60.

36. Mohl ND, McCall WD, Lund JP, Plesh O: Devices for the diagnosis and treatment of temporomandibular disorders, Par I. *Oral Health* June,1990:17-19.

37. Dickinson's FDA Review, "Perverted" FDA officials under criminal probe. 1995;2(8):21.

38. M-D-D-I Reports, "The Gray Sheet" Dental products advisory panel chair resigns following release of IG probe. Oct 20, 1997:6.

39. Dickinson's FDA Review. Biased advisors: FDA slaps staffers as probes continue. Sept 1997:6.

40. *Ibid.*

41. Ferrari R, Leonard MS: Whiplash and temporomandibular disorders: a critical review. *J Am Dent Assoc* 1998;129:1739-1745.

42. Shankland WE: Off come the gloves. *J Craniomandib Pract* 1998;16(4):212-213.

43. Tilley LL, et al.: A look at the facts. *J Craniomandib Pract* 1998;16(4):207-210.

Scientific Rationale for Biomedical Instrumentation

Barry C. Cooper

"If you can measure something, it is a fact; if not, it is an opinion."
—US Supreme Court Justice Benjamin Cardozo

Attempts have been made by dentists to "measure" dental occlusion for decades. Most have utilized various forms of mechanical apparatus, which have added artifact and inaccuracies. All have been static and recorded only the mandibular component of occlusion.

Occlusion Is a Dynamic Phenomenon

Definition: Neuromuscular Occlusion is a stable position of maximum maxillo-mandibular intercuspation, which is synchronized with bilaterally symmetrical elevator muscle activity. The position is achieved by electrical stimulation (TENS) of relaxed masticatory muscles to move the mandible on a trajectory, which originates at a muscularly rested mandibular position.[1]

The concept of Neuromuscular Occlusion and the utilization of biomedical instrumentation in dentistry are inextricably bound. Dr. Bernard Jankelson developed both the occlusal concept and the instrumentation. In order to create a dental occlusion synchronized with healthy mandibular function and a healthy neuromuscular system involving the masticatory muscles, the capacity to relax masticatory muscles must exist. In addition, the capability of objective quantification of all the physical components of mandibular function and dental occlusion must be available. There are significantly more components or parameters to dental occlusion than merely the manner in which the maxillary and mandibular teeth interdigitate.

Dental occlusion is the "end point" of a dynamic activity that involves the mandible, maxilla, dentition, temporomandibular joints, the masticatory muscle system, and the neighboring craniocervical muscle system, as well as the peripheral and central nervous systems. Intimately related to dental occlusion is the resting or postural position of the mandible, which is the "beginning point" of dental occlusion. The neuromuscular system postures the mandible "at rest" and moves the mandible from the rest position to occlusion. Failure to address the dynamic elements of occlusion in creating a therapeutic occlusion may result in a functional compromise. This may predispose to and can ultimately lead to the destruction of the dentition, the supporting structures, the temporomandibular joints, and/or dysfunction in the neuromuscular apparatus.

Fortunately, the human body has the capacity to adapt to imperfection in both form and function in an accommodative manner. The adaptive capacity however has variable limits, which can be exceeded under various circumstances. Sometimes this excess occurs as a direct result of dental procedures or the therapeutic occlusion created. Sometimes, external events or forces, including traumatic injuries, and physical or emotional stresses, can exceed the system's adaptive capacity. The result can be the precipitation of dysfunction and/or pain often associated with temporomandibular disorders. The solution often lies in the improvement of the dental occlusion by the creation of a therapeutic occlusion synchronized with healthy neuromuscular apparatus, a *neuromuscular occlusion.*[2,3]

There are many key elements in dental occlusion, including the interdigitation of the teeth, as well as the path of exit from and entrance into that intercuspation. Equally important is the muscular activity associated with mandibular positions at rest, in occlusion, during opening, and during closing, and also the functioning of the temporomandibular joints during all of the mandible's dynamic activities. These are all key elements involved in dental occlusion.

The Therapeutic Goal

The therapeutic goal of any treatment regimen is to improve health by returning the body to an optimal state of comfort and function. Dental occlusion is purposefully modified for various reasons, including the correction of malocclusion, esthetics, and the restoration of defective or missing dentition. The alteration of the dental occlusion, temporarily or durably, has also been shown to be effective in the relief of certain forms of temporomandibular disorders.

Whatever the reason for alteration of the dental occlusion, justification for the occlusal modification is required, as is the proof of medical necessity of the therapeutic intervention. In current health insurance parlance, two terms are frequently used: outcome measurement and evidence-based care. Analysis of both of these terms reveals the essential role of objective biomedical measurement. In order to justify the medical necessity of any medical or dental procedures, a state of disease must be demonstrable. Disease by definition is a deviation or interruption in the normal structure of a body part or system.[4] In order to measure the outcome of a therapeutic intervention, the status of a patient at initiation of therapy must be measured and recorded. It is the comparison of the functional status pre-treatment and post-treatment that determines the value of a therapeutic intervention. A positive therapeutic result, which is physiological improvement in health, can only be demonstrated with certainty with hard evidence. This hard outcome evidence is obtained, not merely by asking patients how do they feel, but by measuring how form and/or function have been improved. Biomedical instrumentation as utilized as an aid in the creation of neuromuscular occlusion, permits the dentist to objectively evaluate the status of patients' mandibular and masticatory muscle function before and following treatment (outcome measurement). This is evidence-based care.[1]

Biomedical Instrumentation in Medicine and Dentistry

Initial diagnosis in dentistry and in medicine is based on information gained from a carefully obtained history and from a comprehensive clinical examination. Rational treatment is based on an understanding of the pathogenesis of the disease being treated, but it should also be based on an accurate diagnosis. It has been shown repeatedly that clinical examination per se can lead to gross errors in diagnosis.[5,6] The diagnostic process progresses, as additional hard data are obtained.[1] Throughout all disciplines in health care, bioelectronic instrumentation has assumed an essential role. Wherever possible, the computer has been employed to aid the doctor in arriving at a diagnosis, quantifying the parameters of the illness being treated, designing therapy, and evaluating therapeutic outcome. As part of a routine "healthy" medical examination, for example, the internist may prescribe electronic testing of heart function under various conditions, respiratory function, and analysis of blood chemistry. If corrective intervention is undertaken, computerized testing is subsequently repeated to determine whether the therapeutic intervention has been successful and whether any dysfunction or disorder remains. It is no longer reasonable, customary, or acceptable for the physician to rely solely on history and clinical evaluation using only direct visual examination, stethoscopic evaluation of respiration and cardiac function, and palpation. All medical specialty care is likewise dependent upon sophisticated medically necessary biomedical testing modalities. With data obtained from biomedical testing, clinicians can reduce their reliance on subjective symptoms and clinical observations, which are known to often be inaccurate and imprecise.

Within the health care disciplines, dentistry alone with small exceptions has remained reticent to enter the age of electronic measurement. Exceptions include imaging technology as well as endodontic techniques. The field of dental occlusion has remained essentially unchanged in decades, relying on intraoral and extraoral mechanical recording devices to transfer static artificial maxillo-mandibular relationships from the patient to the dental laboratory and then back again to the patient.

The only substantive modification in occlusal concepts within recent years was the change in the designation of the location of the "ideal" centric relation condylar position. Formerly it was considered to be the uppermost/most posterior position in the glenoid fossa, and now it is the uppermost/most anterior position against the slope of the articular eminence with a disk interposed. Even this concept is often appended to mechanical principles and is clinically achieved by artificial manual mandibular manipulations of various forms. With the exception of one, all occlusal philosophies are still without objective dynamic measurement and proof of physiological soundness.

The Role of Electronic Measurement Instrumentation

The capacity to record, scrutinize, and analyze gross and fine movements of the mandible and joint sounds, while monitoring the activity of the masticatory muscles, enables the dentist to create a measured occlusion position with knowledge of the masticatory muscular implications of that occlusion. In the absence of objective measurement, occlusion can indeed be created, as it has historically been done, but the mandibular and muscular functional implications are unknown. Occlusion so created can be beneficial or deleterious to mandibular and masticatory muscle and joint function. Without objective measurement, the dentist cannot know whether the occlusion, which is created, is physiologically sound or not.

Electronic Mandibular Tracking

Electronic instrumentation which tracks the position and movement of the mandible enables the dentist to record and scrutinize in three dimensions the position of the mandible at occlusion and at rest position, as well as during natural and artificially performed movements. Large movements from occlusion to maximum opening and the return to occlusion can be recorded and the data analyzed. This analytical process uses data including maximum range of motion, velocity and fluidity of movement, and directions of movement in frontal and sagittal planes *(Figures 1 and 2)*. Mandibular activity during swallowing and chewing can be simultaneously scrutinized. Small subtle movements can also be scrutinized. The data obtained is significant between the mandibular rest position and occlusion as well as between occlusion and the excursive mandibular movements anteriorly, posteriorly, and laterally[7] *(Figures 3 and 4)*. With accuracy of 0.1 mm in the range between rest and occlusion, the computerized jaw tracking instrument provides essential data for the analysis of occlusion and the mandibular activity associated with reaching the occlusal position.[8]

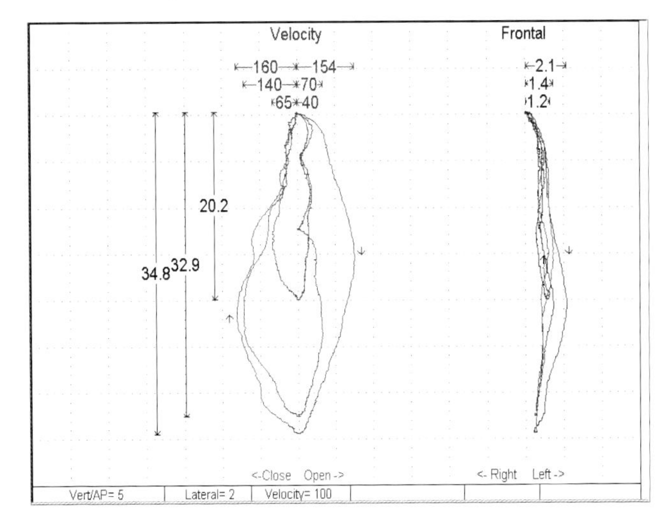

Figure 1. Velocity Pre–TENS Therapy: Opening and closing velocities demonstrate Bradykinesia—patient reports pain on movement.

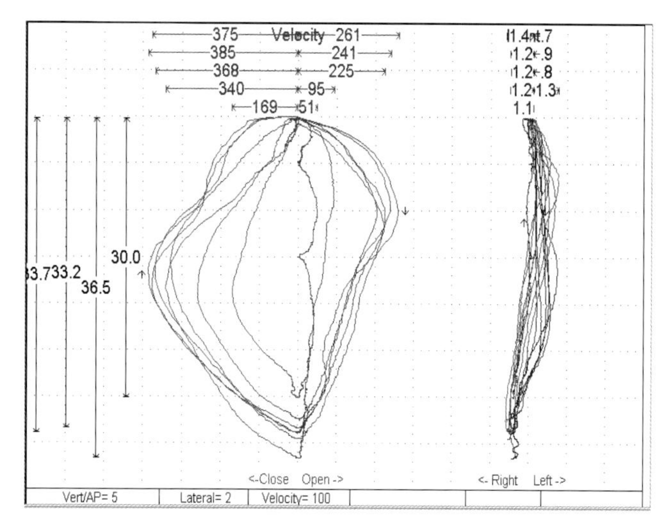

Figure 2. Velocity Post–TENS Therapy: Improved velocity on opening and closing—patient reports less pain on movement.

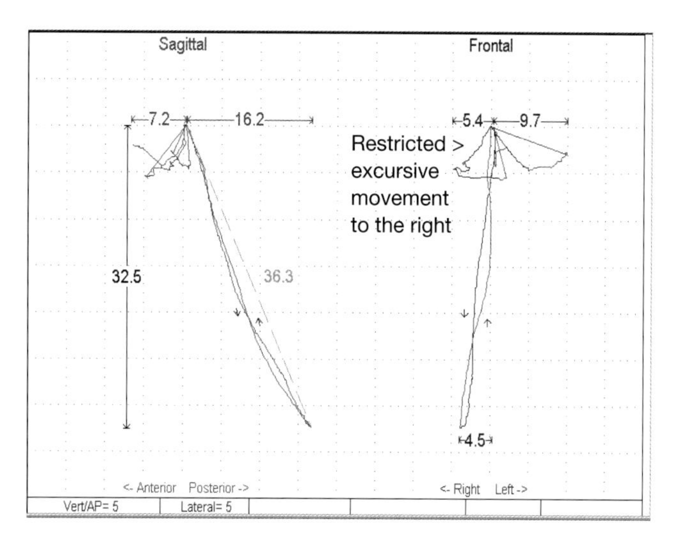

Figure 3. Range of Motion: Pre–TENS therapy.

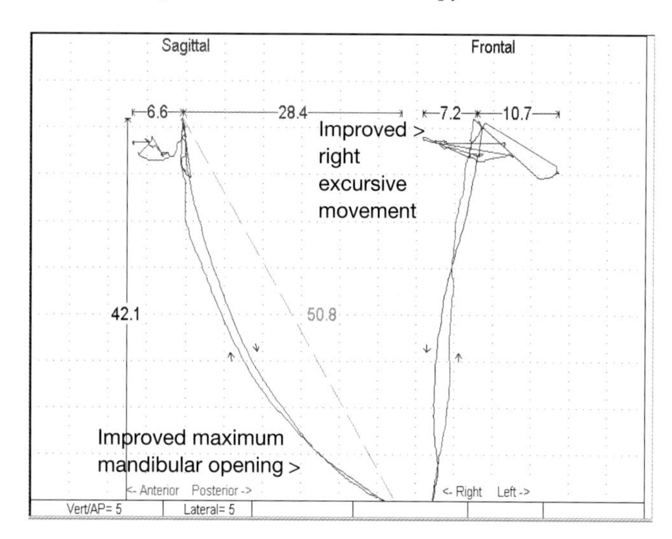

Figure 4. Range of Motion: Post–TENS therapy.

Mandibular tracking is done by recording the movement of a small 0.1 ounce magnet, which is temporarily affixed to the gingiva below the mandibular incisors with an adhesive gel. There is no other device attached to the mandible. In contrast, mechanical tracking devices attach components to the face and mandible, which create both physical and proprioceptive artifacts to the natural resting position and function of the mandible. The further a measurement device is situated from the object being measured, the greater is the measurement error. Therefore, intraoral measurement at the mandibular incisor point is a more accurate position for the recording and analysis of occlusion than a measurement made at some distance from dental occlusion near the lateral poles of the mandibular condyles. Data obtained from electronic tracking can be stored for future analysis and comparative studies. Most importantly, data recorded related to mandibular position and occlusion as well as mandibular movement from rest to occlusion can be displayed with simultaneous electromyographic (EMG) recordings of the electrical activity in "resting" masticatory muscles. This valuable combined data is not available with mechanical jaw tracking devices of any sort.

Electromyography

Temporomandibular disorders (TMD) most often manifest with an abnormality in masticatory muscle resting or functioning activity. In patients who have myogenous TMD, surface electromyography (EMG) has demonstrated elevated resting electrical activity as well as muscular weakness and/or asymmetry during maximum voluntary clenching.[9–16] The latter is a test of maximal muscular activity (force) capability.[12,17–21] Electromyography data are valuable in making a differential diagnosis of muscle dysfunction, with far more reliability and objectivity than merely by the use of reported subjective patient pain report or pain perception on manual palpation. EMG can also be utilized to evaluate the functional outcome of treatment. Ideally, muscle resting electrical activity should become lower and voluntary maximum functional activity more symmetrical and with greater magnitude. EMG function testing of occlusion permits scrutiny of occlusal symmetry and stability.[22–25] Analysis of muscle activity during normal closure into occlusion can be recorded sequentially in time and then scrutinized in order to determine if occlusion is bilaterally balanced or if a unilateral prematurity exists. If one masseter shows a burst of activity before the other, a unilateral prematurity in occlusion exists on the ipsilateral side. This is more precise than information obtained by placement of articulating paper intraorally, for no artifact exists.

Testing Muscular Resting Activity

EMG testing of resting electrical activity can be performed at presentation and following therapeutic intervention to evaluate the therapeutic effect on improvement in resting activity. EMG testing can also be performed at the initial test session to compare the electrical level of activity at presentation and after one hour or more of transcutaneous electrical neural stimulation (TENS). This comparative test provides diagnostically valuable information as it provides a rapid test of the possible hyperactive state of the patient's masticatory muscles, demonstrating a muscular component in that patient's TMD. In addition, the comparative testing demonstrates the capacity to reduce muscle hyperactivity through TENS therapy and the potential for resting activity reduction through therapy designed to improve muscle health[1] *(Figures 5 and 6)*. The ability to lower muscle electrical activity through TENS has been demonstrated to serve in the differential diagnosis of TMD myogenous pain from muscle pain associated with fibromyalgia. TENS neuromuscular stimulation does not lower electrical activity in fibromyalgia patients.[26]

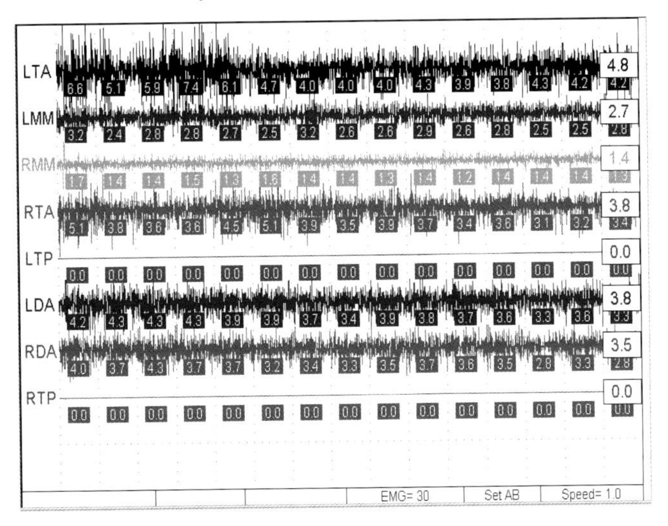

Figure 5. Electromyography of Muscles: Mandible at rest, pre–TENS therapy. Elevated muscle activity at presentation.

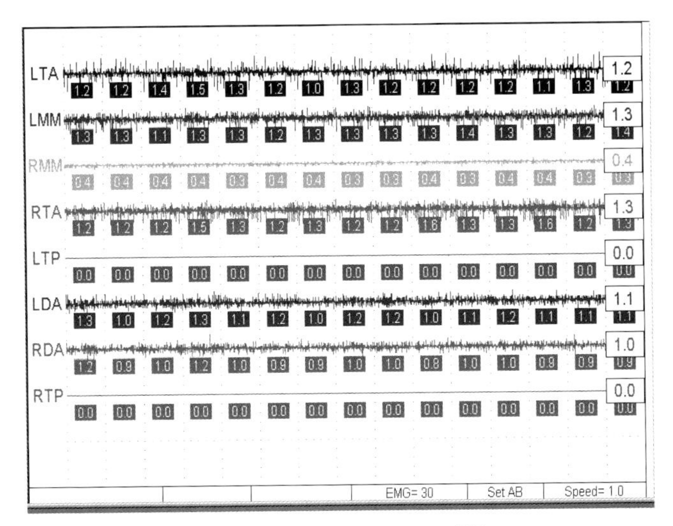

Figure 6. Electromyography of Muscles: Mandible at rest post–TENS therapy. Lower muscle resting levels.

EMG resting electrical activity testing can also be utilized to compare the status of masticatory muscles at initial presentation prior to therapeutic intervention and at presentation at a future visit following a course of therapy. Lowering the resting activity of muscles through therapy is an indication that a more physiological state has been achieved through therapy. *Physiological is defined as ergonomically minimal or economical.* Failure to lower muscle resting activity through therapy, on the other hand, demonstrates the need for further diagnostic assessment and perhaps alteration or augmentation of the therapeutic plan.

Research has demonstrated that resting activity following three months of therapy involving the full-time usage (24 hours per day) of a neuromuscular occlusion orthosis resulted in a significant reduction in resting muscular electrical activity associated with a significant reduction in subjective symptoms[1] *(Table I)*. Quantification of the alteration in a physiologic component or parameter of the TMD is a valuable aid in the ongoing dynamic diagnostic process and in treatment outcome evaluation.

Table I
Table of Average Values for Electromyographic Measurement of Resting Activity TENS Induced Muscle Relaxation Before and In Treatment

(in microvolts)

	Before Treatment			In Treatment (3 months)		
Muscles (bilateral)	Before TENS	After TENS	Change (%)	Before TENS	After TENS	Change (%)
Temporalis Anterior (TA)	2.98±0.15	1.81±0.13	39.3	2.50±0.19	2.10±0.61	15.9
Masseter Middle (MM)	2.22±0.12	1.32±0.11	40.6	1.87±0.12	1.43±0.48	23.3
Digastric Anterior (DA)	2.91±0.55	2.02±0.17	30.6	2.42±0.30	2.24±0.49	7.4
All Muscles	2.70±0.19	1.71±0.08	36.7	2.26±0.12	1.92±0.31	15.2

Level of confidence is 0.001.

Testing Muscle Functional Activity

Functional testing with EMG can also be utilized to test the therapeutic value of occlusal intervention. This can be performed at the initial test visit to evaluate the potential for modification of function through occlusal intervention. This is diagnostically valuable as it "tests" the potential occlusal component in the TMD. Electrical activity during voluntary maximum clench can be recorded on the natural dentition in habitual centric occlusion, which is also known as the intercuspal position or centric occlusion. This can be compared to the electrical activity with maximum voluntary clench into cotton rolls, representing a soft permissive total occlusion. Additional comparisons can be made to maximum voluntary clench into hard acrylic bite registrations made in a selected therapeutic occlusion position. Regardless of occlusal philosophy, any treatment protocol that seeks to produce symmetrical, effective muscle function can be scrutinized with surface EMG. Specifically, the neuromuscular occlusion position has been demonstrated to be associated with improved symmetrical muscle function frequently associated with dominance of masseter over temporalis function *(Figures 7–10)*. Research data demonstrates that the neuromuscular occlusion position is associated with higher levels of muscular activity on maximum clench than occlusion in the bimanual manipulated centric relation position, natural occlusion, or leaf gauge generated occlusions.[27]

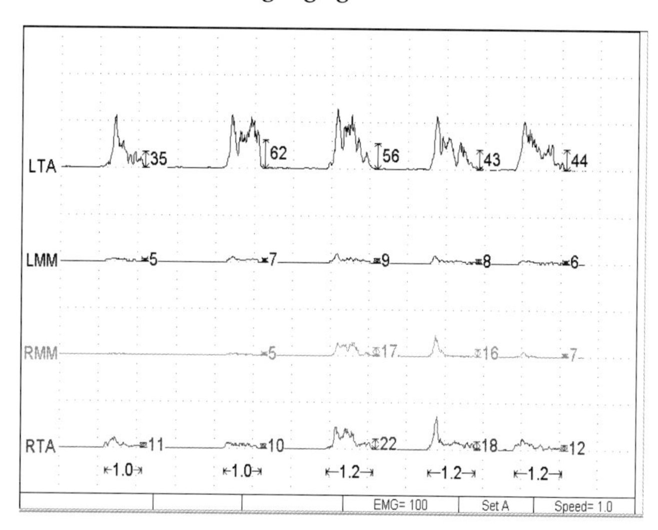

Figure 7. Electromyography of muscles: Maximum Function (Clench). Natural Occlusion: Function is Weak in Natural Dentition.

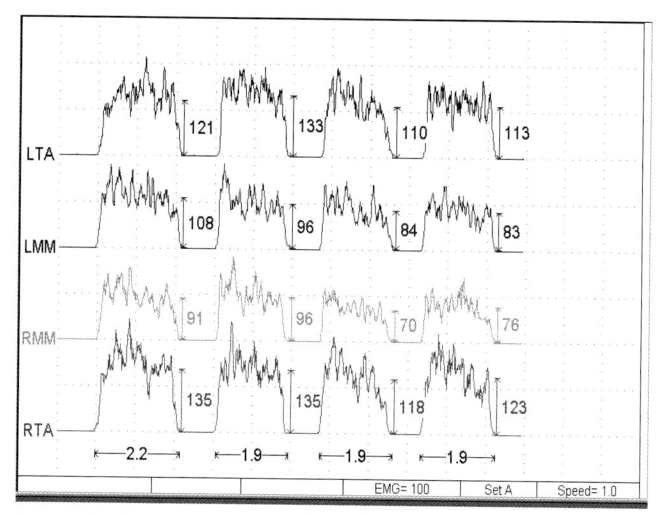

Figure 8. Electromyography of muscles: Maximum Function (Cotton Clench). Cotton Clench demonstrates potential muscle improved function with alteration of occlusion.

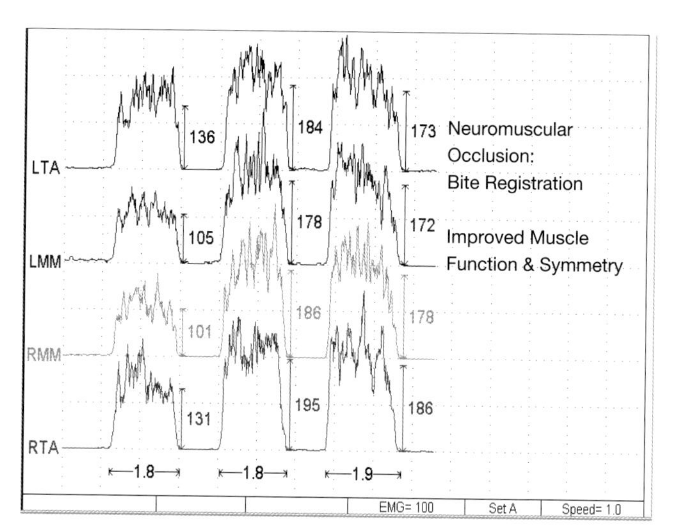

Figure 9. Electromyography of muscles: Maximum Function (Clench).

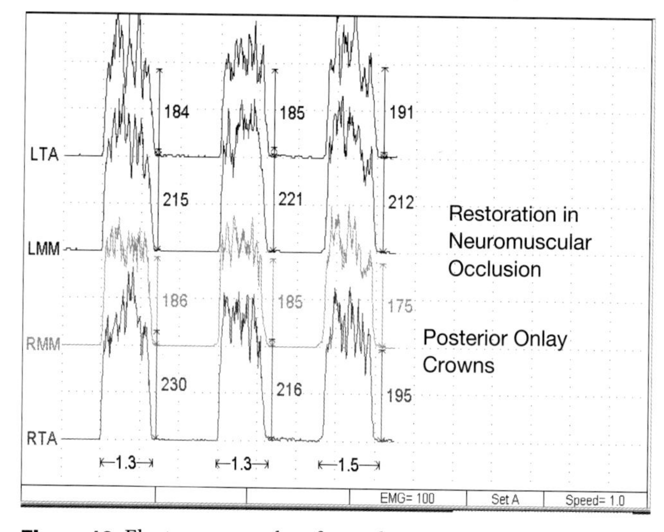

Figure 10. Electromyography of muscles: Maximum Function (Clench).

Table II
Table of Average Values for Electromyographic Measurement of Muscle Activity During Maximum Clench in Natural and Therapeutic Occlusions

(in microvolts)

	Before Treatment			In Treatment (3 months)		
Muscles (bilateral)	Natural Occlusion	Neuromus. Therapeutic Occlusion	Change (%)	Orthotic Occlusion	Neuromusc. Bite Registration	Change (%)
Temporalis Anterior (TA)	77.88±3.66	119.64±4.64	53.6	88.56±6.02	121.91±7.43	37.7
Masseter Middle (MM)	72.57±4.11	137.71±5.17	89.8	94.64±6.60	141.97±8.21	50.0
All Muscles	75.23±2.75	128.67±3.52	71.0	91.60±4.47	131.94±5.62	44.0
% of Subjects TA ⩾ MM	59.3	35.1	–24.2	45.9	34.1	–11.8
% of Subjects TA < MM	40.7	64.9	24.2	54.1	65.9	11.8

Level of confidence is 0.001.

Testing of voluntary maximum clenching activity can be employed after a period of therapeutic intervention to evaluate the long-term effects of the therapy. Research data demonstrate that a therapeutically provided neuromuscular occlusion (provided by an orthosis) used for three months (used full time) maintains improved maximum functional capacity[1] *(Table II).*

Surface vs. Needle Electromyography

The electromyography techniques described above use bipolar (paired) silver-silver chloride *surface electrodes* placed along the long axes of muscles tested. The area covered by each of the electrode pairs provides data related to the collective electrical activity of a large group of muscle fiber units. This is valuable information required to evaluate the type of muscle activity including muscle fiber recruitment involved in the muscle activity associated with dental occlusion whether temporomandibular disorders exist or not.

In contrast, *needle electromyography,* as utilized in medical neurological testing, is employed to test the neural conductive capacity from one point to another. This testing is designed to diagnose neural conductivity. Testing of a single nerve fiber or muscle unit is of no value in the analysis of muscle function/dysfunction associated with myogenous TMD or that which is associated with the analysis of dental occlusion.

Combined Electronic Mandibular Tracking and Electromyography

The ability to simultaneously monitor mandibular position and resting electrical activity of muscles associated with the mandibular "rest" position is valuable in locating the rest position of the mandible *(Figures 11 and 12).* Mandibular rest position serves as a reference point for the selection of a therapeutic occlusion. Physiologic ergonomic principles dictate that muscles function best at their resting length.[28] *The dental occlusion position should, according to this postulate, be located near the mandibular position associated with the postural muscles at their resting length. This should be with the lowest possible postural electrical activity.* EMG spectral analysis has demonstrated that elevated electrical activity of muscles at rest is associated with muscle fatigue, while lower activity is associated with muscle rest.[29] Rest position of the mandible is defined as a position at which there is simultaneous minimal activity in antagonistic muscle groups, mandibular elevators and depressors. For the sake of clinical utility, the anterior temporalis, posterior temporalis, and masseter muscles can be monitored as elevators while the anterior digastric (submandibular) muscles can be monitored as depressors. The rest position of the mandible can exist as an area at which all of these muscles demonstrate minimal activity. This mandibular rest position may represent a small or large area depending on the patient being evaluated. This is significant in the evaluation of a single patient, for it sets the parameters of rest position from which the dentist may select a therapeutic occlusal position.

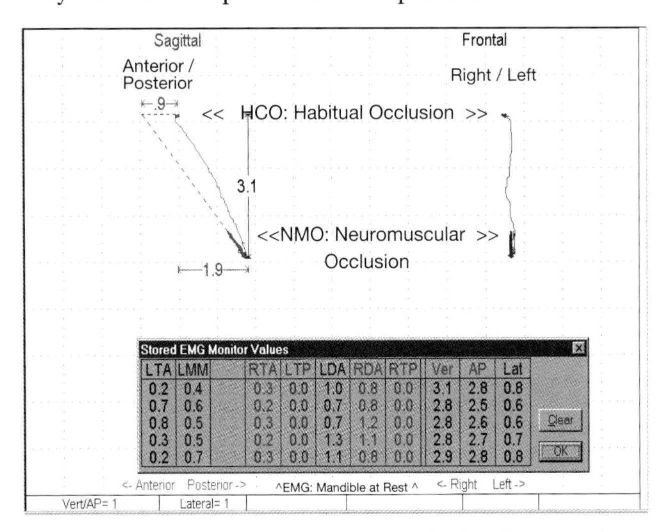

Figure 11. Habitual (Natural) Occlusion is displaced posteriorly and over closed vs. Neuromuscular Occlusion Position.

Finding the Comfortable Bite
Neuromuscular Occlusion

"The Roadmap to Health"

Selection of Rest Position of the mandible as a quiet zone for postural muscle activity.

Combined jaw tracking, Computerized Mandibular Scan and EMG monitoring Rest (below)

From rest position a treatment position is selected which equals the Neuromuscular Occlusion Position: NMO

Figure 12.

With simultaneous recording of the mandibular position of rest and the electrical activity in the postural muscles, the actual resting position of the mandible can be located and confirmed objectively. If voluntary or spontaneous reduction in the vertical freeway space (slight closing) is associated with increased EMG activity in the elevator muscles, rest position has been violated. Similarly, if voluntary or spontaneous increased vertical freeway space (slight opening) is associated with increased EMG depressor activity (anterior digastric), rest position has also been violated. Anterior protrusion of the mandible may also be associated with increased digastric activity and is also a violation of the rest position of the mandible. It is therefore apparent that surface EMG combined with simultaneous 3-dimensional recording of mandibular position is essential in the determination of the parameters of the rest position of the mandible. *Rest position of the mandible is a reference point for the establishment of a therapeutic neuromuscular occlusion*[30,31] *(Figures 13 and 14).*

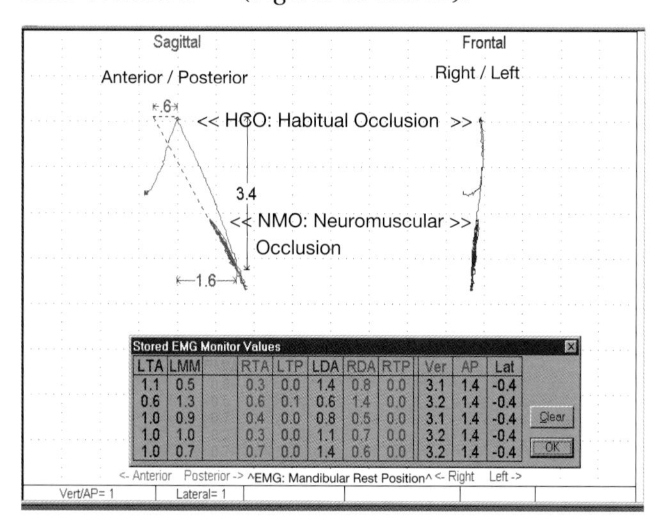

Stored EMG Monitor Values

LTA	LMM	RTA	LTP	LDA	RDA	RTP	Ver	AP	Lat
1.1	0.5	0.3	0.0	1.4	0.8	0.0	3.1	1.4	-0.4
0.6	1.3	0.6	0.1	0.6	1.4	0.0	3.2	1.4	-0.4
1.0	0.9	0.4	0.0	0.8	0.5	0.0	3.1	1.4	-0.4
1.0	1.0	0.3	0.0	1.1	0.7	0.0	3.2	1.4	-0.4
1.0	0.7	0.7	0.0	1.4	0.6	0.0	3.2	1.4	-0.4

Figure 13. Habitual Occlusion is displaced posteriorly and over closed vs. Neuromuscular Occlusion Position.

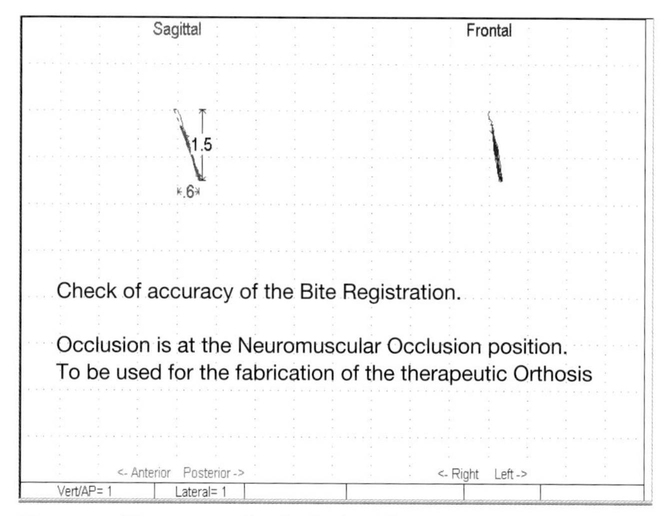

Figure 14. Neuromuscular Occlusion Bite Registration.

The neuromuscular occlusion position is located along a trajectory (arc) of mandibular movement, which begins at rest position of the mandible. With data from electronic jaw tracking and simultaneous electromyography, together with direct visual examination of the patient's maxillo-mandibular relationships, the dentist can determine the rest position of the mandible and select the therapeutic occlusal position. The neuromuscular position is selected by the clinician along the trajectory of mandibular movement beginning at a mandibular rest position. The gentle arc form swinging of the mandible along a trajectory is created by the electrical stimulation provided by the same TENS instrument, which affected muscle relaxation. Customarily, the occlusion position is selected 1 mm above the rest position. This provides one millimeter of vertical freeway space between the therapeutic occlusion and a rest position. This has been demonstrated to be a common functional freeway space. It has been demonstrated to be associated with rested masticatory postural muscles. Note: With the instruments described here, recording of mandibular position and maxillo-mandibular relationships are made at the incisor point.[31,32] The accuracy of the therapeutic occlusal position can be tested in the acrylic bite registration.

A neuromuscular occlusion so created requires no muscle accommodative postural activity with its potential for fatigue and dysfunction, since optimum resting muscle activity is provided for with minimal freeway space. Research data demonstrate that the neuromuscular occlusion position is durable and stable *(Tables III and IV)*. Muscle activity associated with the neuromuscular occlusion has been demonstrated to sustain a rested state at mandibular rest and also provide symmetrically active and strong function when called upon to perform occlusal function.[1] Research data also demonstrate that rest position of the mandible associated with the creation of a neuromuscular occlusion is stable in three dimensions over time *(Tables V and VI)*. These are indicators of physiological health.

Electrosonography

Electrosonography (ESG) is a technique for recording and displaying sounds emanating from the temporomandibular joints bilaterally. The sound produced can be displayed indicating its amplitude (power) and frequency (quality). Although sonographic testing can be performed independently of computerized mandibular tracking, it is significantly more valuable when performed contemporaneously and the data are displayed simultaneously. Combined recording and display of the sound and mandibular opening and closing (with jaw tracking) is extremely valuable as it visualizes the point in the open and close cycle at which a particular type of sound is produced[33] *(Figures 15–18)*.

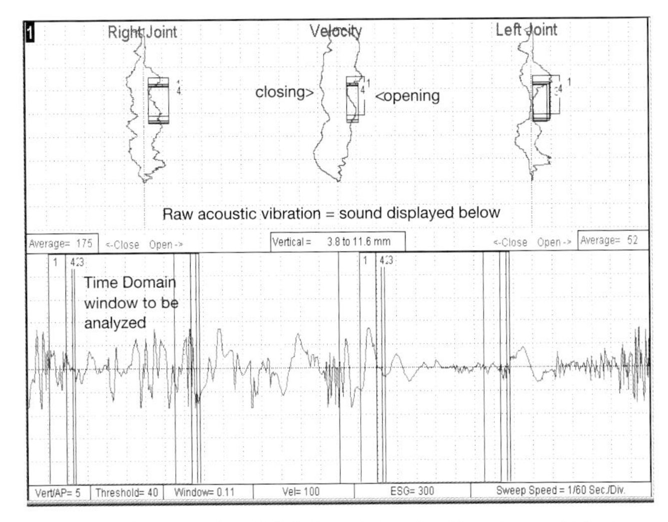

Figure 15. Sonography of TMJ Sounds During Opening and Closing.

Table III
Comparison of Natural Occlusal Position with Neuromuscular Occlusal Position
(in % of subjects analyzed)

Condition	Natural Occlusion	In Treatment with Orthosis	Long Term Treatment
On Neuromuscular Trajectory	19.83	67.00	93.44
Overclosed	77.18	17.85	1.64
Posterior Displacement	65.38	24.07	1.31
Lateral Displacement	25.34	9.43	0.17

Table IV
Comparison of Natural Occlusal Position with Neuromuscular Occlusal Position
(in % of subjects analyzed)

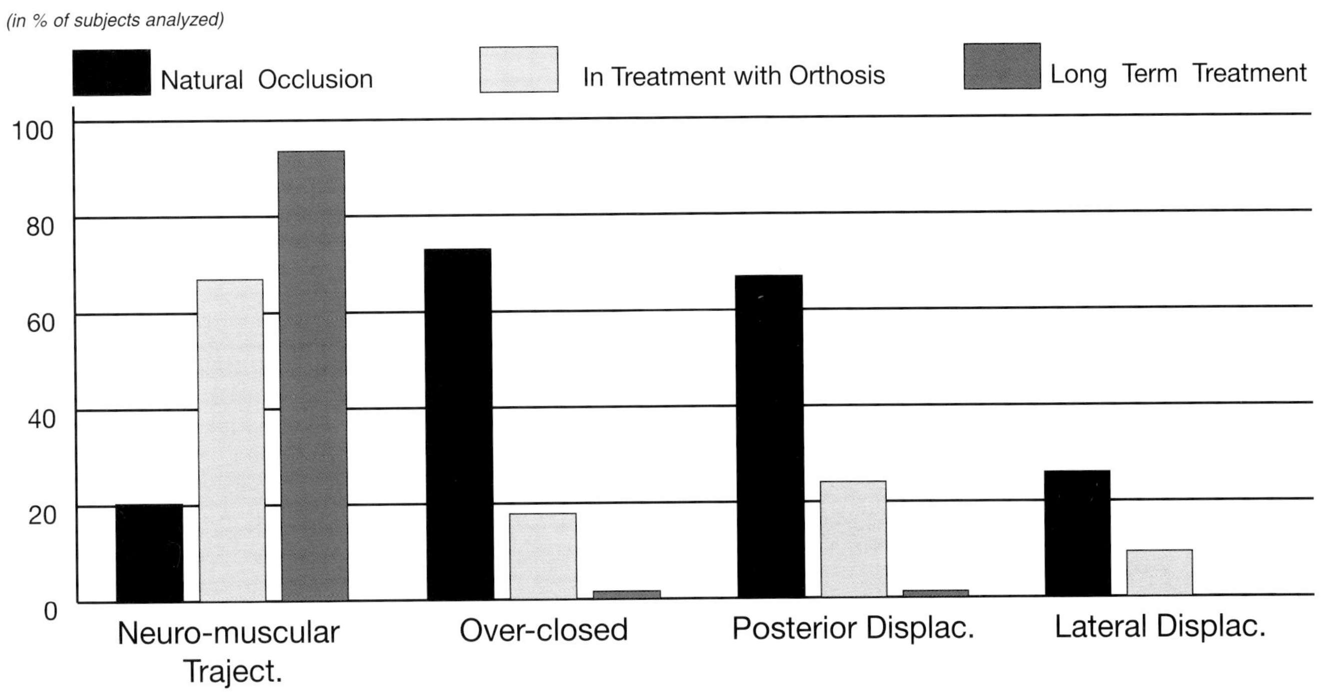

Table V
Electronic Mandibular Tracking of Freeway Space (FWS) Between Rest Position and Occlusion
(in mm)

	Before Treatment		In Treatment with Orthosis		Long Term Treatment
Muscles (bilateral)	Before TENS	After TENS	Before TENS	After TENS	After TENS
Average Vertical FWS	1.89	3.57	1.31	1.69	1.25
Average A/P FWS	0.81	1.29	0.67	0.77	0.62
Average Lateral FWS	0.20	0.36	0.22	0.17	0.09

Recorded at mandibular incisors.

Table VI
Electronic Mandibular Tracking of Freeway Space (FWS) Between Rest Position and Occlusion
(in mm)

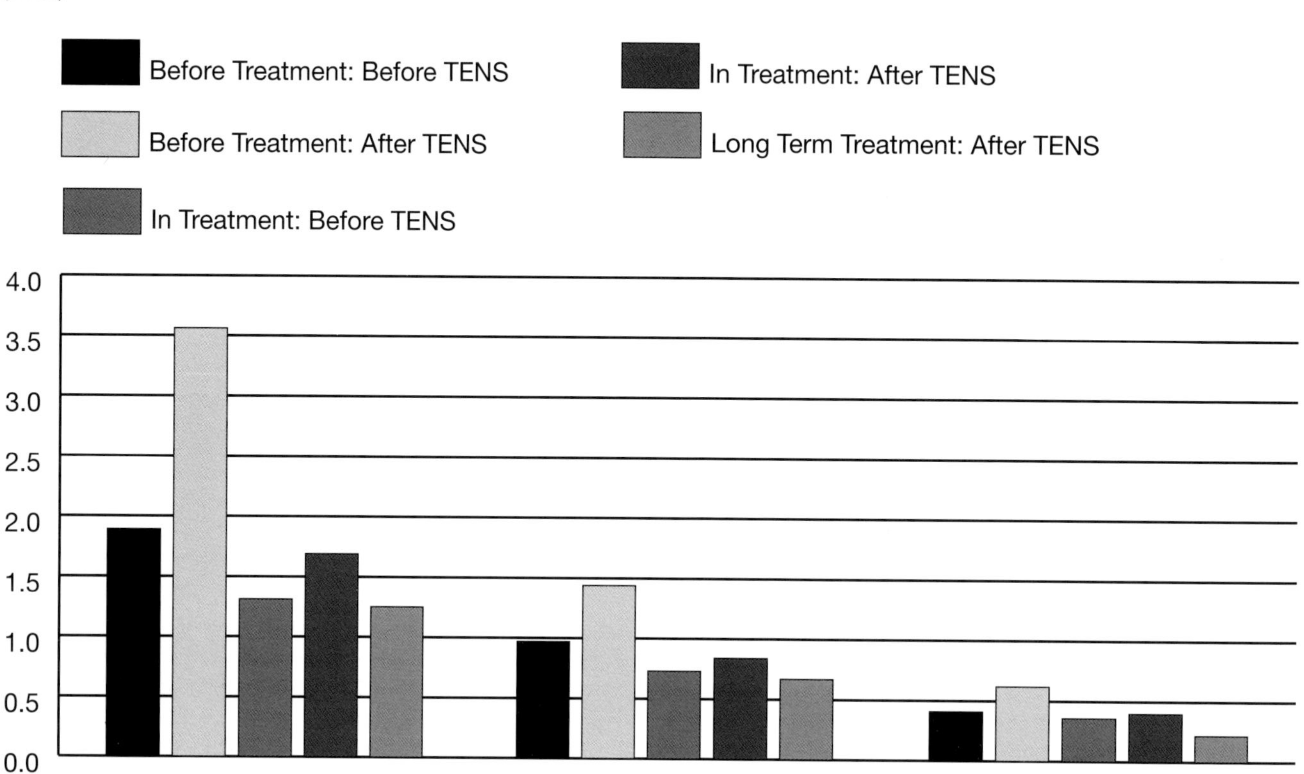

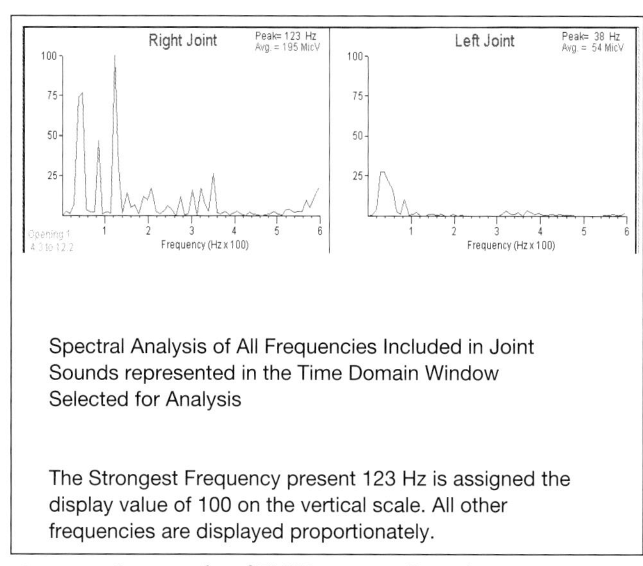

Figure 16. Sonography of TMJ Frequency Domain.

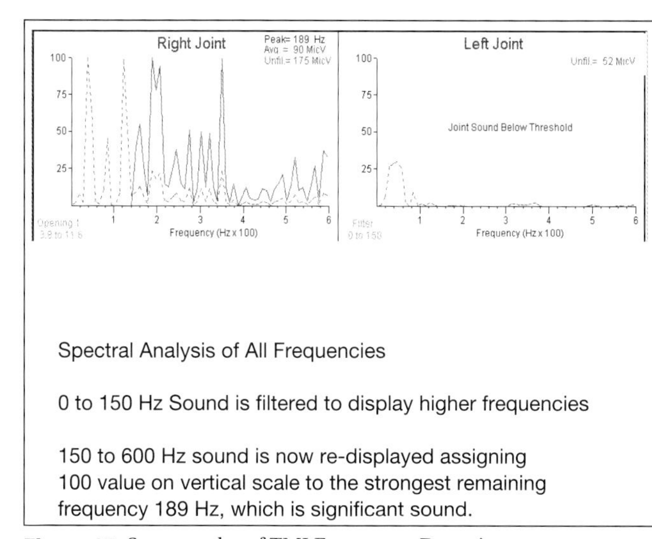

Figure 17. Sonography of TMJ Frequency Domain.

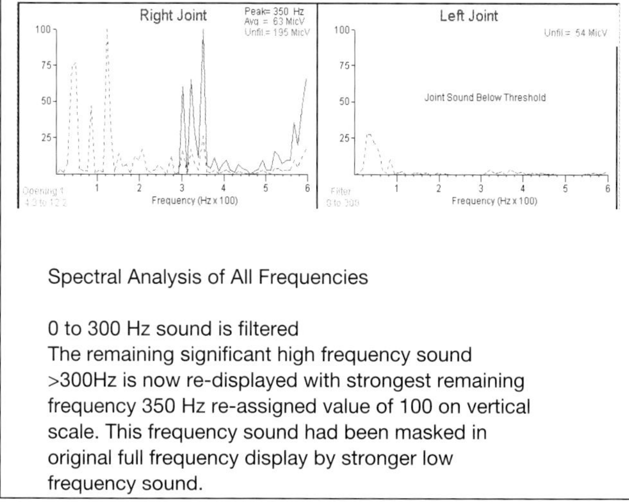

Figure 18. Sonography of TMJ Frequency Domain.

It has long been recognized that recording TMJ joint sounds was valuable in evaluating patients for TMD.[34–39] However, traditional stethoscopic auscultation was often inaccurate, dependent on the acuity of the examiner, the frequency of the sound, and its volume or amplitude. Further observation of sound without accurate determination of the stage of open/closure of the mandible diminishes the diagnostic value of sound observation techniques. Recorded sounds produced in the TMJ can be carefully scrutinized with greater sensitivity and range of frequency than that which can be done with the human auditory system. Storage of data on the computer also permits subsequent re-evaluation and comparison with data obtained after a treatment period. When comprehensive treatment is being undertaken, sonographic analysis is valuable. It is a cost-effective diagnostic aid. The data obtained is useful in concert with other diagnostic tests in determining whether a patient has an intracapsular component in the disease/dysfunction being evaluated and treated.

In its most general interpretation, the presence of sounds in a joint are characteristic of non-optimal function, incoordination of joint structures, alteration in normal anatomy, or disease. Ideally, joints should be sound-free in normal use. The presence of sound does not in and of itself establish the medical necessity of treatment intervention. TMJ sound can exist in an otherwise asymptomatic patient and not serve as a sufficient and necessary criterion for therapeutic intervention. In contrast, the absence of joint sound does not in and of itself demonstrate a state of perfect joint health and function. In the case of a chronically displaced disk, the mandibular range of motion may become normalized, with no joint sounds or discomfort, but the normal joint components are not in their proper place. A patient may report a history of mandibular movement limitation with clicking now resolved. Higher frequency sounds are customarily associated with hard tissue sources and a more advanced degenerative condition. Lower frequency low amplitude sound at early opening has been reported to be typical of sounds in normal joints caused by sudden movement of ligaments, by the separation of articular surfaces, or the sucking of loose tissue behind the condyle as it moves towards the articular eminence.[33,40] Low frequency sound of high amplitude at early opening can reflect soft tissue or fluid changes in the joint.

Clicking is demonstrative of an incoordination between the articular disk and the condyle during mandibular opening and closing. Clicks are usually of shorter duration and higher amplitude than crepitus. A click is a single sound which, if relatively loud, is often referred to as a pop. Ligament laxity, adhesions, and/or muscle spasms that cause incoordination of the disk/condyle movement may cause a click. The condyle is usually posteriorly displaced in the glenoid fossa, and the disk is anteriorly displaced. Clicks of middle range frequency are usually indicative of cartilaginous contact with the condyle. A click early in the open cycle and later in the closing cycle usually represents a reciprocal click in which the disk, having been anteriorly displaced from the condyle at occlusion, is recaptured above the condyle upon opening and is thereafter lost in final tooth closure. This is called a reciprocal click.[33]

The duration of a joint sound is also significant in determining its etiology. Longer duration, high frequency sound is associated with a more chronic condition of crepitus. In this case, bone to bone contact is made with no disk interposed. Crepitation is considered to be a manifestation of structural damage to the articular surfaces, the sound being the result of movement across irregular hard surfaces.[33]

In determining the stage of mandibular movement at which a sound occurs, it is valuable to record the actual contact of teeth in occlusion. This is valuable during the sound recording process and its interpretation by the clinician as it marks the point of dental occlusion. This occlusal signature serves as a reference point for evaluation of the stage in opening/closing at which other specific sound is recorded. Late clicks are more difficult to resolve with treatment than earlier clicks; since the disk is displaced further anteriorly in a late click, morphology of the disk and its attachments can also be altered in this case.

Sound at the end of full opening is significant and may represent the condyle translating beyond the articular eminence upon very large opening of the mouth. This hypermobile state can be of long standing and associated with other hypermobile joints in the patient's body. History is very important in performing an analysis of joint sounds. Depending on the clinician's treatment philosophy, specific sonographic findings may affect the initial treatment decision. Recording of sound following an initial course of therapy is valuable, as data obtained can be compared to data obtained at the initial test at the initiation of treatment. This provides additional outcome evaluation data/evidence. At a post-treatment testing sequence, if sound is recorded in the joint of a patient with significant intracapsular joint pain or a patient with severely restricted mandibular range of motion, either of which is *not* resolved by conservative, noninvasive therapy, referral for further evaluation is usual and customary. This could involve surgical evaluation with appropriate imaging studies, customarily MRI examination. Depending on the status of a patient, such evaluation is sometimes, but rarely, necessary at the initial stage of treatment.

Transcutaneous Electrical Neural Stimulation (TENS)

The term transcutaneous electrical neural stimulation (TENS) describes two distinct types of medical devices. One is a high frequency, low amperage type of stimulation and the other is a low voltage, low frequency stimulator. In addition, there are high voltage stimulators utilized in the management of patients.

High frequency, low amperage TENS is a pain suppressor instrument. Its therapeutic effect, according to the "Gate Theory" of Melzack and Wall,[41] is to block the afferent pain pathways to the central nervous system by flooding the system with a barrage of innocuous low level stimuli.

Low frequency, low amperage TENS on the other hand effects a relaxation of muscles.[42–44] Providing a pumping intermittent stimulation of the nerve innervating the masticatory muscles, the muscles are debrided of waste metabolites (including ADP and lactic acid), circulation is improved with re-stocking of fresh metabolites (ATP), endorphins are released systemically, and muscle contraction released. This is accompanied by neurologenically mediated pain relief and further muscle relaxation.

The specific TENS instrument used by the author, the Myo-monitor (Myotronics-Noromed, Inc.), delivers a repetitive stimulus of 8 to 12 mA for 500 microseconds once every 1.5 seconds. It is applied bilaterally to the area between the temporomandibular joints and the coronoid process of the mandible. A third grounding electrode is placed on the rear of the neck and does not deliver a stimulus. Placement of the bilateral active electrodes is critical, for only at that position is the mandibular division of the trigeminal nerve (V) accessible from the surface of the face. The nerve is located deep to the mandible, but accessible via surface application of the subtle stimulus through the soft tissues.[45] In addition to stimulation of the division of the Vth nerve, the facial nerve (VII), which traverses the same area superficially, is also stimulated. Through this neural route of stimulation, all of the facial and masticatory muscles are stimulated simultaneously[46] *(Table VII)*. This is a very economical and effective device as it employs minimal stimulation and affects significant, but painless, multiple muscle stimulation and muscle relaxation, thereby changing fatigued hyperactive muscles to a state of relaxation.[29]

Table VII
TENS Stimulation for Group Function

Mandibular Nerve V	***Facial Nerve VII***
Masseter	Muscles of the nose
Temporalis	Buccinator
Medial pterygoid	Rhisorius
Lateral pterygoid	Orbicularis oris
Tensor veli palatini	Muscles of lower lip & chin
Mylohyoid	Platysma
Anterior belly of digastric	Posterior belly of digastric

Temporomandibular Disorders

Within the complex of head and neck musculoskeletal disorders there is a group of conditions that involve dysfunction among the temporomandibular joints, masticatory muscles, and dental occlusion. These comprise the temporomandibular disorders (TMD), which are a group of multicausal, multifaceted conditions. TMD can affect the form and function of the temporomandibular joint (TMJ), masticatory muscles, and dental apparatus. Each TMD patient presents with a unique set of symptoms, clinical presentation, and history. Proper management of TMD by the dentist requires accurate appraisal of the status of the patient's dentition, TMJ, and associated muscular apparatus. The dental profession accepts certain predefined standards or parameters of function/dysfunction. Electronic instrumentation provides objective measurement of many of these biological phenomena, and thus can be used throughout treatment for critical analyses that monitor and enhance treatment efficacy.[47-50]

It is universally acknowledged that conservative, reversible therapies should be employed whenever possible in the initial treatment of TMD. The therapies found to have the most clinical success involve alteration in the function of the mandible, TMJ, and masticatory muscles. This is most, though not always, often accomplished through the use of intraoral orthotic appliances, called orthoses or "splints."[51-55] The exception to the prescription of reversible therapy before irreversible is, in the case of certain traumatic injuries or infection, where surgical intervention as a first step may be indicated as the treatment of choice.

Some appliances are specifically designed to alter dental occlusion, others to relax hyperactive muscles, and still others to change the condylar position within the TMJ by repositioning the mandible. Additionally, dentists frequently use other therapeutic modalities to improve the function of the masticatory muscles, by lowering resting activity and improving functioning activity. It is, therefore, because of their intimate knowledge of the structure and function of the mandible, dental occlusion, and masticatory muscles that dentists have rightfully assumed the role of primary TMD therapists.

A TMD Treatment Protocol

A treatment protocol for TMD is presented that has been effectively utilized by this author. It represents a prudent effective use of the electronic devices described above to establish a neuromuscular occlusion initially through an acrylic orthosis and thereafter, if indicated, with various forms of long term durable treatment. This treatment protocol is not presented as a "standard of care." Certainly individual patients require individualized treatment regimens and individualized testing protocols. It is the responsibility of the treating dentist to establish the medical necessity of all diagnostic and therapeutic procedures employed for the specific patient being treated. The following protocol is presented to establish the medical necessity and utility of the three diagnostic instruments (EMG, CMS, and Sonography) and their application in the creation of a neuromuscular occlusion. *Measurement instrumentation provides reliable data, the interpretation of which is the responsibility of the trained dentist.*[30,56]

Treatment of each patient begins with an initial triage and evaluation. After obtaining a careful history and performing a comprehensive head and neck examination related to musculoskeletal and dental/oral structures, the dentist makes a decision as to the patient's treatment needs and, most importantly, the patient's desires for treatment. For some patients, when the examination is in close proximity to a traumatic injury, simple ameliorative therapies are necessary and sufficient, while the natural healing process takes place.

When comprehensive care is indicated by the patient's presentation and the patient agrees to undergo that treatment, comprehensive diagnosis is necessary. Diagnostic testing is medically necessary to provide objective measurement of the specific physical components of the disease processes that are being treated. Imaging techniques and their medical necessity will not be included in this protocol discussion as they are not the subjects of this chapter.

Initial Test Procedure

Bioelectronic testing is performed initially to determine the status of the patient's mandibular and masticatory function at presentation before and after TENS therapy at the same visit. It is the data obtained at this later portion of the test that helps the dentist identify the mandibular rest position. This important position or area serves as a reference point for the selection by the dentist of a Neuromuscular Occlusion (NMO) treatment position. All data recorded are repeated to test for reliability and reproducibility. Obviously aberrant or skewed data are disregarded.

Pre-Tens Testing

- Mandibular range of motion during maximum voluntary opening, lateral, and protrusive excursive movements is recorded *(Figures 3 and 4).*
- Velocity and fluidity of mandibular movement during rapid maximum opening and closing are recorded together with a tracing of mandibular movement in the frontal plane. The later data also provides valuable data related to the quality of final tooth contact on occlusion as being stable (small area of repeated contact) or unstable (broad area of occlusal contact or variable locations) *(Figures 19 and 20).*

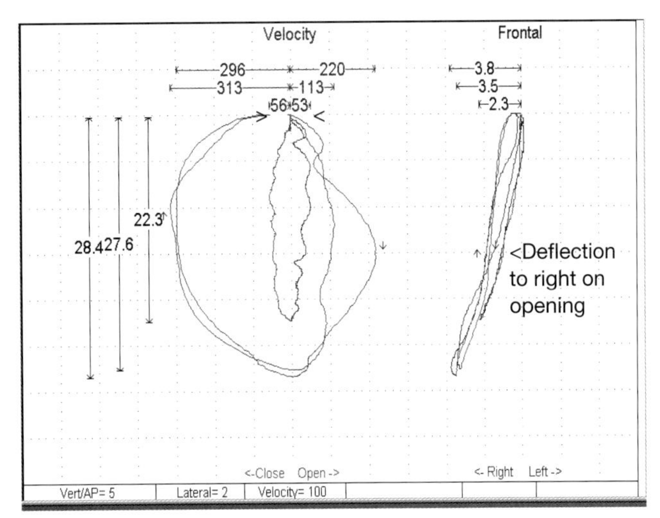

Figure 19. Velocity Pre–TENS Therapy: Opening velocity is initially slow. Two points of closure were observed: unstable occlusion.

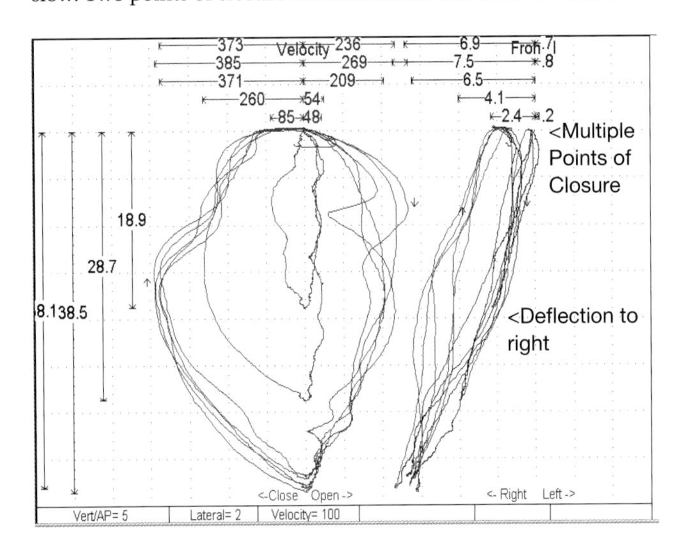

Figure 20. Velocity Post–TENS Therapy: Improved velocity on opening and closing and improved mandibular opening.

- Postural rest position of the mandible in comparison with the habitual or intercuspal occlusion position to evaluate presenting freeway space in the vertical, anterior/posterior, and lateral planes.[57-59]
- Electromyographic recording of resting electrical activity in elevator and depressor mandibular postural muscles.
- Electromyographic recording of electrical activity of elevator muscles during maximum voluntary clench, permitting evaluation of the symmetry/asymmetry and magnitude of muscle activity.
- A second EMG test of electrical activity of elevator muscles with a maximum voluntary clench on cotton rolls provides comparative function testing on a soft permissive substance while voiding the natural occlusion. It is an early pre-treatment test of the potential changes in muscle function, which can be achieved with altered occlusion *(Figures 7 and 8).*
- Electromyographic recording of electrical activity of elevator muscles during normal closure to evaluate symmetry or asymmetry of muscle activity and the chronological order of muscle firing as an evaluation of the dental occlusion symmetry *(Figures 21 and 22).*

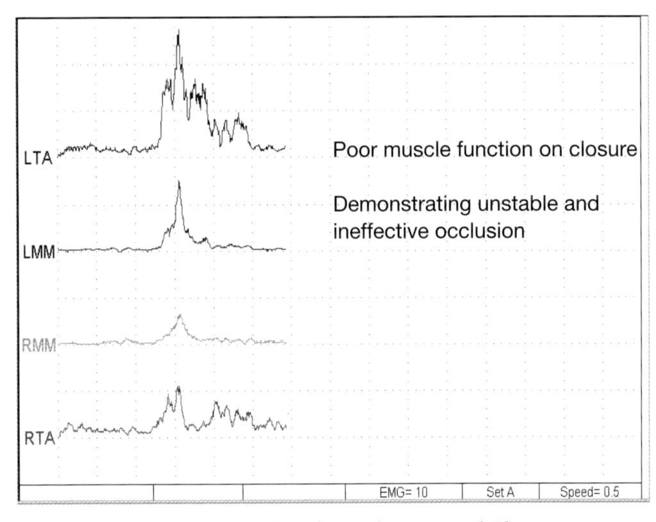

Figure 21. Electromyography of Muscles: Normal Closure

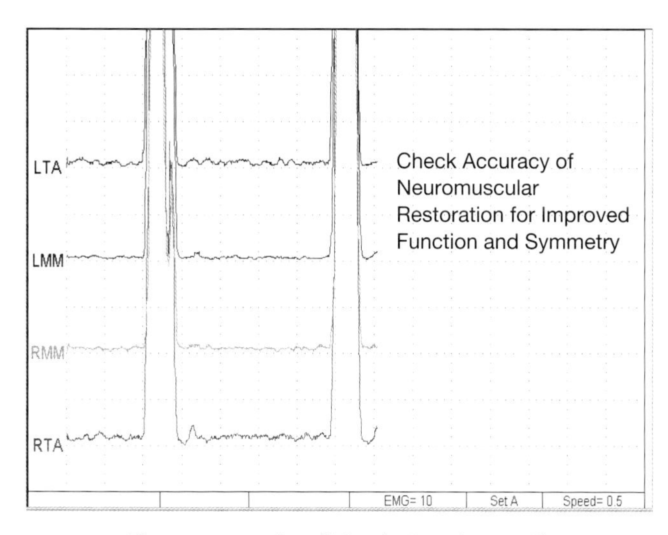

Figure 22. Electromyography of Muscle Function on Closure.

- Sonographic recording of bilateral temporomandibular joint (TMJ) sounds at early, middle, and late opening and the same three positions during closing. With concomitant recording of the actual mandibular open/close movement, data of joint sounds can be identified at the specific position in the open/close cycle. Sound is identified and displayed as frequency and amplitude, permitting qualitative and quantitative evaluation by the dentist of the type of tissue that is suggested as the genesis of the sound. With sequential filtering of lower frequency sounds, which have overshadowed or masked higher frequency sound in the data displayed, the higher frequency sound can be visualized. This is valuable in analyzing the type of sound and its tissue genesis *(Figures 15–18)*. This can obviate the need for MRI examination at this stage of treatment for most patients.

Post–TENS Therapy Testing

- Electromyographic recording of resting electrical activity in elevator and depressor mandibular postural muscles. If resting activity is reduced, it serves to validate a diagnosis of muscle hyperactivity. In addition, the lower values on EMG demonstrate the effectiveness of TENS for that patient and the potential for muscle relaxation through therapy *(Figures 5 and 6)*.
- Electromyographic recording of electrical activity in elevator muscles during maximum voluntary clench to compare with pre-TENS data. This permits evaluation of the effect of muscle relaxation alone of the symmetry and magnitude of elevator muscle activity prior to therapeutic alteration in occlusion.
- Electromyographic recording of electrical activity during normal closure to evaluate the effect of muscle relaxation alone on changes in symmetry or asymmetry of muscle activity which is a function of the dental occlusion.
- Mandibular range of motion, including maximum voluntary opening, lateral and protrusive excursive movements is recorded. Improvement in mandibular range is attributable to relaxation of muscles. Those dimensions that do not normalize can be interpreted as limited by obstruction within the TMJ. Restriction in lateral excursion is customarily attributable to obstruction in the contralateral joint when muscles are relaxed *(Figures 3 and 4)*.
- Velocity and fluidity of mandibular movement during maximum rapid opening and closing are recorded together with a tracing of mandibular movement in the frontal plane. The later tracings also provide valuable data related to the quality of final tooth contact on occlusion as being stable (small area of repeated contact) or unstable (broad area of occlusal contact of variable location) *(Figures 1, 2, 19, and 20)*.
- Postural rest position of the mandible in comparison with the habitual or intercuspal occlusion position to evaluate freeway space in the vertical, anterior/posterior, and lateral planes.[57-59] Change in mandibular rest position after muscle relaxation is significant when associated with documented (EMG) recording of reduced electrical activity in antagonistic muscles bilaterally. This concurrent data acquisition helps identify the mandibular rest position. It serves as a reference position for the selection by the dentist of the therapeutic occlusion position *(Figures 11 and 12)*.

Bite Registration Technique

A therapeutic bite position is determined by the dentist along the trajectory of mandibular movement directed by the TENS stimulus. The treatment position is selected by the dentist as a point along the trajectory, which begins at the mandibular rest position.[30,31] Customarily one millimeter of vertical freeway space is provided for in the selection of a treatment position. This determination is made on the basis of a process in which the range of rest position of the mandible associated with equally low electrical activity in elevator (masseter and anterior temporalis) and depressor (anterior digastric) muscles is established *(Figures 11–14)*. The clinician must evaluate the impact on vertical overbite and posterior vertical freeway space associated with various possible selected treatment positions. The operative guide in the selection of a treatment position is to be on the neuromuscular trajectory, which begins at a muscular "quiet zone" and which causes the minimal alteration of vertical dimension of occlusion consistent with proper perio-prosthetic principles.

- Once selected, the treatment maxillo-mandibular position is recorded in a bite registration material. An ethyl methacrylate acrylic material can be effectively and reliably used for the bite registration (Blue Sapphire, H. Bosworth, Co. Skokie Ill). This material is used because it is passive to imprinting when placed in the mouth as a soft rope placed over the mandibular occlusal surfaces. It requires no voluntary effort to bring the mandible to the neuromuscular occlusal position. The postural activity of the muscles positions the mandible at rest position. While the patient is observed on the computer screen, the doctor can suggest to the patient that the mandible be relaxed further upward if the patient is over-opened due to the presence of the bite registration material. The TENS pulse is sufficient to swing the mandible on the neuromuscular arc or trajectory from the pre-observed rest position to the selected treatment position. The bite registration material is removed from the mouth in a semi-cured, rubbery, non-distortable state. After cutting away excess acrylic, which might lock onto the study casts as it sets, the bite is placed between lubricated study casts and left for final curing. Once cured, it can be replaced in the mouth; its accuracy of fit, position, and associated electrical activity on maximum voluntary clench can be tested.

- EMG testing should demonstrate symmetrical, strong activity. Typically, multiple bite registrations are obtained, and the one which demonstrates the most precision and EMG clench symmetry and magnitude is selected for use in the fabrication of the orthosis. Note: The same bite registration, which remains dimensionally accurate over time, can be re-tested at the three-month re-test. This permits comparison of the originally selected treatment position (the bite registration) with that provided by the orthosis, which has been in use constantly for three months *(Table II)*.
- A mandibular acrylic orthosis is then fabricated using the NMO bite registration to articulate the study casts. The appliance covers the mandibular posterior teeth with an anatomically accurate occlusal surface. This provides a new stable occlusion interdigitating with the maxillary teeth in a maxillo-mandibular position, which is synchronized with balanced muscle function. *This is a neuromuscular occlusion orthosis.*

Additional Testing

- Following the insertion of the orthosis, its occlusal surface is adjusted using TENS therapy to relax muscles and cause the mandible to rotate on a neuromuscular trajectory. Any unilateral marks in the occlusal indicator medium indicate an occlusal prematurity. Occlusal indicator wax (Kerr) is very effective for this process. Following acrylic occlusal adjustment with TENS stimulation, the patient is instructed to voluntarily chew the wax. This natural maneuver demonstrates any inclined destabilizing occlusal contacts. These are then adjusted in the acrylic material. The process is repeated until a stable cusp-fossa occlusion is created. This is used to demonstrate occlusal prematurities.
- The EMG maximum voluntary clench test can then be used to evaluate muscle symmetry and function as an indication of bilateral symmetry of the therapeutic occlusion. Comparisons are made between EMG activity on clenching on the bite registration and on the orthosis, which creates equal test conditions related to electrode placement and skin conductivity on the same date *(Figures 23 and 24)*.

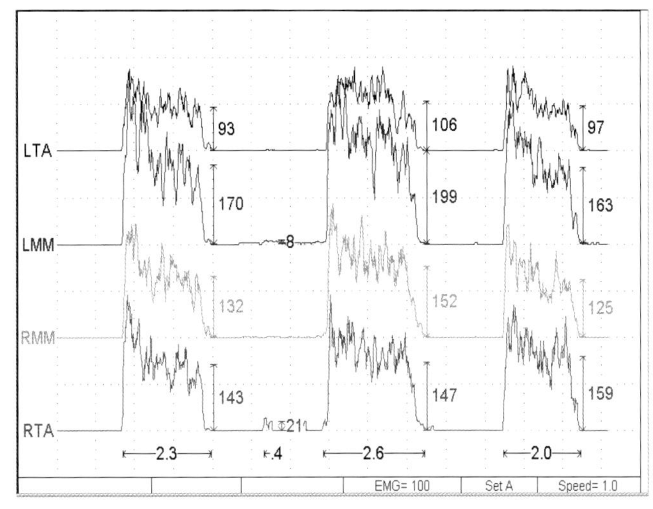

Figure 23. Electromyography of Muscles: Maximum Voluntary Clench on Bite Registration at NMO, Neuromuscular Occlusion.

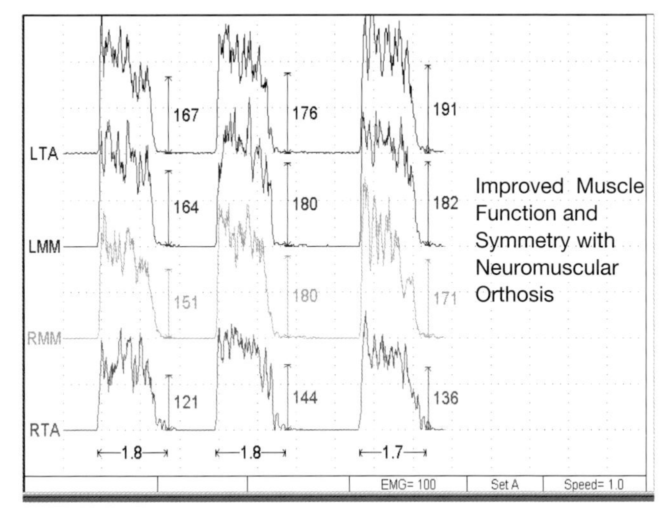

Figure 24. Electromyography of Muscles: Maximum Function (Clench).

Follow-up Testing

After a predetermined treatment period, customarily three months, during which the patient has been wearing the orthosis 24 hours a day, the patient returns for a second complete test. Quite similar to the initial test employing EMG, CMS, and Sonography, the testing protocol includes both pre- and post-TENS data acquisition. A difference between the re-test and the initial test is that at the three-month re-evaluation, the patient wears the orthosis covering the natural mandibular teeth during the portion of the test before TENS.[1] Patients who have worn orthoses full time are not immediately comfortable occluding their teeth in the former habitual occlusion. Note: If patients elect to discontinue wearing the orthosis full time, muscles will retrain through proprioceptive input and the mandible will be brought again to the old occlusal relationship.

After TENS, both the orthosis and then the original bite registration are re-tested for accuracy of the occlusal position at the neuromuscular occlusion position as well as tested for muscle strength and symmetry on clench. This duel re-testing is valuable for several reasons. If the bite registration and orthosis are not at the neuromuscular occlusal position, it can be concluded that during the treatment period the mandibular rest position has moved more anteriorly as muscles continued to relax. A new more accurate bite registration would have to be obtained if additional therapy is undertaken. In a second scenario, if the original bite registration is accurately at the NMO occlusion position, but the orthosis is not, it would demonstrate that attrition of the detailed, precise occlusal surface of the orthosis has occurred. In this case, the initial bite registration could be used for additional prostheses if it is necessary to continue therapy in some form. Finally, if both the bite registration and orthosis are accurate and occlusion is still clearly defined and stable as demonstrated on the computer, the same orthosis can continue to be used if the patient wishes to continue full or part time use of the appliance.

Value of Sonography Re-testing

As previously noted, if re-testing demonstrates the same joint sounds as were recorded at the initial testing, treatment has not removed the cause of the joint sound. If mandibular function is otherwise asymptomatic and normal, the observation joint sound and its characteristics are noted. If sound remains unchanged and the jaw function is symptomatic, referral for an oral surgical evaluation and MRI may be indicated.

Long Term Treatment

If therapy has resulted in significant improvement in function and/or comfort, each patient must decide on their need and desire for continuation of treatment. Long term durable treatment can be instituted in a variety of forms.

Long term treatment should not be performed unless and until reversible treatment has successfully resolved or reduced symptoms and dysfunction to a level that is acceptable to the patient and dentist. Alteration of dental morphology or tooth position should not be performed as an initial course of treatment and should not be employed unless that specific patient experiences re-appearance of symptoms after termination of initial reversible therapy. Such a patient has demonstrated the medical necessity of long term durable treatment.

When initial therapy has affected resolution of a portion of the patient's illness, but significant problems remain, appropriate referral for additional evaluations should be made. This does not imply that the initial treatment has not been successful or that it should be terminated. Patients who ultimately require some form of surgical management, of an intracapsular temporomandibular joint disorder for example, may still benefit from the ongoing use of an appropriate, accurate orthosis to support the mandible, and maintain improved joint relationships and healthy masticatory muscle function.

Part-time Usage of an Orthosis

Some patients maintain comfort and good function by wearing an oral appliance at night and/or during periods of symptom exacerbation. These people are functioning in an adaptive way when the orthosis is not being utilized. Their symptom-free state is maintained by their adaptive capacity. Sometimes, stressors cause an exacerbation of symptoms and increase dysfunction. Patients may return to full time use of an orthosis until symptoms are resolved. If they do not resolve, other forms of long term therapy might be indicated.

A long term durable removable overlay appliance can replace an acrylic orthosis for patients who desire to perpetuate the new occlusal position full time or part time with a more durable appliance. Designed as a mandibular removable partial denture, the anatomical carved occlusal surface can be fabricated with a gold alloy over the cast chrome framework or a processed composite resin or a combination of both.

Orthodontic treatment can be used to alter the natural occlusion, creating the same neuromuscular occlusion that was initially created by the acrylic appliance. A variation of this involves sequential removal of the acrylic of the most posterior tooth covering of the orthosis bilaterally. If the uncovered teeth erupt passively into the new occlusal position, the next most posterior acrylic tooth coverings are removed bilaterally.

Modification of the natural dentition can be performed. The treatment plan must involve an evaluation of the status of the teeth and periodontion, vertical dimension changes, crown to root ratios, and alignment of teeth in both arches. Modification can involve a spectrum of techniques including occlusal equilibration as well as buccal-occlusal onlays and complete coverage restorations. For some patients, long term occlusion changes are accomplished by replacement of removable partial or complete dentures.

Sometimes combinations of therapies are employed to create a stable, durable long term treatment. For example, these combined treatments can include orthodontics and restorative dentistry and orthognathic surgery and orthodontics and sometimes restorative dentistry.

Restorative and Other Dental Applications

The use of bioelectronic measurement instrumentation and the creation of a neuromuscular occlusion have applications in all forms of dental treatment. It is definitely not restricted to those forms of dental treatments associated with the management of temporomandibular disorders. In all areas of dental treatment in which occlusion was to be modified, restored, or replaced, the creation of an occlusion synchronized with healthy masticatory muscle function is of significant physiological value. An occlusion that is associated with healthy, rested, and bilaterally symmetrical muscle function requires no accommodative muscle function. Therefore a potential predisposition to muscle dysfunction has been eliminated. Extensive dental reconstruction via crowns and bridges tooth or implant retained, removable prosthodontics, orthodontics, periodontics, and orthognathic surgery can produce more durable occlusion and supporting structures when neuromuscular occlusion has been created.

Bioelectronic measurement instrumentation provides the roadmap to healthy occlusion and healthy dental/oral structures *(Figures 25 and 26)*. Neuromuscular occlusion is the vehicle by which it is accomplished. The instrumentation can be used with any occlusal philosophy or TMD treatment philosophy as it provides accurate measurement of mandibular and masticatory muscle function.[1]

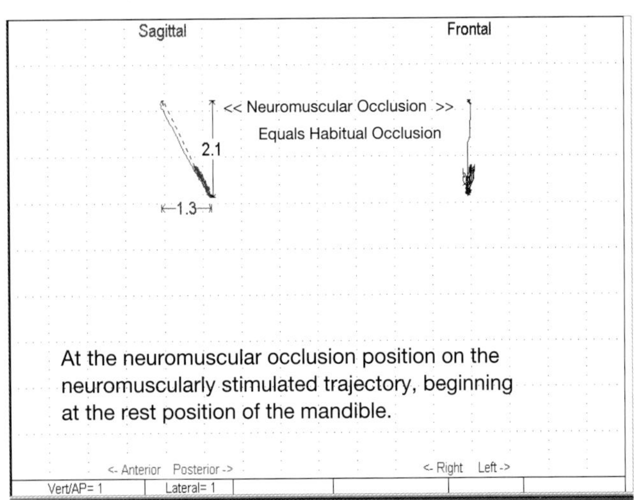

Figure 25. Test of Occlusal Accuracy of Long Term Restorations.

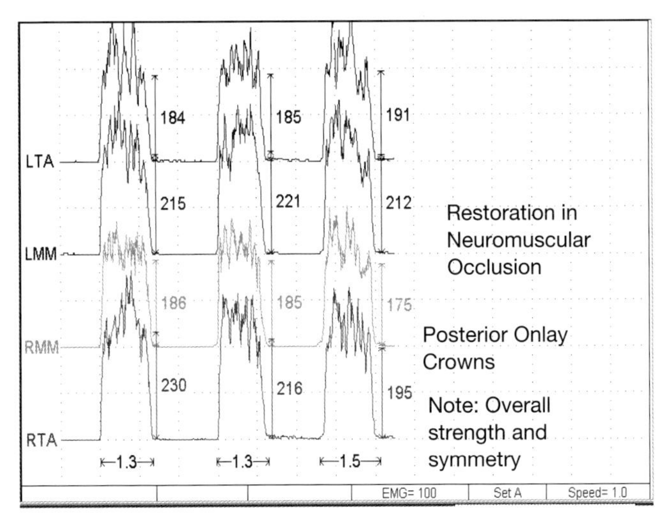

Figure 26. Electromyography of Muscles: Maximum Function (Clench).

References

1. Cooper B: The role of bioelectronic instrumentation in the documentation *Path Oral Radiol* and management of temporomandibular disorders. *Oral Surg Oral Med Oral Endod* 1997;83:91-100.
2. Cooper B: Objective documentation of post-traumatic craniomandibular (TMJ) disorders. *Trial Lawyers Quarterly* 1994;Vol. 24 (4).
3. Moses A, Cooper B: Understanding temporomandibular disorders and whiplash. *Claims Magazine*, July & September, 1993.
4. Dorland, *Illustrated Medical Dictionary, 26th Ed.*, Philadelphia, PA, W. B. Saunders Co. 1985.
5. Paesani D, Westesson PL, Hatala MP, Tallents R, Brooks SL: Accuracy of clinical diagnosis for TMJ internal derangement and arthrosis. *Oral Surg Oral Med Oral Pathol* 1992:73:360-363.
6. Dworkin S, LeResche L, DeRouen T, VonKorff M: Assessing clinical signs of temporomandibular disorders: reliability of clinical examiners. *J Prosthet Dent* 1990;63:574-579.
7. Jankelson R: Anatomy and physiology of the nervous system. In: Jankelson R, ed. *Neuromuscular Dental Diagnosis and Treatment.* St. Louis: Ishiyaku EuroAmerica; 1990;67.
8. Jankelson B: Measurement accuracy of the mandibular kineosiograph: a computerized study. *J Prosthet Dent* 1980;44(6):656-666.
9. Kotani H, Kawazoe Y, Hamada T, et al.: Quantitative electromyographic diagnosis of myofacial pain dysfunction syndrome. *J Prosthet Dent* 1980; 43(4):450-456.

10. Helkimo E, Carlsson G, Carmeli Y: Bite force in patients with functional disturbances of the masticatory system. *J Oral Rehabil* 1975;2:397-406.
11. Kawazoe Y, Kotani H, Mitani T, Yatami H: Integrated electromyographic activity and biting force during rapid isometric contraction of fatigued masseter muscle in man. *Arch Oral Biol* 1981;26:795-801.
12. Cooper B, Cooper D, Lucente F: Electromyography of masticatory muscles in craniomandibular disorders. *Laryngoscope* 1991;101:150-7.
13. Molin C: Vertical isometric muscle forces of the mandible: a comparative study of subjects with and without manifest mandibular pain dysfunction syndrome. *Acta Odontol Scand* 1972;30:485-499.
14. Kotani H, Kawazoe Y, Hamada T, Yamata S: Quantitative electromyographic diagnosis of myofacial pain dysfunction syndrome. *J Prosthet Dent* 1980;43:450-6.
15. Gervais RO, Fitzsimmons GW, Thomas NR: Masseter and temporalis electromyographic activity in asymptomatic subclinical and temporomandibular joint dysfunction patients. *J Craniomandib Pract* 1989:7:52-57.
16. Gervais R, Fitzsimmons G, Thomas N: Masseter and temporalis electromyographic activity in asymptomatic subclinical and temporomandibular joint dysfunction patients. *J Craniomandib Pract,* 1989;7(1):52-57.
17. Milner-Brown HS: The relationship between the surface electromyography and muscular force. *J Physiol* 1975;246:549-69.
18. Bigland B, Lippold OCJ: The relationship between force, velocity and integrated activity in human muscles. *J Physiol* 1954;123:214-24.
19. Ahlgren J, Owall AB: Muscle activity and chewing force: a polygraphic study of human mandibular movements. *Arch Oral Biol* 1970;15:271-280.
20. Kawazoe Y, Kotani H, Hamada T: Relationship between integrated electromyographic activity and biting force during voluntary isometric contraction in human masticatory muscles. *J Dent Res* 1979;58:1440
21. Palla S, Ash M: Effects of bite force in the power spectrum of the surface electromyogram of human muscles. *Arch Oral Biol* 1981; 26:287-295, 547-553.
22. Bakke M, Moller E: Distortion of maximal elevator activity by unilateral premature tooth contact. *Scand J Dent Res* 1980;80:67-75.
23. Riise C, Sheikloleslam A: The influence of experimental interfering occlusal contacts on the activity of the anterior temporal and masseter muscles during mastication. *J Oral Rehabil* 1984;11:325-333.
24. Jarabak JR: An electromyographic analysis of muscular and temporomandibular joint disturbances due to imbalances in occlusion. *Angle Orthod* 1956;26:170-190.
25. Jankelson B: Neuromuscular aspects of occlusion: effects of occlusal position on the physiology and dysfunction of the mandibular musculature. *Dent Clin North Am* 1979;23:157-68.
26. Bergamini M, Prayer-Galletti S: Fibromyalgia and myofacial pain. *Proceedings of the International College of Cranio-Mandibular Orthopedics,* Washington, DC., 1996.
27. Hickman D, Cramer R, Stauber W: The effect of four jaw relations on electromyographic activity in human masticatory muscles. *Arch of Oral Biol* 1993;38(3):261-264.
28. Guyton AC: *Textbook of Medical Physiology, 6th Ed.* Philadelphia: W.B. Saunders Co.; 1981;137.
29. Thomas NR: The effect of fatigue and TENS on the EMG mean power frequency. In: Bergamini M, ed. Pathophysiology of head and neck musculoskeletal disorders. *Frontiers of Oral Pathology.* Basil, Switzerland: Karger; 1990;7:162-170.
30. Cooper B: The role of bioelectronic instruments in the management of TMD. *NY State Dent J* 1995;61:48-53.
31. Cooper BC: Craniomandibular disorders. In: Cooper BC, Lucente FE, eds. *Management of Facial, Head and Neck Pain.* Philadelphia: W.B. Saunders; 1989:153-254.
32. Cooper B, Alleva M, Cooper D, Lucente F: Myofacial pain dysfunction: analysis of 476 patients. *Larnyngoscope* 1986;96(10):1099-1106.
33. Jankelson RR: *Electrosonography (ESG) of the temporomandibular joint: clinical manual.,* Publ. Robert R. Jankelson, DDS, Chelan, WA, 1995
34. Ishigaki S, Bessette R, Maruyama T: A clinical study of temporomandibular joint (TMJ) vibration in TMJ dysfunction patients. J *Craniomandib Pract* 1993;11(1):7-13.
35. Combadazou JC, Combelles R: The efficacy of sonography in the diagnosis of joint disorders. In: Coy R, ed. *Anthology of Craniomandibular Orthopedics.* Int'l. College of Craniomandibular Disorders, Collinsville, IL: Buchanan Pub., 1992.

36. Heffez L, Blaustein D: Advances in sonography of the temporomandibular joint. *J Oral Surg Oral Med Oral Path* 1986;62:486-495.

37. Ovellette PL: TMJ sound prints: electronic auscultation and sonographic audiospectral analysis of the temporomandibular joint. *J Am Dent Assoc* 1974;89:623-628.

38. Drum R, Litt, M: Spectral analysis of temporomandibular joint sounds. *J Prosthet Dent* 1987;58(4):485-494.

39. Gay T: The acoustical characteristics of the normal and abnormal temporomandibular joint. *J Oral Maxillofac Surg* 1987;45:397-407.

40. Watt DM: Temporomandibular joint sounds. In *Gnathosonic Diagnosis and Occlusal Dynamics.* New York, NY: Praeger Publishers, 1981.

41. Melzack R, Wall PD: Pain mechanisms: a new theory. *Science* 1965;150:971-973.

42. Jankelson B, Swain C: Physiological aspects of masticatory muscle stimulation: the myomonitor. *Periodont Oral Hyg* 1972;12.

43. Wessberg GA, Carroll WL, Dinham R, Wolford LM: Transcutaneous electrical stimulation as an adjunct in the management of myofacial pain dysfunction syndrome. *J Prosthet Dent* 1981;45:307-314.

44. Kawazoe Y, Kotani H, Mitani T, et al: The slopes of the fatigued muscle voltage tension curves decreased to a greater degree with percutaneous stimulation than with rest alone. *Arch Oral Biol* 1981;26:796-801.

45. Jankelson B, Radke J: The myomonitor: its use and abuse. *Quintessence Int Dent Digest* 1978;9:35-39,47-52.

46. Jankelson B, Sparks S, Crane P, Radke JC: Neural conduction of the myomonitor stimulus: a quantitative analysis. *J Prosthet Dent,* 1975;34:245-53.

47. Kuwahara T, Miyauchi S, Maruyama T: Clinical classification of the patterns of mandibular movements during mastication in subjects with TMJ disorders. *Int J Prosthod* 1992; 5:122-129.

48. Kuwahara T, Bessette R, Maruyama T: Chewing pattern analysis in TMD patients with unilateral and bilateral internal derangement. *J Craniomandib Pract* 1995;13(3):167-172.

49. Tsolka P, Fenion M, McCullock A, Preiskel H: A controlled clinical, electromyographic and kinesiographic assessment of craniomandibular disorders in women. *J Orofacial Pain* 1994;8(1):80-89.

50. Tsolka P, Preiskel H: Kinesiographic and electromyographic assessment of the effects of occlusal adjustment therapy on craniomandibular disorders by double-blind method. *J Prosthet Dent* 1993;69(1):85-92.

51. Christiansen LV: Effects of an occlusal splint on integrated electromyography of masseter muscle in experimental tooth-clenching in man. *J Oral Rehabil* 1980;7:281.

52. Sheikholeslam A, Holmgren K, Riise C: A clinical and electromyographic study of the long-term effects of an occlusal splint on the temporal and masseter muscles in patients with functional disorders and noctural bruxism. *J Oral Rehabil* 1986;13:137-145.

53. Hamada T, Kotani H, Kawazoe Y, Yamada S: Effect of occlusal splints on the EMG activity in masseter and temporal muscles in bruxism with clinical symptoms. *J Oral Rehabil,* 1982;9:119-23.

54. Kawazoe Y, Kotani H, Hamada T, Yamada S: Effect of occlusal splints on the electromyographic activities of masseter muscles during maximum clenching in patients with myofascial pain dysfunction syndrome. *J Prosthet Dent,* 1980;43:578-80.

55. Mann A, Miralles R, Cumsille F: Influence of vertical dimension on masseter muscle electromyographic activity in patients with mandibular dysfunction. *J Prosthet Dent* 1985;53(2):243-247.

56. *ICCMO Protocol for the Management of Temporomandibular disorders.* International College of Cranio-Mandibular Orthopedics, Seattle, WA, 1998.

57. Konchak P, Thomas N, Lanigan D, Devon R: Freeway space measurement using mandibular kinesiograph and EMG before and after TENS. *Angle Orthodont* 1988;58(4):343-350.

58. Lous I, Sheikholeslam A, Moller E: Postural activity in subjects with functional disorders of the chewing apparatus. *Scand J Dent Res* 1970;78:404-410.

59. Shpuntoff H, Shpuntoff W: A study of physiologic rest position and centric position by electromyography. *J Prosthet Dent* 1956;6(5):621-628.

PHYSICAL ASSESSMENT

Upper Airway Compromise and Musculoskeletal Dysfunction

James F. Garry

Part I: The Head and Neck

Introduction

This paper presents a limited overview of the anatomy and physiology of the upper (nasal) respiratory tract and its relationship to airway obstruction. The correlation between airway obstruction and musculoskeletal dysfunction of the neck will become evident as the paper progresses. This paper cannot be truly comprehensive. Judgements were made as to what to exclude, as well as what to include, and what is likely to be of greatest interest to the practitioner. For example, this paper will not cover congenital anomalies such as clefts or other dysfunctions of the nose such as choanal atresia, midline nasal dermoids, encephaloceles, congenital hemangiomas, neoplasms, etc., which result in airway obstruction. The primary emphasis will be on airway obstruction most commonly encountered by the dentist. Orofacial deformities that result from airway obstruction have been misunderstood by a vast majority of the dental profession. The interrelationship of upper airway compromise to three dimensional craniofacial growth and development has been neglected in the dental curriculum. The dentist should be able to recognize chronic nasal blockade resulting from a deviated septum, inferior turbinate hypertrophy, and/or marked adenotonsillar hypertrophy. If a patient presents to the office with a history of nasal blockade nine to twelve months out of the year, chronic open mouth habitus, and a history of mouth-breathing and/or nocturnal snoring, immediate consideration should be given to nasal airway obstruction.

Orthodontic literature is replete with articles referring to airway compromise, but it is unfortunate that undergraduate literature is sparse and in most universities nonexistent. The majority of published articles relate airway compromise to the long face syndrome resulting in the dolichocephalic (narrow faced) child with a steep mandibular plane angle.

It has been the author's clinical experience that most malocclusions and orofacial deformities are the result of noxious environmental influences that disturb an optimal genetic growth potential. It is too simplistic to relate upper airway obstruction only to the long face syndrome. This paper is intended to stimulate each reader to recognize chronic upper airway obstruction and its relation to musculoskeletal dysfunction of the head and neck.

The concept that the stomatognathic system is subject to constant interactions between soft tissues in functional motion and its influence upon the forming skeletal structures has been well documented by Van Der Klaauw[1] and Moss.[2,3] This concept clarifies the role of the tongue and posture of the mandible in the morphogenesis of the facial structures. In addition, clinical observation supports this functional matrix theory. For example, in *Figure 1*, it is obvious that a pathological morphogenesis has evolved due to non-physiologic posturing of the tongue between the dental arches. Some would classify the etiology of the dental deformity as an enlarged tongue and would fear relapse of orthodontic treatment. Some may recommend orthognathic surgery, and others may recommend a partial glossectomy. Consideration must be given to airway obstruction as playing a pathologic role in tongue posture, and its size influencing the resultant dentofacial deformity.

Review of the Literature

Magendie, in 1829, was the first to refer to the nose as part of the respiratory tract that helps warm and moisten inspired air.[4] "The adenoidal face" was first described as early as 1872 by Tomes,[5] who noted that patients with V-shaped contracted maxillas had a long narrow face. Angle[6] included airway obstruction as an important etiologic factor in the development of malocclusion in 1907. The first multidisciplinary approach to treatment of malocclusion and airway obstruction was suggested by Ketchum[7] in 1912. He recommended that patients seek an opinion by both a rhinologist and an orthodontist to receive the full benefit of modern science. In 1935, McCoy[8] related naso-respiratory function to craniofacial growth. He noted an increase in Class III malocclusions in patients with partial airway obstruction. Balyeat and Bowen,[9] in 1934, noted facial and dental deformities resulting from perennial nasal allergies in childhood. In 1939, Todd and Broadbent[10] described the role of allergy in the etiology of orthodontic deformity.

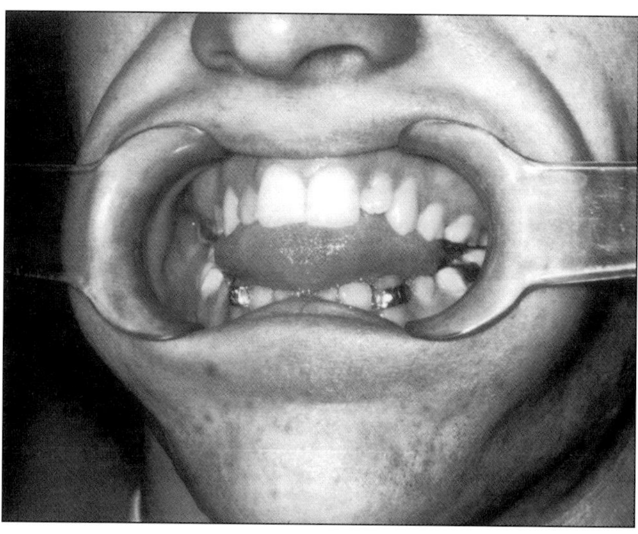

Figure 1. Teeth in occlusion. Note: Only posterior teeth are contacting (full fan open bite), steep mandibular plane angle, poor tongue posture, and dolichocephalic long face syndrome (dentofacial deformity).

The significance of adenoid and tonsillar tissue in orthodontics was described by Subtelny[11] in 1954 as it related to facial growth. This concept was supported by Ricketts[12] in 1958. Nasal obstruction was related to orofacial deformities in children by Marks[13] in 1965. The same year a significant study was done by Bushey[14] on monozygotic twins which confirmed alterations in certain anatomical relations accompanying a change from oral to nasal breathing. This study gave credence to the "Functional Matrix Theory" of Moss in 1962.[15] The functional matrix theory simply stated that the skull consists of a series of bones. The forms of these bones (where form = size and shape), as well as their position in space, have no obligatory relationship to each other. They are, in fact, relatively independent, both phylogenetically and ontogenetically. The functional matrix theory was originally proposed by Van Der Klaauw[1] and was expanded by Moss, Dunn, Green, and Cunat[16] in 1973. They reported a relationship between the variation of mandibular morphology and the variation of nasopharyngeal airway size in monozygotic twins, thus confirming the study by Bushey.[14] The classic primate research by Harvold[17] published in 1972 demonstrated skeletal changes, as well as soft tissue changes, when the nasal air passage became restricted. In 1974, Subtelny[18] described the influence of hypertrophied tonsils and adenoids on facial growth. In 1975, Linder-Aronson[19] reported the effects of adenoidectomy on the dentition and facial skeleton over a period of five years. He noted that a group of post-adenotonsillectomy patients who became nasal respirators later experienced significant changes toward normalization of craniofacial growth, whereas there was no change in the persistent mouthbreathers and unoperated controls. Quinn,[20] in 1978, reported the influence of airway on the growth and development of the face, jaws, dentition, and associated parts. In 1979, Linder-Aronson and Woodside[19] did a comparative study of the upper and lower anterior face heights compared to a standard population and concluded that airway was an important influence on facial form. In 1980, Rubin[21] supported the view that the mode of respiration has an effect on facial growth. This viewpoint was shared by McNamara[22] in 1981. That same year, Hannuksela[23] reported craniofacial changes in children with allergic rhinitis, which predisposes children to hypertrophied tonsils and enlarged adenoids. The children developed steep mandibular plane angles as seen on lateral headplates. McNamara noted a change in two cases. After nasal airway obstruction was corrected, there was a change in facial form to a more brachycephalic (wide maxilla and mandible) form in both cases.

There is an attempt by many researchers to find a formula that will justify the need for adenotonsillectomy and/or surgery. However, the complexity of human physiology will leave the researcher with more questions than answers. Clinical observation and treatment is considered anecdotal or purely empirical by the researcher. Yet, the consensus of clinicians who have been aware of airway obstruction for several decades clearly favors a functioning airway and recommends adenotonsillectomies as early as necessary to reduce pharyngeal obstruction when chronic mouthbreathing is evident.

Etiology of Upper Airway Obstruction

There are a myriad of factors causing upper airway obstruction. It would be presumptuous of this author to state that the etiology of airway obstruction is engraved in stone; it is not. However, the obvious should be pointed out. What is the primary etiology? When can it begin? What abnormal conditions are associated with prolonged impairment of nasal respiration? How can we recognize the impairment? What effect does the impairment have on orofacial development? What can or should we do to improve the airway impairment?

The most common etiology of upper airway obstructions is respiratory tract allergies. Inhalants are the most common nasal allergens. Food allergens are also important but are difficult to trace. The sensitive patient will develop chronic rhinitis, polypoid changes in the mucosa, and chronic nasal obstruction. The most common inhalant agents are pollens, animal dander, fungal spores, house dust, feathers, and detergents. House dust is a particularly active inhalant which consists of many substances such as spores, dander, fabric dust, mites, and so on. Allergy to house dust causes perennial symptoms, whereas allergy to pollens is seasonal. Hypersensitivity reactions release chemical mediators such as histamine, kinins, slow reacting substance of anaphylaxis (SRA-A), and eosinophilic chemotactic factor (ECF) into the microcirculation, resulting in venous congestion. Allergic edema of the mucous membranes of the nasal and paranasal cavities results in "venous pudding."[24] The interior of the allergic nose characteristically shows boggy, grayish-pink inferior turbinates with glistening mucoid secretions. One or both swollen, mucous-covered turbinates often occlude the nostril. Marks[25] points out that nasal septal deviations are not uncommon and occur in over one-third of children afflicted with persistent perennial allergic rhinitis. In addition, maxillary sinus polyps often accompany severe and chronic allergic rhinitis.

The IgE Connection

Researchers have noted that there is a relation between hypersensitivity or allergic reaction and the amount of immunoglobulin E (IgE) found in the blood.[25] A study by Sassouni et. al.[26] suggests that perennial rhinitis with an allergic reaction can lead to chronic mouthbreathing, which can alter the development of the midface. There was a definite correlation between the IgE level and airway blockage. It has been estimated that obstructions in the nasal cavity exist in 85% of all children. Increased resistance within the nasal airway may be due to edema of the turbinates, hypertrophied adenoidal tissue, marked deviation of the nasal septum, chronic purulent rhinitis, nasal polyposis, narrow nostrils, etc.

The focus of this paper will be on the most common result of nasal obstruction, nasopharyngeal obstruction, and hypopharyngeal obstruction resulting from allergy of the upper respiratory tract.

Function and Anatomy of the Nose

The function of the nose is to warm, humidify, and filter the air in preparation to enter the lungs and bronchi. Olfaction and phonation are also a function of the nose and can give the dentist a clue regarding the patency of nasal function. Nasal obstruction can result in hyposmia (abnormally decreased sensitivity to odors).

The external nose consists of two fused nasal bones superiorly and four alar cartilages inferiorly. There are two nasal passages which are separated by a central vertical septum containing cartilage anteroinferiorly and bone posterosuperiorly (perpendicular plate of the ethmoid and vomer). Both passages have anterior and posterior openings, the choanae. Both passages are lined with mucoperchondrium that contains mucous secreting goblet cells and glands. The cribriform plate forms the roof of the nose, while the hard palate forms the floor.

Turbinates

There are three turbinates on each lateral wall; superior, middle, and inferior. The inferior is the largest and most vascular. The entire inferior turbinate and lower two-thirds of the middle turbinate are responsible for heating and moistening the passing air. Mouthbreathers lose this capability as the mouth and trachea do not heat and moisten passing air.

Turbinates are scroll-like thin plates of bone that are covered by a thick mucosa. The bone and mucosa contain longitudinal blood vessels, resembling channels, through which blood flows rapidly. The volume of air that passes through the nose is controlled by the size of turbinates, which fluctuate every one to four hours from one nasal passage to the other. This is called the nasal cycle and results from cyclic engorgement of the turbinates.[27]

Turbinates are extremely responsive to allergens and non-allergic vasomotor rhinitis and, as a result, are a major cause of airway obstruction. Nasal resistance will change in response to hormones, inhaled allergens and irritants, and various pharmacologic agents.

Liminal Valve

A liminal valve located at the junction of the hard and soft nose regulates the overall resistance throughout the nasal respiratory system. During normal inspiration, muscles within the liminal valve become rigid to allow a more patent airway. However, during rapid inspiration, the liminal valve collapses against the septum, regulating airflow. Damage to the valve, soft tissue, or bony deformities within the nose can produce significant elevations in nasal resistance and result in airway obstruction.

Clinical Evaluation of the Nose

Observe the external architecture of the nose. Asymmetry is obvious, i.e., depressed nasal fracture. The nose should be straight, the nasal bridge should not be obviously narrow. The columela (tissue between the nares) should not be thick, the alae should not be collapsed, the tip of the nose normally is not hooked (distorts air flow) or not typically at an acute angle (indicative of microrhinic dysplasia). Lift the tip of the nose and observe if the cartilagenous septum is displaced to the right or left of the midline. Internal nasal inspection can be done with a nasal speculum and a good light source. The tips of the blade should not touch the sensitive mucosa. The septum should not be deviated, as small deviations in the valve area are significant in terms of airway obstruction. The nasal mucosa in an allergic nose characteristically show boggy, grayish-pink, inferior turbinates covered with glistening mucoid secretions.[13] One or both swollen, mucous-covered turbinates often occlude the nostrils. Nasal polyps are difficult for the dentist to view; however, P-A cephalograms are of value. Intranasal spurs (usually at the vomer junction) are rarely diagnosed by the dentist, but the dentist should understand that spurs can cause chronic irritation to the nasal mucosa resulting in airway obstruction. If the nose is open for respiration, a strip of soft tissue paper in front of the nares moves with the airflow. Keep in mind that both nares do not function simultaneously due to the nasal cycle. If the patient is a habitual nose breather, the alae nasi show only slight movement as respiration is increased. Transient oral respiration resulting from a cold or allergy must be ruled out. If mouthbreathing is the dominant function, the alae nasi do not move. A limited inspection of the nose will enable the dentist to make an intelligent referral to the physician.

Anatomy of the Pharynx

The pharynx extends from the base of the skull to the beginning of the esophagus, and it is divided into the nasopharynx above the soft palate, the oropharynx between the soft palate and base of the tongue, and the laryngopharynx or hypopharynx below.

Waldeyer's Ring

Waldeyer's ring is a band of lymphoid tissue that encircles the nasopharynx and oropharynx. The main components are the adenoids and faucial tonsils. The lingual tonsils, pharyngeal lymph nodes, and lymphoid aggregations above and behind the openings of the eustachian tubes complete the ring. It serves as a protective organ at the ingress of the body, and it frequently is the site of acute and chronic infections or other abnormalities. It is frequently involved in airway obstruction, which can lead to mouthbreathing and poor tongue repose.

Adenoids

The adenoids are situated on the posterior wall of the nasopharynx and are thrown into a series of longitudinal ridges enlarging their surface area. The tissue immediately beneath the surface epithelium is lymphoid and arranged in nodules, some with germ centers, and loose lymphoid tissue separates the nodules. The surface epithelium is infiltrated with lymphocytes.

Adenoiditis usually occurs concomitantly with acute tonsillitis. Symptoms resemble those of acute tonsillitis, but nasal obstruction may also be evident. Involvement of the eustachian tube causes earaches and fullness in the ear, and may develop into otitis media.

Adenoid hypertrophy can result from chronic allergies in the upper respiratory tract. Chronic nasal allergies cause a reduction of ciliated columnar epithelium, an increase in nasal mucous secretions, and inspissated nasal mucous secretions. This reduces the efficiency of cilia locomotion, which results in stagnation of bacteria, viruses, and foreign bodies in the nasal cavities. The resultant enlarged nasopharyngeal structures obstruct the posterior nares and eustachian tubes and may cause nasal speech, postnasal discharge, cough, vomiting, oral fetor, an alteration of facial expression (open mouth habitus), and chronic mouthbreathing. On examination of the oral cavity, a high arched palate and dental malocclusion are usually evident.

The adenoids grow at an accelerated rate from six months until two or three years of age when they occupy approximately one-half of the nasopharyngeal cavity.[28] Gray[29] has stated that, in his clinical experience, adenoids begin to involute at approximately four years of age. However, it is not uncommon to see enlarged tonsils in older children. Most tonsils and adenoids have regressed by puberty. Rarely, hypertrophied lingual tonsils and adenoids are evident in adults. He further stated that there is a general consensus among rhinologists that the regression is due to a maturing bone marrow in the growing child which produces lymphocytes, taking over the role of tonsils and adenoids.

Faucial Tonsils

The faucial tonsils lie in a triangular fossa formed by the palatoglossal and palatopharyngeal folds and the base of the tongue. The palatoglossal fold may largely conceal the tonsil but during contraction of the superior constrictor muscles during swallowing the tonsils are "extruded" into the pharynx. Between 10 and 30 crypts descend from the surface of the tonsil, penetrating almost to its base. Epithelial lined extensions project from these structures, greatly increasing the epithelial surface area. Subepithelial lymphoid tissue is thus brought into contact with the environment of the oral and pharyngeal cavities. As well as organisms, the crypts contain desquamated cells and debris. Lymphocytes from the lymphoid tissue escape into the mouth. Although mucous glands are present, their ducts do not open into the bases of the crypts, so that stagnation and infection at the bottom of the crypts are prone to occur. Diseased tonsils or adenoids may cause local, constitutional, focal, or allergic disturbances. Local symptoms include recurrent sore throat, halitosis, chronic nasal discharge, and cervical lymphadenopathy. These patients have a tendency to develop frequent colds. Constitutional symptoms are asthenia, low grade fever, lassitude, and failure of growing children to gain weight. Infected tonsils and adenoids have been regarded as responsible for bacterial allergy and for many systemic disorders on the grounds that improvement of the disorders followed tonsillectomy or adenoidectomy. The dentist must be cognizant of the proprioceptive effect of an enlarged tonsil or tonsils on the dorsum of the tongue. The proprioceptive effect postures the tongue away from the enlarged tonsil, resulting in a non-physiologic tongue posture within the dental arches *(Figure 2)*. The result is orofacial deformity.

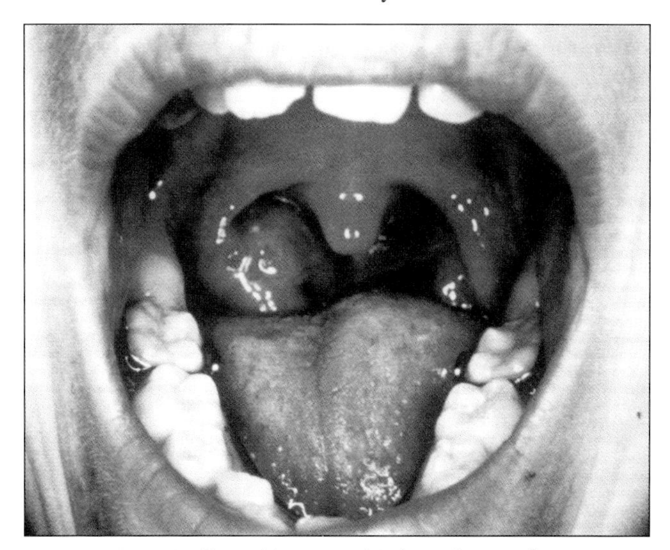

Figure 2. Note: Unilateral hypertrophied tonsil. Note the proprioceptive effect of the right dorsum of the tongue, resulting in a narrow pointed tongue. The tongue deviates away from the hypertrophied tonsil at its dorsum, forcing the tongue into a deviant orientation, and distorting the dentition, which results in malocclusion and dentofacial deformity.

The role of lymphoid tissue antibody formation in the early years is understood; however, the resultant orofacial deformities that occur from the proprioceptive effect of retained enlarged obstructive tonsils and adenoids is poorly understood by the physician. Quality of life is threatened by retaining tonsils and adenoids that are not only obstructive but that create abnormal tongue posture via proprioception. The dogmatic dictum that tonsils and adenoids must not be removed unless a patient has three episodes of recurrent tonsillitis in each of three years seems to be one of the most unscientific and unreasonable dictums that has dominated the medical scene for years. One basis for the contraindications of adenotonsillectomies resulted from a study that indicated that patients who had had tonsillectomies were more apt to develop bulbar poliomyelitis than patients who have not undergone such surgery. Wholesale removal of tonsils and adenoids is unwarranted. However, when a child is a chronic mouthbreather, day and/or night, and facial deformity is evident, serious consideration must be given to adenotonsillectomy. Poor tongue repose resulting from enlarged tonsils and/or adenoids does not allow the maxillary and mandibular arches to develop properly. The patient may develop chronic mouthbreathing, which lowers alveolar oxygen saturation (PaO_2) and increases $PaCO_2$ which alters the pH of the blood. Some bizarre by-products are sleep apnea, dysphagia, pulmonary hypertension, cor pulmonale, enuresis, bruxism, behavioral disorders, hyperkinesis, etc. The dentist and physician need to observe patients and make an intelligent, reasonable evaluation of their presenting facial asymmetries and correlate the deformities to upper airway obstructions. The adult patient will usually give a history of sore throats and/or earaches as a child. Many adults have had their tonsils and adenoids removed; however, if they were removed after a prolonged series of "sore throats," the dental arches may have already been malformed, creating an environment too small to accommodate the tongue which, in turn, acts as an obstructor to proper arch development and tooth eruption. This can ultimately result in craniomandibular dysfunction.

Lingual Tonsil

The lingual tonsils are a collection of lymphatic tissue at the root of the tongue resembling the faucial tonsils grossly and microscopically, but possessing mucous glands with duct openings at the crypt bases.

Lymphoid nodules are inconspicuous in health but may become prominent in Waldeyer's ring when an infection is present.

There are basically five functions of the lymphoid tissue in Waldeyer's ring: (1) antibody synthesis, (2) cellular defense against infection, (3) formation of lymphocytes, (4) removal of microorganisms, bacterial toxins, extravascular proteins, and foreign particles from lymphatic fluid, and (5) phagocytosis. It would seem that removal of lymphoid tissue with the functions listed above would be criminal. However, these tissues begin to regress as early as four years of age and typically regress by puberty. To what extent antibody formation is jeopardized by adenotonsillectomy is still uncertain, and the possible deleterious effects of chronic tonsil infections have not been documented in large groups of patients in longitudinal studies. An accurate medical history and a careful clinical examination can determine when an adenotonsillectomy is indicated.

T & A Morbidity and Mortality

The risk of morbidity and mortality from tonsillectomy and adenoidectomy (T & A) ranges postoperatively from throat discomfort to death.[30]

In one of the largest studies of T & A, consisting of 6,175,729 cases, Pratt[31] showed a mortality of 1 in 16,381 (0.006%). This study showed that anesthesia was responsible for 139 deaths, or 1 in 44,429 (0.002%). Cardiac arrest occurred in 0.002 per cent and hemorrhage in 1 in 55,637 (0.002%). These percentages were compiled without regard to the skill of the surgeon and anesthesiologist. Many surgeons who deal with a skilled anesthesiologist have very few complications. The question now becomes: is the risk worth the result? Consideration must be given to quality of life. If quality of life is improved significantly by a T & A, and a skilled surgeon and anesthesiologist perform the procedure, the patient stands to benefit with little risk.

Respiration

The process of respiration can be divided into four major categories: (1) pulmonary ventilation, which means the inflow and outflow of air between the atmosphere and the alveoli, (2) diffusion of oxygen and carbon dioxide between the alveoli and blood, (3) transport of oxygen and carbon dioxide in the blood and body fluids to and from the cells, and (4) regulation of ventilation and other facets of respiration.

Respiration is controlled in cerebral centers, which send signals to medullary and pontine centers. Breathing is constantly monitored by receptors in the brain, which monitors pressure, airflow, and resistance along the respiratory tract. For example, if airway resistance increases due to nasal obstruction, or there is an increased need for oxygen due to excessive exercise, impulses from the respiratory centers descend within the spinal cord. These impulses reach the diaphragm through phrenic innervation and intercostal muscles via intercostal nerves, resulting in an increase in rate and amplitude of respiration. Accelerated respiration improves ventilation and thus tends to normalize the PaO_2, $PaCO_2$, and pH of the blood. Chronic nasal airway resistance will result in chronic mouthbreathing to lower airway resistance along the respiratory tract.

On inspiration, air flows to the lungs by virtue of contraction of the intercostal muscles. This expands the chest cage, enlarges the lungs, and stretches the elastic fibers within the lungs and thoracic cage in conjunction with the diaphragm. The resultant negative pressure allows air to rush into the lungs via the nose and/or mouth. There are three types of airflow in the nose: laminar, turbulent, and transitional flow. Anatomic constrictions change airflow from laminar, which is characterized by streamlined planes of air traveling parallel to the sides of the tube and capable of sliding over one another. Turbulent flow, which occurs at high flow rates, is characterized by a complete disorganization of streamlining. Transitional flow is created when laminar flow becomes blunted and the streamlined planes of air separate from the walls of the tube, resulting in minor eddy formations. A combination of all three patterns of airflow occurs throughout the respiratory system. The amount of turbulence depends on the number of sizes of anatomical structures through which the air must pass. In turbulent airflow, the air passing through the nasal passages strikes many obstructing vanes: the turbinates, the septum, and the pharyngeal wall. Each time air strikes an obstruction, it changes the direction of movement. The particles suspended in the passing air, having far more mass and momentum than air, cannot change their direction of travel as rapidly as air. Therefore, they continue forward, striking the surfaces of the obstructions.

The turbinates play an essential role as resisters to pulmonary air loss during expiration. They resist the loss of air within the lung when the elastic fibers in the thoracic cage and lung recoil to compress the heated and humidified air against the pulmonary vascular bed. This enables an optimal absorption and transfer of oxygen at the pulmonary level. It is important to understand that the body is not oxygenated during inspiration. Oxygen enters the vascular system during expiration. The turbinates resist a rapid recoil of the lungs, resulting in better ventilatory compliance for optimal absorption and transfer of oxygen. The body requires optimal resistance from the turbinates on expiration.[32]

Mucociliary Function, Turbinate Responsiveness, and Airway Resistance

All surfaces of the nose are coated with a thin layer of mucous which is secreted by the mucous membrane covering these surfaces. It has been postulated that the secretory IgA, which is present in the mucous, defends against airborne disease.[33] Furthermore, the epithelium of the nasal passageways is ciliated, and the cilia constantly oscillate, carrying mucous toward the pharynx. Therefore, after particles are entrapped in the mucous, this mucous is moved like a sliding sheet toward the pharynx at a rate of approximately 5.7 mm per minute and finally is either expectorated or swallowed. The entrapment of airborn allergens within the nasal passageways makes this region most susceptible to an allergic response (allergic rhinitis). The most common obvious response is an engorgement of the turbinates, resulting in a restricted nasal airway with concomitant mouthbreathing. When nasal respiration is circumvented by oral respiration, the passing air is not filtered, heated, or humidified; the mandible drops, increasing the mandibular plane angle; and the tongue is no longer in an optimal physiologic relationship to the developing dental arches. The result is lowered pulmonary oxygen saturation and abnormal orofacial development. However, when the nasal airway becomes obstructed due to engorged responsive turbinates, beyond the so-called "norm," expiration and inspiration become difficult, and mouthbreathing occurs to keep the airflow within "normal" limits. A study by McCaffrey and Eugene Kem[34,35] at Mayo Clinic established a relationship of increased nasal resistance and the presence of nasal obstruction symptomatology. Their rhinometric study of one thousand asymptomatic patients established asymptomatic normal nasal resistances to be from 2.5 cm H_2O/liter/sec to 3.5 cm H_2O/liter/sec. It is interesting to note that newborns have resistances from 10 cm H_2O/liter/sec to 12 cm H_2O/liter/sec, and, as we grow older, nasal resistance decreases.

According to Gray, a rhinologist,[29] it is extremely difficult to establish "norms" of airway resistance with any biomedical instrumentation currently in use. The proprioceptive effect of the instrumentation to which the patient is attached changes the airflow significantly, compared to the patient who is not attached to instrumentation. An example of the variation in normal values of airway resistances was described in a study by Adams[36] in 1978. He found that resistances of 3 cm H_2O/liter/sec to 4.5 cm H_2O/liter/sec were normal and resulted in a higher velocity of airflow. This provided more oxygen to the peripheral alveoli of the lungs. Nasal blockade resulted in mouthbreathing, which affects airflow (lowers velocity of incoming air), pulmonary mechanics, and gas exchange.

The efficiency of the nose is incredible. Imagine a system capable of heating, moistening, filtering the passing air, and, in addition, regulating airway resistance and providing olfaction. By the time passing air reaches the nasopharynx, it is heated to body temperature, 90% humidified, and virtually free of solid particles. No engineer has been able to design such an efficient system. When airway resistance is detrimental to the quality of life, impulses from respiratory centers descend within the spinal cord and increase or decrease the amplitude of respiration to normalize the pH of the blood. An increase in amplitude improves ventilation and, in cases of nasal obstruction, results in mouthbreathing bypassing the nasal blockade.[37]

Chemical Control of Respiration

Inadequate ventilation for bodily needs may depress PaO_2 and/or elevate PaO_2 in the blood. Elevated PaO_2 leads to lower pH. Lowered PaO_2 of blood affects chemoreceptors of carotid and aortic bodies, which are also responsive to markedly lowered pH. Elevated PaO_2 (lowered pH) of blood and cerebral spinal fluid affects central chemoreceptors. There are two types of receptors that sample pH changes in the blood: (1) those in the vicinity of the bifurcation of the carotid artery with its internal and external branches which send signals to the brain via the 9th cranial nerve and (2) those in the aortic arch which signal the brain via the 10th nerve. The receptors seem to respond directly to changes in arterial PO_2. If the receptors are removed, hypoxia exerts a depressant effect on central neurons and decreases ventilation. Receptors located in the ventrolateral surface of the medulla account for approximately 80% of the increase in ventilation produced when carbon dioxide is inhaled. Impulses from the respiratory centers descend within the spinal cord to reach the diaphragm via phrenic nerves and the intercostal muscles via intercostal nerves. This increases the rate and amplitude of respiration. Accelerated respiration improves ventilation and thus tends to normalize PaO_2, $PaCO_2$, and pH of the blood.[38]

Limited History

When upper airway compromise is suspected, a limited history should be taken prior to referral to the otolaryngologist and/or allergist. Observing the patient as he or she enters the operatory and when he or she is unaware of the observation will enable the dentist to decide whether to pursue a more detailed allergy history. *Figure 3* is an example of an unposed allergic child. Edematous nasal and paranasal mucous membranes restrict airway, and mouthbreathing is a compensatory result. Note the open mouth habitus, dry large bulbous lips, pseudocheilosis, allergic shiners, tearing from eyes, head tilted to the left, short upper lip, right eye higher than left eye, nose tilted upward, and a hypertonic mentalis.

A family history may reveal that the parents or a sibling suffer from frequent sore throats, colds, or sinus pain. If so, there is a 40% chance that the child will be allergic.[39] Sleep patterns should be investigated. It is pathologic for a patient to be a chronic nocturnal mouthbreather or snorer, or to have sleep apnea.

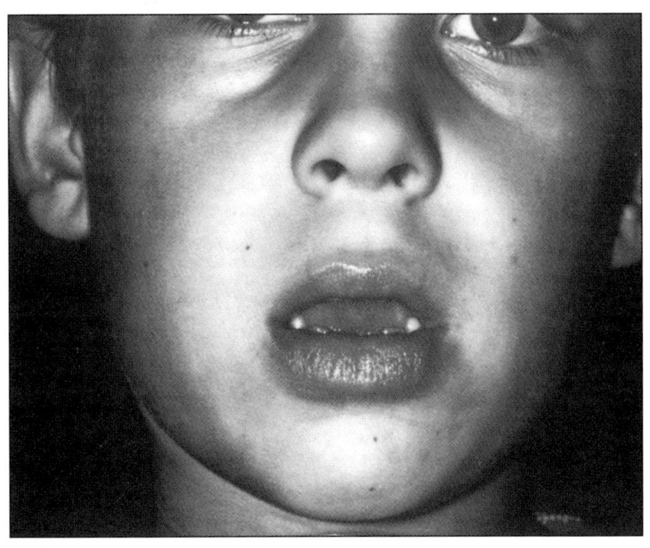

Figure 3. Typical appearance of a child with upper airway obstruction resulting from chronic upper respiratory allergies. Edematous nasal and paranasal mucous membranes restrict airway, and mouthbreathing is a compensatory result. Note: Open mouth habitus, dry large bulbous lips, allergic shiners, tearing of the eyes, radiating lines in the lower oribopalpebral groove extending from the corner of the eye with a downward slant and an upward swing (Dennie's sign), deep labiomental fold, and a hyperactive mentalis.

Have someone observe the patient after they have gone to sleep and take note of breathing patterns. It is essential that the history of an airway-obstructed patient include any medications that he or she is currently taking. Prescribed medications can be the source of "rebound rhinitis" similar to that which follows the use of a vasoconstrictor.[40] A decrease in sympathetic stimulation or increase in parasympathetic stimulation usually results in the engorgement of sinusoidal venous spaces and edema in the turbinates.[41]

Medications prescribed for hypertension generally reduce sympathetic activity, although the modes of action are variable. Non-select beta blockers (e.g., Propanolol and Madrolol) generally induce nasal stuffiness since they block the response to the sympathetic nerve impulses equally at all sites of the body.[42] On the other hand, cardioselective beta blockers (e.g., Metaprolol, Antenolol, and Toamoial) normally do not produce nasal stuffiness because they selectively block nerve impulses only to the cardiac muscle.

Antipsychotic drugs possess alpha-antiadrenergic action to some degree, which decreases sympathetic stimulation and leads to turbinate engorgement.[42]

Nasal stuffiness can occur during pregnancy because of increased estrogen titers. Nasal stuffiness can occur as a result of contraceptive pills. It appears as though a direct hormonal effect on the turbinate stroma is likely.[42] In most cases, the symptoms subside with the withdrawal of the medication. However, in some cases, permanent stromal hypertrophy may occur. This may be treated with corticosteroids[38] or may require surgical reduction.[43]

Clinical Signs of Upper Airway Obstruction

The following are the stigmata of upper airway obstruction that will enable the dentist to make an intelligent preliminary diagnosis: (1) chronic open mouth habitus, (2) lip pursing during a swallow, (3) lip habitus (lower lip postured behind maxillary incisors), (4) facial asymmetry, (5) dry lips (usually resulting from chronic mouthbreathing), (6) deep labiomental fold due to overclosure, (7) commissural cheilitis occurring with no vitamin B deficiency or herpetic lesions, usually prevalent with chronic nocturnal mouthbreathing and concomitant drooling, (8) dished out or flat labial profile, (9) rolled hypotonic lower lip, (10) prognathic maxilla or mandible, (11) retrognathic maxilla or mandible, (12) TMJ noise (popping or crepitus), (13) bruxism, (14) cervical erosion, (15) mobile teeth, (16) headaches in the frontal, temporal, parietal, and/or occipital regions, (17) dysphagia (difficulty in swallowing), usually due to a lack of volume for the tongue within the dental arches resulting from early airway obstruction, (18) open bite, (19) closed bite, (20) high V palatal vault, (21) narrow maxillary arch, (22) crowded anterior teeth, (23) pain in maxillary teeth with no evident pathology (usually due to maxillary sinusitis, referred soft tissue pain, or neuralgia of the maxillary branch of the trigeminal nerve, (24) scalloped tongue (tooth imprints on borders of the tongue due to lack of intra-oral volume for the tongue), (25) cheek chewing, (26) dry mouth in the morning (resulting from nocturnal mouthbreathing), (27) drooling during sleep (open mouth), (28) snoring or mouthbreathing during sleep, (29) chronic asymptomatic hyperemia of the pharynx, (30) enlarged tonsils, (31) enlarged adenoids, (32) constant fatigue resulting from anemia or hypoxemia, (33) injected conjunctiva, (34) pectus excavatum, (35) chronic earaches, (36) chronic recurrent throat infections, (37) obstructive sleep apnea, (38) maxillary diastema, (39) hyperactivity, (40) severe fatigue after exercise, (41) constantly tired (malaise), (42) tinnitus, (43) fullness in the ears, (44) difficulty in nasal breathing, (45) lisping, (46) postural problems such as forward head posture, side bending of head, etc., (47) steep mandibular plane angle (adenoidal face), (48) chin deviation, (49) allergic shiners (dark circles below the eyes), (50) infraorbital edema (bags below the eyes), (51) allergic pseudopannus (bilateral asymptomatic opaque supracomeal patch), (52) marginal upper eyelid eczema, and (53) enuresis due to nocturnal arousals as a result of a drop in blood oxygen saturation.[44,45]

Airway Obstruction and Quality of Life

Airway obstruction results in mouthbreathing. Later the relationship of mouthbreathing to orofacial deformity resulting from mandibular posture and tongue repose will be discussed. Mouthbreathing can lead to lowered oxygen saturation (hypoxemia), resulting from a decreased resistance of the turbinates on expiration, lowered humidification, and a lack of optimal warming of the air on inspiration. Blood gas studies by Ogura[46] revealed that mouthbreathers have 20% more carbon dioxide and 20% less oxygen in the blood than non-mouthbreathers. A reduction in oxygen saturation has been reported to cause "cor pulmonale,"[47] which is an enlargement of the right ventricle secondary to malfunction of the lungs. This can result from intrinsic pulmonary disease, an abnormal chest bellow, or a depressed ventilatory drive (airway obstruction). Cor pulmonale (CP) is directly caused by alterations in the pulmonary circulation leading to pulmonary hypertension and, thereby, an increased mechanical load on right ventricular emptying.[48]

Many mouthbreathers complain of a dry mouth and/or recurrent infections of the throat. This, in part, may be attributable to the fact that the esophagus contains no mucous glands and is lubricated by mucous from the nose and pharynx, which denies the esophagus essential lubrication resulting in low grade esophagitis. Lowered humidification of respired air[49] also results in drying of the protective pharyngeal mucoid secretions, leading to recurrent infection in the throat, gingivitis, and halitosis due to the so-called "putrefaction" of dried saliva.[50] The amount of mucous secreted per day is approximately one pint.[51]

Airway obstruction causes a change in naso-central reflexes[52] which can cause lowering of confidence and feeling of well-being, impairment of concentration, and an increase in incidence of headaches.

An interesting study was done in Europe in 1966 showing a lowering of production of the pituitary growth hormone in airway obstruction.[53]

Sleep apnea is defined as a cessation of breathing for ten seconds or longer and at least five episodes per hour. Sleep apnea syndrome, particularly the obstructive type, has been found in patients with hypertrophied adenoids and tonsils.[54,55,56] Sleep apneic children have more episodes of enuresis than non-apneic children as a result of restless sleep.[57]

The most important substance a patient needs for an improvement in the quality of life is not food or water, it is oxygen. Lowered blood oxygen saturation can result in malaise during quiet periods, lowered exercise tolerance, below average intellectual achievement, behavioral disorders, pulmonary hypertension, and cor pulmonale.

Enlarged tonsils and/or adenoids can result in dysphagia, which leads to poor eating habits and nutritional depletion.

A correlation was found between upper airway obstruction and pectus excavatum by Fan and Murphy.[58]

Common upper airway obstructors are:

1. Mucosal swelling, resulting in a normal compensatory turbinate hypertrophy of the lateral wall of the nose opposite any concavity of the septum, or as the result of an allergic rhinitis or infection causing temporary swelling.

2. Septal deformity, occuring in about 80% of adults and in 60% of infants.[59,60] If present at birth, septal deformities do not straighten with growth. Septal deformity is the major cause of obstruction from birth to 18 months, and can be readily straightened by manipulation.[61]

3. Enlargement in lymphoid tissue of Waldeyer's ring, particularly the adenoids.

4. Polyps, which may occur with edema and prolapse of sinus mucosa into the nasal cavity. This is usually seen below the middle turbinate since they commonly originate in the maxillary and ethmoid sinuses. Among the most common are allergic or inflammatory polyps.[62]

Nasal and Sinus Headache

Although acute or chronic inflammation and neoplasms of the paranasal sinuses can cause a headache, most patients who have seen a physician or self-diagnosed as having sinus headaches are in fact suffering from either vascular or muscle contraction headache.[63] Most true paranasal sinus headaches result from acute inflammation of the paranasal sinuses, which produce pain localized over the involved sinus. These headaches are associated with the stigmata of acute infection, including fever, swelling, and tenderness over the sinus and engorgement of the turbinates, ostia, nasofrontal ducts, and superior nasal spaces. Most of the discomfort comes from the ostia, which are frequently much more sensitive than the poorly innervated walls of the sinuses. The sinuses may be radiographically clear; however, the patient complains of pain in the sinus region. The pain may result from vacuum sinusitis that results from blocked ostia.[64] The pain may be the result of inflammation in the region of mucosal nerve endings.

Most patients with chronic sinusitis complain of nasal obstruction, but their obstruction is often due to other factors such as septal deviation and/or hypertrophied turbinates. Bony spurs within the nasal cavity can result in chronic sinusitis.

Chronic sinusitis may predispose to recurrent tonsillitis, pharyngitis, laryngitis, otitis media, airway obstruction, and chronic mouthbreathing.

Partial Resection of Inferior Turbinates

It is not uncommon for nasal obstruction to recur months or years after adenotonsillectomy. Often pediatricians and allergists incorrectly diagnose this as regrowth of adenoids. Unless an inadequate adenoidectomy was performed initially, adenoidal tissue generally does not "regrow." Instead, this problem is that of the allergic target organ shifting from the faucial tonsils and adenoidal pad to the inferior turbinates.[65] There are a number of adult studies that clearly demonstrate that the symptom complex associated with allergic, as well as non-allergic, vasomotor rhinitis and inferior turbinate hypertrophy significantly improves following partial resection of the inferior turbinates.[66-68]

You may hear of horror stories resulting from overjudicious removal of turbinates resulting in an overly patent nasal airway. The deleterious effects can be rhinitis sicca or dryness attributed to excessive airflow and a subsequent reduction of the mucosal area, destruction of cilia secondary to scarring, tissue atrophy, and endstage infection.[69] The loss of cilia function is suspected of causing ozena, a foul smelling nasal discharge. However, the current state of modern surgical procedures has virtually eliminated the overjudicious resection of turbinates. My experience favors partial resection of the inferior turbinates when they are chronically obstructive. Success rates of 86% have been reported with no detrimental effects such as a paradoxical sensation of nasal blockage, ozena, loss of ciliary function, etc.[70]

Deviated Septum

Septal deformities are a particular common cause of nasal congestion. They may occur as a result of acute trauma or growth disturbances. Septoplasty, which is a surgical reconstruction of the nasal septum, should be considered when there is evidence of chronic upper airway obstruction concomitant with a deviated septum. Usually, the convex side of the septum is reduced along with a partial resection of the contralateral turbinate. The turbinate on the concave side of the septum usually hypertrophies into the concavity over a period of years. Every dentist should have a nasal speculum and examine the interior of the nose in order to make an intelligent referral to an otorhinolaryngologist.

Although not the most common etiology for nasal obstruction, significant nasal septum deviation can be seen in the pediatric group. This condition can and should be corrected in the more advanced cases of septal deflection with impaction. A considerable volume of literature is devoted to nasal septal surgery in children.[71,72] When approached properly, nasal septal deviation can indeed be surgically corrected in the child using safe and effective conservative techniques.

Airway Obstruction and Dentofacial Development

Common sense dictates that when upper airway obstruction occurs there is a concomitant lowering of the mandible, increasing the mandibular plane angle. The autonomic nervous system constantly monitors pressure, airflow, and resistance along the respiratory tract. As stated previously, increased nasal resistance beyond the "norm" results in mouthbreathing, just enough to keep the airflow within "normal" limits. Linder-Aronson's study of adenoids and their effect on mode of breathing, nasal airflow, and their relationship to characteristics of the facial skeleton and the dentition is a classic.[73] His study revealed that nasal obstruction is related to increased facial height, increased mandibular plane angle, increased angulation of the mandible to sella nasion line, retrognathic mandible, short sagittal depth of the nasopharynx, long and narrow face, and a non-physiologic tongue position (low tongue position measured at rest). Marks noted that children with an open mouth habitus had a high arched palate, and one-third of the patients had a deviated septum.[74] It is important to understand that the septum is above the palate, and, as growth occurs, the palate drops in normal unobstructed children. The lowering of the palate allows the septum to develop vertically without bowing. If the palate does not drop, a deviated septum may occur.

Lips and Cheeks

Mouthbreathers have a lips-apart posture, whereas nasal breathers have their lips together with a relaxed facial musculature. When the lips are separated, the tongue no longer has the same force vectors relative to the teeth and dental arches as when the lips are together.[74]

It is essential to understand that teeth seek a neutral position within a system of forces acting upon them. The cheek and lip muscles exert positive pressure on the dental arches, and they tend to move the teeth toward the tongue. This movement is counteracted by optimal tongue posture exerting an equilibrium between extraoral and intraoral force vectors. This only occurs with nasal respiration with the lips together. Breathe through your mouth and notice that your tongue does not contact the lingual surfaces of your maxillary teeth. Next, breathe through your nose with your lips together and notice the light contact between your tongue and the lingual surfaces of the maxillary teeth. The light pressure of the tongue against the lingual surfaces of maxillary teeth offsets the pressure of the cheeks and lips against labial and buccal surfaces of the dentition. The tongue changes in tonus due to a lack of proprioception from the teeth.[74] This is extremely evident in children who suffer from a central nervous system disorder. These children usually have a chronic open mouth habitus with a concomitant hypotonic tongue referred to as "macroglossia" along with a malocclusion which is usually an open bite. The chronic lips-apart posture, whether it be from airway obstruction or a central nervous system disorder, results in a hypotonic large rolled dry lower lip with the upper lip curling upward. Such lips are usually associated with a past or present respiratory problem.[45]

Tongue

Harvold, in his research with primates, demonstrated that a reduction of tongue size is followed by a corresponding collapse of the dental arches. He found that the tongue could change shape with a plastic insert in the palate. This demonstrated that the shape of the tongue partially depends on its contact with surrounding structures. He found that when a tongue is carried into a new position the distribution of its forces will be altered against the teeth for several months. The teeth, in turn, changed position in response to the new force system with concomitant dental arch changes. Harvold concluded that the extent to which the tongue alters its shape to fit the dental arches depends upon the relative significance of the particular sensation of tooth contact compared with other sensory inputs. The proprioceptive response of the dorsum of the tongue from hypertrophied adenoids and/or enlarged tonsils may elicit dominant sensory stimuli resulting in a non-physiologic position of the tongue within the dental arches.[74] It has been the author's clinical experience that all chronic mouthbreathers develop a malocclusion.

It is essential that the tongue has optimal volume within the dental arches, as well as within the oropharynx and hypopharynx to avoid abnormal forces being placed upon the developing arches and dentition by tongue displacement. It is noteworthy to repeat that there must be a balance between intra- and extra-oral forces to allow for an optimal genetic growth potential to occur. The tongue is an intra-oral activator and influences growth and development of the dental arches, as well as the position of teeth within the developing arches. Our form and function was developed over centuries with a lips-together posture confining the tongue within the dental arches. When upper airway obstruction occurs, the mandible will drop and the lips will separate to initiate mouthbreathing. When mouthbreathing occurs, the tongue no longer contacts the lingual surfaces of the maxillary teeth. The result is an imbalance between intra-oral and extra-oral forces on the dental arches and dentition, and these abnormal force vectors will result in a malocclusion. During growth, tongue posture has a profound effect on the developing craniomaxillary complex (skull) and mandible which can result in orofacial deformity. It is essential that patients treated orthopedically and orthodontically have a functioning airway if the treatment result is to be stable. The genetic potential for optimal growth and development of the orofacial complex can be influenced by environmental influences on the immune system lowering resistance to allergies with resultant enlarged tonsils, enlarged adenoids, and/or responsive turbinates. The result can be chronic upper airway obstruction with concomitant mouthbreathing.

Most common clinical signs of non-physiologic tongue posture are: (1) depressed curve of Spee or bicuspid dropoff (lateral borders of the tongue posture over the posterior teeth during repose and prevent full eruption of posterior teeth), (2) micrognathia and/or macrognathia, (3) high V palatal vault (usually associated with a narrow maxillary arch), (4) maxillary protrusion with or without diastema, (5) Class II Div. I, Class II Div. II, Class III, and Class I malocclusions, (6) crossbite (posterior and/or anterior), (7) full fan open bite (only the most posterior teeth occlude in centric occlusion), (8) premature contact in CO, (9) midline discrepancy, (10) anterior and/or posterior facets, (11) anterior keys (notch area on cingulum of maxillary anterior teeth caused by the incisal edge of the mandibular incisors striking the cingulum), (12) posterior cusp wear, (13) rotated teeth, (14) tilted teeth, (15) fremitus (palpable vibrations in teeth as they occlude), (16) tooth mobility, (17) cervical erosion (notching at the cemento-dentinal junction), (18) open contacts between teeth, (19) sensitivity to percussion, and (20) thermal sensitivity (hot and/or cold). These are the most common clinical signs; however, the list is by no means complete.

Head Posture and the Neuromuscular System

The head, as a whole, is a lever system with the fulcrum at the level of the occipital condyles. The center of gravity lies near the sella turcica, which is anterior to atlas and axis. This anterior position of the center of gravity of the head explains the needed strength of the posterior neck muscles relative to the flexor muscles of the neck. In fact, the extensor muscles counteract gravity, whereas the flexors are aided by gravity. The constant tone of posterior neck muscles prevents the head from dropping forward. When one sleeps while sitting, the tone of these muscles is reduced and the head falls forward toward the chest.

The head is balanced on the cervical vertebral column and is in equilibrium with the bipupilar and occlusal planes *(Figure 4)*. The neuromuscular system is in a state of constant activity to maintain these planes in an optimal physiologic relationship to one another when standing or sitting. Two planes are used to establish the bipupilar plane: (1) the sagittal plane (a line drawn from the superior border of the external auditory meatus to the nasal spine called the auriculo-nasal plane) and (2) the frontal plane (a line drawn through the center of the pupils which should be parallel to the horizontal plane with respect to the earth's surface). The next plane is the otic plane. The three semicircular canals in each vestibular apparatus are arranged at right angles to each other so that they represent all three planes within space. Any disruption of the optimal relation of the canals relative to the surface of the earth transmits a volley of nerve impulses to the central nervous system. The maculae, located in the wall of the utricle and saccule of the vestibular system, is a sensitive area for detecting the orientation of the head with respect to the direction of the gravitational pull or other acceleratory forces. As postural changes occur throughout life, there is a constant struggle to maintain the vestibular system in an optimal relation to the surface of the earth. This requires constant neuromuscular accommodation. When the head no longer maintains an optimal physiologic relation to the gravitational pull of the earth, a patient's equilibrium is disturbed, resulting in vertigo, nausea, and frequent myalgia in the posturing musculature. The third plane is the transverse mandibular plane. This plane should be parallel to the auriculonasal (AN) plane sagittally and parallel to the bipupilar plane anteriorly.

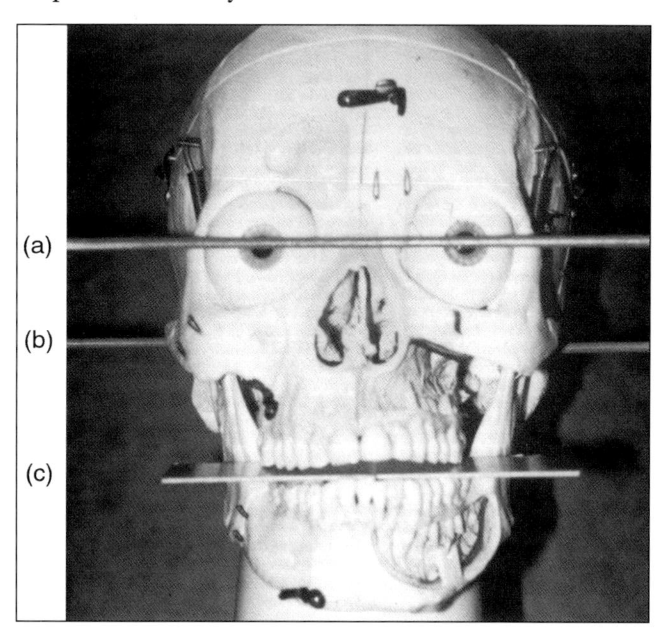

Figure 4. The three planes maintain a horizontal and parallel relation to each other and to the ground: (a) the bipupilar plane; (b) the otic plane; (c) the transverse occlusal plane.

The cervical vertebral column is not straight, but is concave posteriorly, described as a cervical lordosis. Any change in cervical concavity results in a neuromuscular response in order to maintain the three planes (otic, bipupilar, and transverse mandibular) of the head in an optimal relation to the earth's surface. A change in head posture can be devastating to the neuromuscular system. The average weight of the head is 14 to 17 pounds. An 8 degree forward head posture requires 35 to 40 pounds of pull in the posterior muscles to maintain the head in an optimal posture relative to the earth's surface. This explains the consistent occipital pain, tension, and headaches that are so common among patients with musculoskeletal dysfunctions of the head and neck.

Head Posture and Airway Obstruction

Many investigators[75-77] have shown that head posture is extended in persons with oral respiration. As the head postures forward, usually resulting from nasal airway obstruction, the posterior cranio-cervical muscles shorten and the anterior prevertebral, infrahyoid, and suprahyoid muscles are stretched. The stretched infrahyoid and suprahyoid muscles pull the mandible posteriorly and inferiorly, resulting in musculoskeletal dysfunction of the head and neck. The shortened suboccipital muscles and/or sternocleidomastoids can extend the occiput to the extent that the posterior tubercle of C1 approximates the occiput, which can create compression pathology in the high cervical region. The result can be pain in the suboccipital musculature radiating down the back and as high as the vertex of the cranium.[78] An evaluation of forward head posture is essential when treating musculoskeletal disorders of the head and neck. The anteroposterior (A-P) posture of the head in relation to the cervical spine can be determined by dropping a plumb line that touches the most dorsal thoracic spine. A perpendicular measurement can be made from the plumb line to the deepest curvature of the cervical spine. The optimal distance, according to Rocabado,[79] is 6 cm. An increase in the A-P measurement indicates a forward head posture, and a decreased measurement indicates a lack of optimal lordosis and a possible kyphotic cervical curve. In either case, the patient should have an ear, nose, and throat evaluation for nasal obstruction and a postural analysis by a physical therapist, orthopedist, or chiropractor.

Shoulder Protraction

Forward head posture is usually concomitant with shoulder protraction (forward, rolled shoulders). This results since the shoulder girdle relates to the position of the head and neck in the same way that the sacral base rules the position of the lumbar spine. The ala of the scapula will protrude (winging) and can be easily palpated. The primary retractors of the scapula are the rhomboids major, rhomboids minor, and trapezius. Shoulder protraction angulates the clavicle laterally and elevates the first rib. The diminished space impinges the subclavian vessels and nerves. The patient may complain of paresthesia, pain, and/or coldness in the arm and fingers. This is further confirmation of a postural asymmetry. It must be pointed out that there are other medical conditions that can give rise to these same sensations. However, consideration must be given to body asymmetry. Neuromuscular compression of the shoulder girdle is known as thoracic outlet obstruction syndrome. It is characterized by subjective complaints of pain and paresthesias in the neck, shoulder, arm, and hand. As in so-called "TMJ," the condition is more common in women than men and most frequently occurring between the ages of 35 and 55. The pathogenesis is believed to be due to compression of the subclavian vessels and sometimes the lower medial trunks of the brachial plexus against a cervical rib or an entrapment of the brachial plexus between the anterior and middle scaleni muscles as a result of forward head posture. When complaints such as these occur, the dentist must consider postural dysfunction that may involve posture of the head on atlas with concomitant muscle accommodation in an attempt to maintain the bipupilar, otic, and transverse mandibular planes in an optimal position. The resultant neuromuscular response can cause symptoms the dentist has labeled as myofascial pain dysfunction and/or TMJ dysfunction. Keep in mind, an obstructed airway will cause a forward head posture with a simultaneous forward shoulder posture, which will foreshorten the suboccipital musculature and elongate the prevertebral musculature. A simple demonstration is to move your head forward without tilting it upward, enabling one to feel the contraction of the suboccipital muscles and stretching of the prevertebral muscles.[80]

Scoliosis and Head Posture

Scoliosis is a lateral deviation of the vertebral column. It is best examined with the patient bending forward, because the spinal curve is more pronounced in that position. Most curves are convex to the right in the thoracic area and to the left in the lumbar area.[81] A spinal curvature may render one shoulder lower than the other, with the dominant side being more muscular. The result is usually a lateral tilt of the head to the side opposite the lower shoulder and a slight rotation to the side opposite the head tilt. The patient may complain of occipital headaches or pain radiating from occiput to the vertex. Palpation of the suboccipital muscles will usually elicit pain. The patient may complain of nausea and/or vertigo due to tilting of the vestibular system. If head tilt results from pain and muscle splinting within the masticatory musculature, an orthotic will usually correct the head tilt. However, if the tilt results from body asymmetry (leg length discrepancy, scoliosis, etc.), the patient will need correction of the body asymmetry by an appropriate health provider prior to completion of the orthotic phase of treatment.

Leg Length Discrepancy and the Mandible

It is essential to determine if a leg length discrepancy exists and whether it is structural or functional problem. A structural limb length discrepancy is one in which there is an actual shortage in bone length. A functional shortage is one that is caused by muscle spasm and tightness that influences the position of the extremity and causes it to function as a shorter limb. Leg length discrepancy should be determined by an appropriate health provider. Structural leg length is determined by measuring the distance from the anterior superior iliac spine (ASIS) to the medial malleoli of the ankles. Unequal distances between these fixed points verify that one leg is shorter than the other.

Functional leg length discrepancy can result from pelvic obliquity, adduction, or a flexion deformity in the hip joint. Pelvic obliquity manifests itself as uneven anterior or posterior superior iliac spine while the patient is standing. Structural and functional leg length discrepancies cause an imbalance of the pelvis.[82] Determination of the pelvic level may be made from the relative heights of the anterior superior iliac spines (ASIS). A pelvi-rule is an excellent screening instrument. It has a level bubble in the center, and the lateral wings can be placed against the ASIS. If there is a tilt between the right and left ASIS, the patient should be referred to an appropriate health provider. An ASIS tilt affects the vertebral column and may result in scoliosis, which can affect head and shoulder posture and lead to an orthopedic malalignment of the mandible to the craniomaxillary complex (skull).

Flat Feet (Pes Planus) and the Mandible

In pes planus, the talar head displaces medially and plantward from under cover of the navicular and stretches the spring and the tibias posterior ligaments, resulting in a loss of the medial longitudinal arch.[83] A loss of arch unilaterally will reduce the distance from the ASIS to the floor when standing. In addition, there is a medial rotation of the tibia and fibula which rotates the femur medially. The result is an anterior and inferior rotation of the ASIS on the affected side as the head of the femur rotates in the acetabulum. The effect is body asymmetry from the foot to the head. Pain may be referred to the knee from the hip, lumbar spine, and the foot and ankle.[84] Pronation or supination of the foot affects the ankle, knee, hip, spine, and head posture. Head posture affects mandibular posture; therefore, a limited postural examination is essential when treating musculoskeletal dysfunction of the head and neck. The statement that we hear so often, "a splint will correct posture and reduce pain in the head, neck, shoulders, and back," is only partially correct. If the pain results from an anatomical asymmetry of the foot, leg, or spine, no splint will correct the musculoskeletal dysfunction. It is essential to understand that the approach to treatment may be multidisciplinary.

The Mandibular Connection

It is clear that mandibular posture, as it relates to the craniomaxillary complex (skull), is influenced by postural changes distant from the head and neck. The musculoskeletal system must be fully understood in its static anatomical sense and in its kinetic function before abnormality and the mechanism of pain production can be recognized and understood. Pathologic changes may be prevented, and, when a complete reversal of abnormal changes is impossible, at least the symptoms and disability caused by these changes may be ameliorated.

Part II: The Ear Connection

Eustachian Tube Dysfunction

The three functions of the eustachian tube are aeration, clearance, and protection of the middle ear. Normally, the eustachian tube is closed, open only when there is positive pressure in the nasopharynx or by muscle action of the tensor veli palatini, levator palatini, or salpingopharyngeous. Although controversial, most anatomic and physiologic evidence supports the belief that the tensor veli palatini muscle is solely responsible for active tubal dilation on swallowing.[85] Patients suffering from craniomandibular disorders often complain of a hearing loss, fullness in the ears, and hyperacusis (hypersensitivity to sounds).

There is a causal relationship that has been absent in dental and medical literature, yet correction of a craniomandibular disorder often eliminates the aforementioned ear complaints.

The tensor veli palatini muscle is innervated by a segment of the trigeminal nerve. When deep somatic and visceral pain occurs from a primary pain source such as the temporalis, masseter, and medial pterygoid muscles, the effects spread to other divisions of the same neural segment. Central excitatory effects are frequently observed accompanying deep somatic and visceral pains. The effects relate to both the intensity and duration of primary pain. When interuncial neurons are secondarily stimulated via efferent motor neurons, the effect of such excitation can be muscular contraction. The clinical effect will depend upon which muscles are affected and to what degree, as well as the constancy and duration of such contraction. If skeletal muscles are involved, some clincal dysfunction may be observed such as movement, rigidity, displacement, or swelling.[87] Excitatory patterns spread to other main divisions of the same segment. Secondary effects from primary trigeminal pain therefore would be expected to remain confined within the trigeminal distribution.[88]

Since the tensor veli palatini muscle (TVPM) is a division of the same neural segment as the muscles of mastication, excitation of efferent motor neurons can result in muscle contraction, causing the lumen of the eustachian tube to remain patent at rest and pressure from the nasopharynx to be transmitted to the middle ear. The patients complain of a sensation of fullness or pressure in the ear (autophony) and their voices sound hollow, as though one is talking in a drum or echo chamber. Hearing, however, is unaltered.[86]

The TVPM originates from a flat lamella of the scaphoid fossa at the base of the medial pterygoid plate, from the spine of the sphenoid, and from the lateral wall of the cartilage of the eustachian tube. It descends vertically between the pterygoid plate and the medial pterygoid muscle and ends in a tendon that winds around the pterygoid hamulus. The TVPM is retained in this position by fibers of origin from the medial pterygoid and inserts into the aponeurosis of the soft palate *(Figure 5)*. It is supplied by a branch of the mandibular nerve, the medial pterygoid nerve, hence, the Trigeminal Connection.

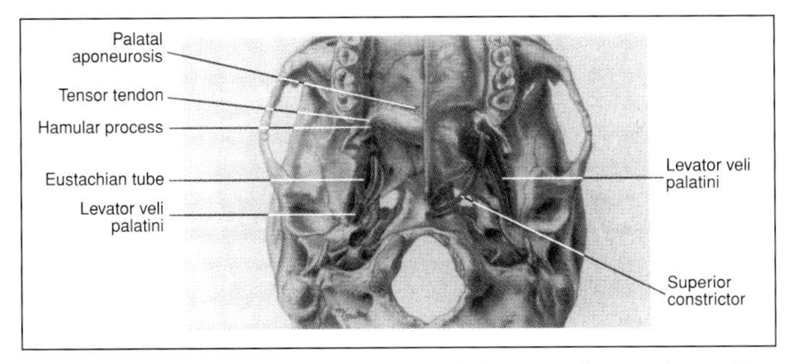

Figure 5. Anatomy and relationships of the eustachian tube and paratubal musculature in the adult human.

Approximation of the TVPM to the medial pterygoid muscle is of paramount importance. Chronic contracture of the medial pterygoid can impair normal function of the TVPM muscle as it descends vertically between the medial pterygoid plate and pterygoid muscle and can be entrapped when the medial pterygoid is in dysfunction, preventing normal dilation of the eustachian tube lumen *(Figure 6)*. The result is an inability to equalize middle and outer ear pressure. Patients may complain of pain in rapidly descending airplanes and when scuba diving. This explains why many patients who complain of ear pain, fullness, and/or pressure are relieved of symptoms following successful resolution of craniomandibular disorders.

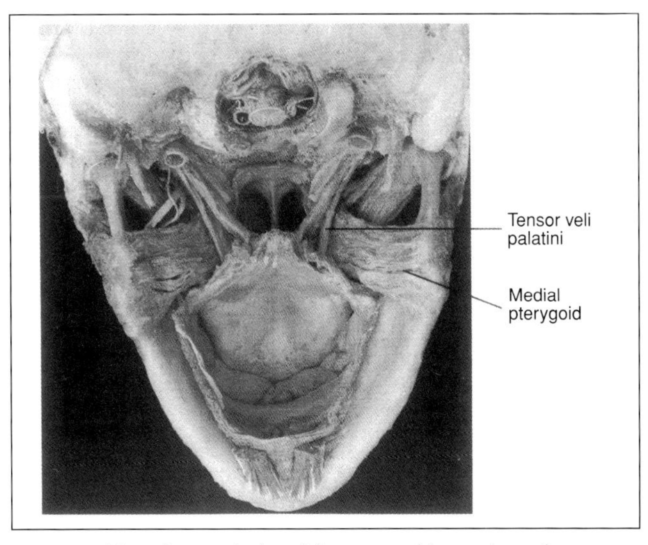

Figure 6. Note the proximity of the pterygoid muscle to the tensor veli palatini muscle (posterior aspect).

Condylar Retrusion and Mandibular-Malleolar Ligament Ear Connection

Craniomandibular articulation is bilateral, forming a functioning unit. They cannot function separately. What affects one temporomandibular joint must also influence the other.

Each of the two joints is a compound and classified as a ginglymoarthrodial (hinge-sliding) joint. A change in vertical dimension affects condylar position within the glenoid fossa. There is no rotation without translation. An increase in vertical dimension translates the condyle anteriorly, and a decrease of vertical dimension translates the condyle posteriorly. Teeth dictate the relationship of the mandible to the maxilla when teeth are in contact. Teeth are, in essence, an articulating extension of the bony skeletal structures. For example, occlusion resulting in an overclosure or distalization of the mandible will translate the condyles posteriorly within the glenoid fossa resulting in compression of the retrodiscal tissues. The degree of compression dictates the patient's response. Retrusion of the mandible, whether it be iatrogenically induced, traumatically induced, or a result of malocclusion, often results in otalgia due to excessive compression of the neurovascular retrodiscal tissues. The patient's impression is otalgia. The mandibular-malleolar ligament *(Figure 7)* also plays a role in ear complaints. This ligament is composed of fibroelastic tissue with ligamentous qualities and connects the neck and anterior process of the malleus to the medioposterosuperior part of the capsule, the articular disc, and the sphenomandibular ligament through the petrotympanic fissure.[89] A change in mandibular posture can affect the tension of the ligament, which in turn affects movement of the ear ossicles and may result in a medial displacement of the tympanic membrane. Many patients will complain of pressure and/or ringing in the ears when protruding the mandible, demonstrating the viability of the petrotympanic fissure.

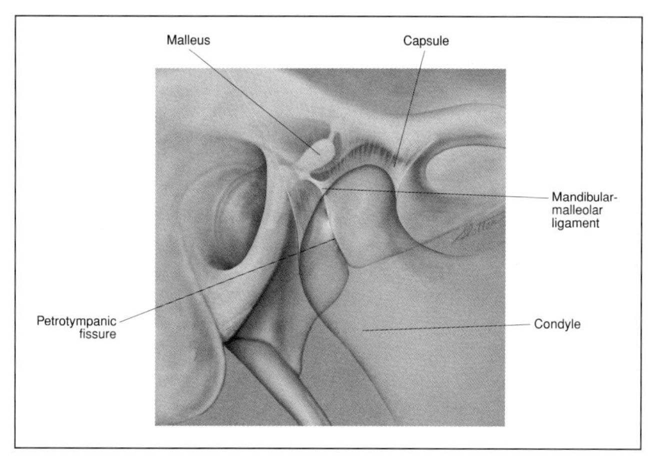

Figure 7. Mandibular-malleolar ligament.

The petrotympanic fissure is a communication from the middle ear to the glenoid fossa and is located posterior to the condyle *(Figure 7)*. In addition to the mandibular-malleolar ligament, the fissure contains the anterior tympanic artery which supplies the anterior two-thirds of the tympanic membrane and the chorda tympani which passes between the malleus and incus.[90] It also transmits the tegman tympani, which contains lymph channels from the petrous bone. The tympanic bone, forming the posteromedial boundary of the glenoid fossa, contains similar lymph channels.[89] Posterior displacement of the condyle such as evidenced by changes in vertical dimension or anterior condylar displacement due to malocclusion results in a decided increase of tinnitus and vertigo.[91] This suggests that a mechanical impingement of retrodiscal tissues could be capable of impairing normal balance as well as sounds. Bleiker[90] related ear disturbances of temporomandibular origin to pressure on neighboring blood vessels and nerves.

Tympanic Muscles and Protection of the Middle Ear

Mechanisms exist that protect the inner ear from excessive sound energy. This protection is achieved by contraction of the intratympanic muscles and by slippage of the incudomalleolar joint that occurs primarily at low frequencies. Sound is the stimulus for activity of the stapedius muscle by way of a reflex arc through the cochlea, cochlear nuclei, and 7th cranial nerve. This is a bilateral phenomenon that can be excited by a stimulus of adequate intensity to the ipsilateral or contralateral ear (the stapedial reflex). The tensor tympani muscle responds to sound stimuli with a comparatively long latency period. The tensor tympani is contained in a bony canal above the osseous portion of the auditory tube. It arises from the cartilagenous portion of the auditory tube and the adjoining part of the greater wing of the sphenoid, as well as the osseous canal in which it is contained. It then passes posteriorly through the canal. Here it exits as a slender tendon and is inserted into the manubrium of the malleus. It is supplied by a branch of the mandibular nerve that passes through the otic ganglion *(Figure 8)*.

The stapedius arises from the wall of the conical cavity inside the pyramid. Its tendon is inserted into the posterior surface of the neck of the stapes. It is supplied by a branch of the facial nerve.

The tensor tympani draws the tympanic membrane medially and thus increases tension. The stapedius pulls the head of the stapes posteriorly, tilting the base and increasing the tension of the fluid within the internal ear. Both muscles have a dampening action, reducing oscillations of the ossicles and protecting the inner ear from injury from loud noises such as that produced by a riveting machine.[85] The stapedius muscle, innervated by the facial nerve, may also be involved if it is in dysfunction.

The tensor tympani is innervated by the mandibular branch of the 5th cranial nerve. This can be affected by a primary pain source depending on its intensity and duration, as described previously. The clinical manifestation observed is muscle dysfunction. Clinically, the patient may complain of sensitivity to sounds when the tensor tympani can no longer dampen loud sounds. This is a common complaint of many patients suffering from myofascial pain dysfunction.

It is possible to provide therapy to all muscles that are supplied by the 5th and 7th cranial nerves by low frequency stimulation of the nerve trunks as they pass through foramen ovale and foramen spinosum. There is no other modality that will stimulate the tensor veli palatini, tensor tympani, lateral pterygoid, and stapedius muscles due to a lack of anatomic access. The Myo-monitor is a low frequency transcutaneous electrical neural stimulation (TENS) unit that acts on small afferent and motor efferent muscle fibers. The electrical stimuli inhibit impulses from associated muscle spindles. This stimulation takes tension off of the nuclear bag, thereby allowing the contractile protein fibrils to assume their passive resting length. This has been verified with electromyographic (EMG) recordings.[92-95] Clinically, the patient will report that the chief complaints of myofascial pain have been eliminated or substantially reduced and, as a result, the fullness in the ears, sensitivity to sounds, pain in the ears, etc. are eliminated.

Complaint of subjective hearing loss usually accompanies fullness in the ears. It is possible to differentiate true hearing loss from subjective hearing loss using a Welch Allyn Audioscope that measures sound frequencies in the range of 500, 1000, 2000,

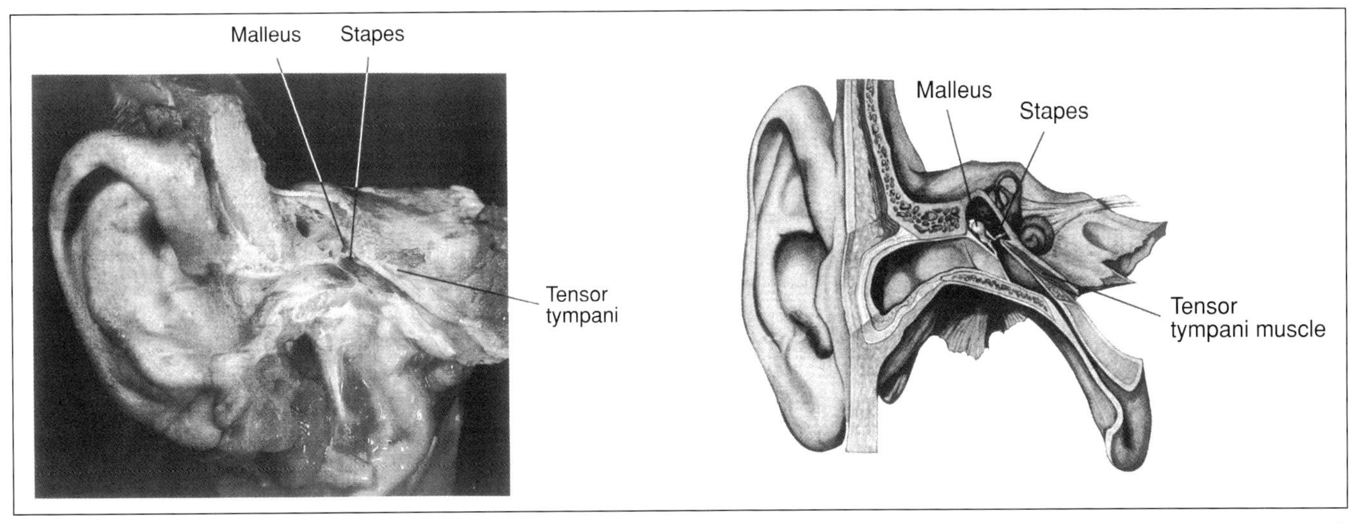

Figure 8. Note the tensor tympani muscle arising from the cartilagenous portion of the auditory tube and its insertion into the manubrium of the malleus.

and 4000 Hz at 25 decibels. The scope also allows the dentist to examine the external ear for excessive cerumen, which gives the patient an impression of subjective hearing loss, and allows the dentist to view the tympanic membrane for inflammation that is associated with otalgia. It is an excellent instrument to aid in the development of a differential diagnosis.

Hearing Loss and Craniomandibular Disorders

There are two general types of hearing loss, conductive and sensorineural. Conductive hearing loss results from disruption in the passage of sound from the external ear to the oval window. Anatomically, this pathway includes the ear canal, tympanic membrane, and ossicles. Such loss may be due to cerumen impaction, tympanic membrane perforation, otitis media, osteosclerosis, intraaural muscle dysfunction, or displacement of the ossicles by the malleolar ligament. Sensorineural hearing loss results from otologic abnormalities beyond the oval window. Such abnormalities may affect the sensory cells of the cochlea or the neural fibers of the 8th cranial nerve. Hearing loss with age (presbycusis) is an example. Eighth cranial nerve tumors may also lead to such hearing loss. The Audioscope is an excellent screening instrument for the two types of hearing loss.

The frequency range for normal hearing is 20–20,000 Hz. However, the typical adult can only detect frequencies between 20–10,000 Hz. The speech frequency range is from 400–3,000 Hz. Intensity is measured in decibels. A hearing threshold of <20 decibels is considered to be within the normal hearing range.[85]

Hearing loss resulting from eustachian tube dysfunction, initiated by craniomandibular disorders, is usually subjective, and the Audioscope is an excellent screening instrument for differential diagnosis. Prognosis for successful resolution of subjective hearing loss is excellent, providing the craniomandibular disorder is resolved.

A thorough ENT examination should be performed by an appropriate health provider when no pathology exists and when there is no apparent etiology for the patient's otalgia and/or eustachian tube dysfunction. A craniomandibular disorder must be considered.

Tinnitus—the Great Quandary

Tinnitus is a spontaneous, internally generated noise which is usually heard in one ear but can be heard in both ears. It is primarily a subjective complaint, and the severity is dependent primarily on the patient's description.[96] Almost any condition that causes malfunction of the auditory end-organ might cause tinnitus, but the most common cause is age degeneration (presbycusis). Other causes are biochemical changes, e.g., from aspirin, Meniere's disease, trauma (acoustic or chemical), and labyrinthitis.[97] It may occur alone or in concert with other symptoms such as head, neck, and back pain; dizziness (vertigo); otalgia; impaired hearing; stuffy sensations in the ears; double and blurred vision; various TM joint noises during chewing; maximum voluntary clenching; maximum jaw protrusion; mouth opening against resistance; and pressure applied to the ipsilateral temporomandibular joint.

As many as one-third (32%) of all Americans experience tinnitus sometime in their lives. These data are supported by similar studies performed in Europe. It is estimated that approximately 18 million Americans seek medical attention for their tinnitus.[98] Nine million report being seriously affected by their condition, and two million are disabled because of elusive sounds.

There are two historical classifications for tinnitus. Objective tinnitus refers to a noise that can be heard by both the patient and physician. This form of tinnitus is usually derived from one of two sources: the vascular system or from muscle contraction.[97] Vascular tinnitus is usually pulsatile and synchronous with the pulse. Glomus tumors, aneurysms along the carotid system, and other vascular malformations cause a pulsatile tinnitus that can be heard with a stethoscope and that abates when pressure is applied to the feeding vessels. The tinnitus of muscle contraction is usually a most annoying ringing sound caused by clonic activity of the tensor veli palatini (palatal myoclonus). Treatment has been frustrating for the treating physician who often prescribes tranquilizers and muscle relaxants in an effort to control muscle contraction. Although there is no specific medical or surgical therapy for tinnitus, many patients find relief by playing background music to mask the tinnitus. A hearing aid for the associated hearing loss often results in suppression of the tinnitus. Some patients benefit from use of a tinnitus masker, a device worn like a hearing aid that presents a noise more pleasant than tinnitus.[99]

The current medical theory is that the majority of cases of tinnitus have no detectable acoustic basis, but instead arise from anomalies in one or more of the elements of the neural chain that constitutes the auditory nervous system.[100] In the past few years, experts treating patients from a stomatognathic approach have had success in alleviating tinnitus. However, since tinnitus can be a symptom of serious ear disease, it is recommended that an ENT or neurological evaluation be performed prior to initiating dental treatment.

For more than half a century, investigators have attempted to explain the association between TMJ and tinnitus in the dental otologic literature. One of the first was Costen, who speculated that pressure from the condyle could cause eustachian tube blockage, thereby producing tinnitus. A second hypothesis, which is implicated with eustachian tube, was based on the common nerve supply to the masticatory muscles and tensor veli palatini muscle. These researchers speculated that hyperactivity of the masticatory muscles could induce a secondary reflex contraction of the tensor veli palatini muscle, congestion of the middle ear, and consequently tinnitus.[101-104] Others have proposed the concept that the middle and inner ears receive input from the trigeminal nerve and sympathetic nerves of the middle ear through the tympanic plexus, thus speculating these combined inputs might be responsible for tinnitus.[105] Chan and Reade[104] speculated that a masseter muscle trigger point may cause tinnitus and referred pain at distant locations. Other investigators speculated that inflammation within the TMJ could be a source of tinnitus.[101,106]

Dissection through the TMJ and middle ear has documented that some people have a structural connection between the two.[103,107,108] Alkofide and others found that, in 68% of their specimens, the sphenomandibular ligament passed through the petrotympanic fissure into the middle ear, and in 8% of the specimens it is attached to the malleus.[107] Pinto found that moving the capsule or disc appeared to cause the chain of ossicles in the middle ear and tympanic membrane to move, suggesting this action as a basis for tinnitus in patients with TMD.[109]

Despite the many diverse hypotheses that have been proposed, the clinical improvement or resolution of tinnitus has been anecdotally noted in clinical practice when TMD symptoms are significantly improved.

Arlen's clinical impressions were that tinnitus is present in approximately one-third of patients who present with ear pain, fullness, hearing loss, etc. The patients complain of a high frequency hissing sound, not the roaring type. In older patients exhibiting a high frequency sensorineural hearing loss, tinnitus could be attributed to a degenerative process in the cochlea by most patients seen under 50 years of age. After proper dental therapy was performed, tinnitus was generally relieved.[110]

The etiology of tinnitus has been reported as being caused by everything from impacted earwax (cerumen) to virtually every known disease or pathologic condition.[101]

Patients with temporomandibular disorders report a higher prevalence of tinnitus than do age matched controls.[101] Also, TMD has been implicated as a cause of tinnitus.[111-113] It has been reported that TMD therapy improves tinnitus in 46–96% of patients who have TMD and coexisting tinnitus.[114,115]

Vernon and Griest, using a questionnaire at an otolaryngology clinic, divided tinnitus patients into two groups, those with TMD and those without TMD. Significantly more patients with TMD reported alterations in their tinnitus as a result of jaw movement.[116] Other researchers divided patients with tinnitus into TMD and non-TMD groups and found that patients with TMD experienced a gradual onset of tinnitus more often than the subjects without TMD.[101] Shulman found TMD patients could intensify tinnitus by clenching their teeth, and concluded that TMD was contributing to their tinnitus.[113] Rubenstein et.al. reported an alteration in tinnitus when pressure was applied to the ipsilateral TM joint, when the ipsilateral TMJ was loaded, and when resistance was applied against opening or protruding the mandible.[101] It has been reported that palpation of the deep masseter, medial pterygoid, lateral pterygoid, and sternocleidomastoid muscles can reproduce or intensify a patient's tinnitus.[117,118] The neuromuscular dentist has the ability to measure masticatory muscle activity at rest and in function, thereby obtaining quantitative objective data from which therapy can be instituted. It has been this author's clinical experience that when masticatory and associated muscle activity are optimally at rest and in function, TMD/MSD complaints of tinnitus usually resolve. However, when the only complaint is tinnitus with no TMD/MSD complaints, resolution of tinnitus is poor. It has been reported that younger patients with TMD/MSD were more likely to report that their tinnitus improved than did older patients. Most patients with TMD are between the ages of 24 and 40, whereas most patients with tinnitus are between 40 and 80 years of age.[105,119] It appears that the cause of tinnitus in the younger patients is related to TMD, whereas the cause in older patients tended to be from other sources (most likely presbycusis).

In a study by Wright and Bifano,[120] no single question or test identified patients with TMD and coexisting tinnitus who may have experienced improvement or resolution of their tinnitus with treatment. However, questions associated with tinnitus were statistically significant as an aid in identifying patients who have the greater likelihood of experiencing tinnitus improvement.

The following data derived from this study will help practitioners determine which TMD patients have the greatest likelihood of experiencing tinnitus improvement. The patients reported that:

1. The age range in this population was 18 to 67 years.
2. Tinnitus occurs less frequently, that is, on a monthly basis rather than on a constant basis.
3. Tinnitus lasts for a short period of time, seconds rather than continuously.
4. Hearing is normal.
5. They have pain in their ipsilateral ear.
6. Tinnitus began approximately when TMD symptoms began.
7. Tinnitus is more intense when their TMD symptoms increase.
8. Tinnitus appeared to be related to stress.
9. They experience changes in tinnitus (such as intensity) when they move their jaw.
10. Tinnitus is reproduced or intensified when they clench their posterior teeth as hard as possible.

It is unfortunate that the medical profession has little or no knowledge in the field of craniomandibular orthopedics. The literature is sparse, and most medical health providers have little or no understanding of the necessity for a multidisciplinary approach to the treatment of patients suffering from eustachian tube dysfunction, otalgia, and/or tinnitus. After medical treatment options have been exhausted, it is essential that craniomandibular orthopedics be considered.

References

1. Van Der Klaauw: Size and position of functional components of the skull. *Arch Germany, Neerl Jour* 1948-1952;9:1-559.
2. Moss ML: Vertical growth of the human face. *Am J Orthod* 1964;50(5):359-376.
3. Moss ML: The Functional Matrix. In: Kraus BS, Riedel RA, eds. *Vistas in Orthodontics.* Philadelphia: Lea and Febiger; 1962;85-98.
4. Olmstead JM: Francois Magendie. New York: *Shuman's*, 1829.
5. Tomes CS: On the developmental origin of the V-shaped contracted maxilla. *Monthly Rev Dental Surgery* 1872:1-25.
6. Angle EH: *Treatment of Malocclusion of Teeth, 7th ed.* Philadelphia: SS White Dental Mfg. Co., 1907.
7. Ketchum AH: Treatment by the orthodontist supplementing that of the rhinologist. *Laryngoscope* 1912;22:1286-1299.
8. McCoy ID: *Applied Orthodontics.* Philadelphia: Lea and Febiger, 1935.
9. Balyeat RM, Bowen R: Facial and dental deformities due to perennial nasal allergy in childhood. *Int J Orthod* 1934;20:445-449.
10. Todd TW, Cohen MD, Broadbent BH: The role of allergy in the etiology of orthodontic deformity. *J Allergy* 1939;10:246-249.
11. Subtelny JD: The significance of adenoid tissue in orthodontia. *Angle Orthod* 1954;24:59-69.
12. Ricketts RM: Respiratory obstructions and their relation to tongue posture. *Cleft Palate Bul* 1958;8:3-6.
13. Marks MB: Allergy in relation to orofacial dental deformities in children. *J Allergy* 1965;36:293-302.
14. Bushy RS: *Alterations in Certain Anatomical Relations Accompanying the Change From Oral to Nasal Breathing.* M.S. Thesis, University of Illinois, Chicago: 1965.
15. Moss ML: The functional matrix: Functional cranial components. In: Kraus BS, Reihel R, eds. *Vistas of Orthodontics.* Philadelphia: Lea and Febiger; 1962;85-98.
16. Dann FG, Green LJ, Cunat JJ: Relationship between variations of mandibular morphology and variation of nasopharyngeal airway size in monozygotic twins. *Angle Orthod* 1973;43:129-135.
17. Harvold EP, et al.: Primate experiments on oral respiration. *Am J Orthod* 1981;79:359-372.

18. Subtelny JD: Workshop on tonsillectomy and adenoidectomy. *Rhinol Laryngol* 1974;84(19):250-254.

19. Linder-Aronson S: Effect of adenoidectomy on the dentition and facial skeleton over a period of five years. In: Linder-Aronson S, ed. *Transactions of the Third International Congress.* St. Louis: C. V. Mosby Co.; 1975;85-100.

20. Quinn GW: Airway interference and its effect upon growth and development of the face, jaw, dentition, and associated parts. *N C Dent J* 1978;60:28-31.

21. Rubin RM: Mode of respiration and facial growth. *Am J Orthod* 1980;78:504-510.

22. McNamara JA: Influence of respiratory pattern on craniofacial growth. *Angle Orthod* 1981;51:269-299.

23. Hannuksela A: The effect of moderate to severe atrophy on the facial skeleton. *Eur J Orthod* 1981;3:187-193.

24. Marks MB: *Stigmata of Respiratory Tract Allergies.* A Scope Publication. Kalamazoo, NJ: Upjohn Co., 1977.

25. Waldman TA, et al.: The metabolism of IgE. Studies in normal individuals and a patient with IgE myeloma. *J Immunol* 1976;117:1139-1144.

26. Sassouni V, et al.: The influence of perennial allergy rhinitis on facial type—a pilot study on the effect of allergic management on facial patterns. *Annal Allergy* 1985;54:493-497.

27. Van Cauwenberge PB: Nasal cycle in children. *Arch Otolaryngol* 1984;110:118-120.

28. Subtelney JD: A cephalometric study of the growth of the soft palate. *Plast Reconstr Surg* 1957;19;49-62.

29. Gray V: Update 86 TMJ Seminar. Myotronics Inc. Seminar, Seattle, WA., 1986.

30. Tate H: Deaths in tonsillectomies. *Lancet* 1963;7:1090-1091.

31. Pratt OW: Tonsillectomy and adenoidectomy mortality and morbidity. *Trans Am Acad Opthalmol Otolaryngol* 1970;74:1146-1154.

32. Gray V: Upper airway and dento-facial deformity. In: Coy R, ed. *Anthology of Craniomandibular Orthopedics.* Collinsville, IL: Buchanan Publishing; 1991;57.

33. Abrahamson M, Harker LA: Physiology of the nose. *Otolaryngol Clinic N Am* 1973;6:623-635.

34. McCaffrey TV, Kem EB: Response of nasal airway to hypercapnia and hypoxia in the dog. *Acta Otolaryngol* 1979;87:545-553

35. McCaffrey TV, Kem E: Clinical evaluation of nasal obstruction: A study of 1000 patients. *Arch Otolaryngol* 1979;105:542-545.

36. Adams GL, Boles LR, Paparella MM: *Fundamentals of Otolaryngology.* Philadelphia: W. B. Saunders Co., 1978.

37. Cherniak NS, Lahiri S: Respiratory system. In: Netter FH, ed. *The CIBA Collection of Medical Illustrations.* West Caldwell, NJ: CIBA; 1980;7:75-77.

38. Cherniak NS: Control and Disorders of Respiration. In: Netter NS, ed. *The CIBA Collection of Medical Illustrations.* West Caldwell, NJ: CIBA; 1980;77-82.

39. Nelson WE, Vaughn VC: *Textbook of Pediatrics.* Philadelphia: W B Saunders, 1969.

40. Mabry RL: Rhinitis medicamentosa: The forgotten factor in nasal obstruction. *South Med J* 1982;75:817-819.

41. Scott-Brown WG, Ballantyne J, Groves V: *Diseases of the Ear, Nose and Throat.* London: Butterworth and Co., 1965.

42. Ballin JC: *AMA Drug Evaluations 4th Ed.* American Medical Association; 1980.

43. Mabry RL: Nasal stuffiness due to systemic medication. *Otolaryngol Head Neck Surg* 1983:91;93-94.

44. Marks M: *Stigmata of Upper Respiratory Tract Allergies.* A Scope Publication; Kalamazoo, NJ: Upjohn Co.; 1967;16-32.

45. Garry JF: Early iatrogenic muscle, skeletal and TMJ dysfunction. In: Morgan D, ed. *Diseases of the Temporomandibular Apparatus.* St. Louis: C. V. Mosby Co.; 1982;59.

46. Ogura JH: Physiologic relationships of the upper and lower airways. *Ann Otol Rhin Laryngol* 1970;70:495-501.

47. Menashe WD, Feffehi C, Miller M: Hyperventilation and cor pulmonale due to chronic upper airway obstruction. *J Pediatr* 1965;67:198-203.

48. *The Merck Manual, 15th ed.* Rathway, NJ; Merck & Co.;1987;29.

49. Liese W, Joshi RA, Cummings G: Humidification of respired gas by nasal mucosa. *Ann Otol Rhin Laryngol* 1973;82:330-352.

50. Morris PP, Reid RR: Halitosis and variations in the mouth and total breath odor intensity resulting from prophylaxis and antisepsis. *J Dent Res* 1949;28:324-333.

51. Lawlor GL, Fisher TJ: *Manual of Allergy and Immunology.* Boston: Little Brown and Co., 1981.

52. Wachsberger TA: The deviated septum. *Arch Otolaryngol* 1942;37:789.

53. Markwardt A: *Verlanfige Erfahrungen Uber die Auswirking De Gaumennatherweitenmg Auf Des Helfsachallkinde.* Forsch Kieferorthop; 1966; 22:359-361.

54. Eliaschar L, Lavie P, Halperin E, Gordon C, Elroy E: Apneic episodes as indications for adenotonsillectomy. *Arch Otolaryngol* 1980;8:492-496.

55. Kravath RF, Pollak RC, Borwiecki B: Hypoventilation during sleep in children who have lymphoid airway obstruction treated by nasopharyngeal tube and T & A. *Pediatrics* 1977;59:865-871.

56. Mangat D, Orr WC, Smith OR: Sleep apnea, hypersomnolence and upper airway obstruction secondary to adenotonsillar enlargement. *Arch Otolaryngol* 1977;103:383-386.

57. Weider DJ, Hauri PJ: Nocturnal enuresis in children with upper airway obstruction. *Int J Pediatr Otorhinolaryngol* 1985;9:173-182.

58. Fan L, Murphy S: Pectus excavatum from chronic upper airway obstruction. *Am J Dis Child,* 1981;135:550-552

59. Gray LP: Deviated septum, incidence and etiology. *Ann Otol Rhin Laryngol* 1978;87:50.

60. Gray LP: The development and significance of septal and dental deformity from birth to eight years. *Int J Ped Otorhinolaryngology* 1983;6:265-277.

61. Gray LP: Septal manipulation in the neonate, methods and results. *Int J Ped Otorhinolaryngology* 1985;8:195-209.

62. Karmony CC: The nose and the paranasal sinuses. In: Karmony CC, ed. *Otolaryngology.* Philadelphia: C. V. Mosby Co.; 1974;116.

63. Posner JB: Disorders of Sensation. In: Wyngaaden JB, Lloyd SH, eds. *Cecil's Textbook of Medicine, 17th ed.* Philadelphia: W B Saunders; 1985;2058.

64. Drettner B, Lindholm CE: *Acta Otolaryngolica Stockholm* 1967;64:508.

65. Meredith G: Airway and dentofacial development. *Am J Rhin* 1988;3:33-41.

66. Shapiro G, Shapiro PA: Nasal airway obstruction and facial development. *Clin Rev Allergy* 1984;2:225-235.

67. Fry HJH: Judicious turbinectomy for nasal obstruction. *Aus J Surg* 1976;42:291-294.

68. Pollock R, Rohring RJ: Inferior turbinate surgery. *Plast Reconstr Surg* 1984;74:227-236.

69. Courtiss EH, Goldwyn RM, O'Brian JJ: Resection obstructing inferior nasal turbinates. *Plast Reconstr Surg* 1978;62:249-257.

70. Mabry RL: Nasal stuffiness due to systemic medication. *Otolaryngol Head Neck Surg* 1983:91;93-94.

71. Crysdale WS, Tatham B: External septal rhinoplasty in children. *Laryngoscope* 1985;95:211-216.

72. Crysdale WS: Septorhinoplasty in children. *Can J Otolaryngol* 1973;2:211-216.

73. Linder-Aronson S: Adenoids, their effect on mode of breathing and nasal airflow relationship to characteristics of the facial skeleton and the dentition. *Acta Otolaryngol Suppl* (Stockholm) 1970:265;1-132.

74. Harvold BP: *The Activator in Interceptive Orthopedics.* St Louis: C. V. Mosby Co.;1964;57-63.

75. Woodside DG: The channelization of upper and lower face heights compared to population standards in males between 6 and 20 years. *Eur J Orthod* 1979;1:25-40.

76. Linder-Aronson S: The growth in the sagital depth of any bony nasopharynx in relation to some other facial variables. In: McNamara, ed. *Naso Respiratory Function and Craniofacial Growth Series.* Ann Arbor, MI. Center for Human Growth and Development: University of Michigan; 1979.

77. Vig PS, Showfety K, Phillips C: Experimental manipulation of head posture. *Am J Orthod* 1980;77:258-268.

78. Rocabado M: Head, Neck and Temporomandibular Joint Dysfunction. Lecture at Phoenix Academy Meeting. May 27-29, 1982.

79. Rocabado M: Biomechanical relationship of the cranial, cervical and hyoid regions. *J Craniomandib Pract* 1983;3:64.

80. Rocabado M: Physical therapy and dentistry: An overview. *J Craniomandib Pract* 1982; 1:46-49.

81. *The Merck Manual 15th Ed: Idiopathic Scoliosis.* Rahway, NJ: Merck, Sharp, & Dome Research Lab; 1987;2121.

82. Blustein SM, D'Amico JC: Limb length discrepancy. *J Am Pod Med Assoc* 1985;75:200-206.

83. Kapandji IA: *The Physiology of the Joints, 2nd Ed,* Vol. 2. New York: Churchill Livingston, 1970;216.

84. Travell JG, Simons DG: *Myofacial Pain and Dysfunction: The Trigger Point Manual.* Baltimore: The Williams and Wilkins Co., 1883.

85. Jafek, BW, Stark AK: *ENT Secrets.* St. Louis: C. V. Mosby Co.; 1996.

86. Karmody, CS: *Textbook of Otolaryngology.* Philadelphia: Lea & Febiger, 1983.

87. Bell WE: *Orofacial Pains and Differential Diagnosis.* Chicago: Year Book Publishers, 1983;47-48.

88. Bell, 81-82.

89. Young M: Wharton Deformities. *Anat Rec* 1950:106,130.

90. Bleiker, R: Ear disturbances of temporomandibular joint origin. *J Am Dent Assoc* 1983;107(3):25.

91. Murray M, Stewart WR: An explanation of pathogenesis physiology and therapy in Mieniere's disease. *Arch Otolaryngol* 1958:67:184-196.

92. Fujii H, Mitani H: Reflex response of masseter and temporalis muscle in man. *J Dent Res* 1973;52:1046-1051.

93. Jankelson B, Radke J: The Myo-monitor: its use and abuse. *Quintessence Int Dent Digest* 1978;9(2):47-52.

94. Jankelson B, et al.: Neural conduction of the Myo-monitor stimulus: a quantitative analysis. *J Prosthet Dent* 1975;3:245-253.

95. Jankelson RR: *Neuromuscular Dental Diagnosis and Treatment.* St. Louis: Ishiyaku EuroAmerica, 1990.

96. Wagner M: The relationship of tinnitus to craniocervical mandibular disorders. *Dental Annual* 1989;149-160.

97. Karmody C: *Otolaryngology.* Philadelphia: Lea & Febiger, 1983;87.

98. Jafek BW: *ENT Secrets.* Philadelphia: Hanley & Belfus; 1996;58.

99. Lucente, F: *The Merck Manual, 16th Ed.* 1992;2324-2325.

100. Dovek, E: Classification of tinnitus. In CIBA Foundation Symposium. London: Pitman Press, 1991.

101. Rubenstein B: Tinnitus and craniomandibular disorders—Is there a link? *Swed Dent J Supply* 1993;95;1-46.

102. Chole KA, Parker WS: Tinnitus and vertigo in patients with temporomandibular disorders. *Arch Otolaryngol Head Neck Surg* 1992:118(8);817-821.

103. Ash CM, Pinto OF: The TMJ and the middle ear; structural and functional correlates for aural symptoms associated with temporomandibular joint dysfunction. *Int J Prosthodont* 1991:4(l):51-57.

104. Chan SW, Reade P: Tinnitus and temporomandibular pain dysfunction disorders. *Clin Otolaryngol* 1994:19;370-80.

105. Meyerhoff WL, Cooper JC, Padarella MM, Shumrisk DA, Gluckman JL: *Tinnitus in Otolaryngology 3rd ed.* Philadelphia: W.B. Saunders Co.; 1991; 1169-79.

106. Myers LJ: Possible inflammatory pathways relating temporomandibular joint dysfunction to otic symptoms. *J Craniomandib Pract* 1998;6:64-70.

107. Alkofide EA, Clark E, Bermani W, Kronman JH, Mehta N: The incidence and nature of fibrous continuity between the sphenomandibular ligament and the anterior malleolar ligament of the middle ear. *J Orofacial Pain* 1997;4;7-14.

108. Eckemal O: The petrotympanic fissure: A link connecting the tympanic cavity and the temporomandibuar joint. *J Craniomandib Pract* 1991;9(1):15-22.

109. Pinto OF: New structure related to the temporomandibular joint and middle ear. *J Prosthet Dent* 1962;12(1);95-103.

110. Arlen, H: The otomandibular syndrome. In: Gelb H, ed. *Clinical Management of Head, Neck and TMJ Pain and Dysfunction.* Philadelphia: W.B. Saunders Co.; 1985;181-185.

111. Ren YF, Isberg A: Tinnitus in patients with temporomandibular joint internal derangement. *J Craniomandib Pract* 1995;13(2):75-80.

112. Cioncaglini R, Loreti P, Radaeli G: Ear, nose and throat symptoms in patients with TMD: The association of symptoms according to the severity of arthropathy. *J Orofacial Pain* 1994;8(3):293-297.

113. Shulman A: The temporomandibular joint. In: Shulman A, ed. *Tinnitus: Diagnosis and Treatment.* Philadelphia: Lea & Febiger; 1991;387-90.

114. Bush FM: Tinnitus and otalgia in temporomandibular disorders. *J Prosthet Dent* 1987:58(4):495-498.

115. Bernstein JM, Mohl ND, Spiller H: Temporomandibular joint dysfunction masquerading as disease of the car, nose and throat. *Trans Am Acad Opthalmol Otolaryngol* 1969;73(6):1208-1217.

116. Vernon J, Griest S, Press L: Attributes of tinnitis that may predict temporomandibular joint dysfunction. *J Craniomandibid Pract* 1992;10(4):282-287.

117. Okeson JP: *Bells Orofacial Pain 5th ed.* Carol Strem, IL: Quintessence; 1995;269.

118. Fricton JP, Kroening RJ, Haley D: Muscular disorders: The most common diagnosis. In: Fricton J.D. ed. *TMJ and Craniofacial Pain: Diagnosis and Management.* St. Louis: Ishiyaku Euro America; 1988;67-83.

119. National Institutes of Health Technology Assessment Conference Statement. Management of Temporomandibular Disorders. *J Am Dent Assoc* 1996;127:1595-1606.

120. Wright E, Bifano S: Tinnitus improvement through TMJ therapy. *J Am Dent Assoc* 1996:128:1424-32.

Figure 5 is reprinted, with permission, from *Hearing Loss and Dizziness* by Nomura (Williams and Wilkins). Figures 6 and 8 are reprinted, with permission, from *Color Atlas of Anatomy* by J. W. Rohen and C. Yokochi (Igaku-Shoin, 1988). Figure 7 is reprinted, with permission, from *Diseases of the Temporomandibular Apparatus - A Multidisciplinary Approach.* St. Louis. C.V. Mosby Co.; 1982.

TMD—An Upper Quarter Condition

Larry Tilley and David M. Hickman

Understanding the complex interrelationship of craniomandibular disorders (CMD) to overall health requires a broad understanding of not only the anatomy and physiology of the head and neck but also the cervical spine and upper quarter complex. To understand neuromuscular dentistry one is required to consider maxillo-mandibular relationships from a different perspective and its relationship with the head and neck. This is paramount for the practitioner treating head, neck, and face pain, and/or dysfunction. Only recently has dentistry begun to think of the mandible and its association to the cranium as a three-dimensional relationship, rather than only considering it as an isolated structure and evaluated within two dimensions as has been taught traditionally. We understand that the mandible can move in all planes of space or in a combination of planes.[1] These movements are relatively small and limited by many structures, but the implications are significant.

To properly evaluate maxillo-mandibular relationships, one must begin by considering physiologic rest. Physiologic rest is a basic axiom and may be defined as that mandibular position that allows mandibular elevators and depressors to function from a position requiring a minimum of muscle activity.[2-4] Physiologic rest is a physiologic concept that is applicable to all muscles throughout the body, the stomatognathic musculature is no exception.[5] As stated, when maxillo-mandibular relationships are evaluated, one must consider mandibular position spatially or three dimensionally, not solely in an anteroposterior and/or lateral plane(s). This implies that, when accessing these relationships, the added dimension within a vertical plane must be evaluated, as well as a combination of planes or torque.

Considerable accommodative or postural influences may occur within the stomatognathic neuromusculature in pathologic/dysfunctional conditions, such as with a malocclusion. In a normal physiologic state, engrams, or habitual muscle patterns, develop as result of a balanced occlusion. Malocclusion, however, alters these normal muscle patterns resulting in habitual postural changes and persistent muscle tension preventing the mandible from returning to physiologic rest. This explains much about the muscle and joint pathology commonly observed.[6,30,31] In many cases, centric occlusion, temporomandibular joint function and/or position, and neuromuscular function may not be compatible, resulting in structural breakdown or pathology as adaptive mechanisms are overcome. The end results are typically seen in the CMD patient[1] and may be exemplified in the developing child who has a chronic mouth breathing habit resulting from chronic allergies or nasal pathology.

A compromised nasal airway not only provides an environment allowing for the development of a dental malocclusion, but also a spatial malrelationship of the mandible to the cranial base. Garry stated that it is essential to understand that teeth seek a neutral position within a system of forces acting upon them.[7] Where imbalances exist, the resultant occlusal manifestations may be a crossbite, bicuspid drop-off, deep curve of Spee, lingually tipped mandibular posterior teeth, etc. This is well described by Linder-Aronson, Garry, Rubin, Meredith, and others.[8-17] Very typically seen in the patient with a compromised nasal airway is a resultant head forward posture. A forward head posture will always influence the resting posture of the mandible.[18] Furthermore, and of equal importance, is the influence that changes in mandibular posture have on the upper quarter.[19-22] Accommodative capacities vary from person to person, but when surpassed, pain and/or dysfunction develop. It is crucial for the dentist to evaluate the upper quarter when assessing the patient with craniomandibular disorders. Evaluation and concurrent treatment of craniomandibular, as well as the cranio-cervical, apparatus, is a necessity to maximize treatment efficacy and long-term results in the pain and/or disfunction patient.

Etiology of Head, Neck, and Face Pain

When evaluating head, neck, and face pain, there are multiple conditions that must be considered in developing a differential diagnosis. Pain of the head, neck, and face may be attributed to: sinus pathology, myofascial pain, dental pathology, craniomandibular disorders, cavitational osteonecrosis (NICO), temporal tendinitis, lesser and greater occipital neuralgias, Ernest syndrome (stylomandibular ligament injury), and cervical-sacral disorders, as well as neurologic, vascular, and systemic disorders.[23-37]

In the management of pain patients, we as dentists must first rule out dental pathology. Many times complicated treatment has been undertaken only to find that the presenting condition resulted from pulpal pathology, a cracked tooth, periodontal pathology, etc. Next, one must evaluate intracapsular temporomandibular joint pathology as a source of pain. Much has been written about anterior disc displacement, the resultant bony changes which may occur, and the compression of the sensitive retrodiscal tissue.[38] The temporomandibular (TM) joint may be the source of pain, and it is important to include in your differential diagnosis; however, joint pathology typically does not exist without concomitant involvement of associated muscles which move the joint. Muscles serve multiple functions, and one function is to protect a damaged joint. Further, it is *crucial to understand* that masticatory muscle pathology may frequently exist without intracapsular TM joint pathology.

The stomatognathic neuromusculature has complex peripheral and/or central involvement when considering its role in respiration, chewing, speaking, and swallowing. Understanding the role of the muscles, the pathology that may develop within these structures, the resulting myofascial pain, and the referred pain patterns that may result is paramount in understanding head, neck, and face pain. Travell, Simons, and others have clearly demonstrated that myofascial trigger points may have far-reaching pain patterns within the head, neck, and temporomandibular region.[30,31] Every dentist or health care provider who treats such patients must be thoroughly familiar with the diagnosis and treatment of myofascial trigger points and their referral patterns. To insure treatment success, however, it is necessary to also evaluate and treat the many perpetuating factors that may influence effective management of trigger points, i.e., nutritional, metabolic, and endocrine inadequacies; psychological factors; chronic infection; allergies; impaired sleep; radiculopathy; and chronic visceral disease.[30] These perpetuating factors must be considered in formulating a differential diagnosis and may require an appropriate referral.

Mechanical stressors may include poor posture, abuse of muscles, constricting pressure on muscles, and prolonged immobility. Travell stated that "the most common source of mechanical stress perpetuating trigger points is skeletal asymmetry and disproportion." Such skeletal problems may include a short leg (functional or structural), a small hemipelvis, long second metatarsal (Morton's foot), or short upper arms.[39]

Many agree that the most significant and profound structural asymmetry or disproportion is an anomalous relationship of the mandible to the cranial base.[30] Unlike other asymmetries which affect one only when sitting, standing, or walking, a disruption of normal mandibular orthopedics has continuous effects resulting from neurologic controls which constantly affect mandibular position/malposition.[40]

One of the most significant considerations when developing a differential diagnosis and treatment is to understand the interrelationship between the craniomandibular complex and the "upper quarter" (i.e., cranium, mandible, cervical spine, shoulder girdle, 1st and 2nd ribs).

The interrelationship of posture and TMD was first introduced to dentistry in 1949 in an article entitled "Current Advances in Dentistry" published by the University of Illinois College of Dentistry. The muscular balance of the head and neck is made clear with the example in *Figure 1*, which illustrates this complex interrelationship.

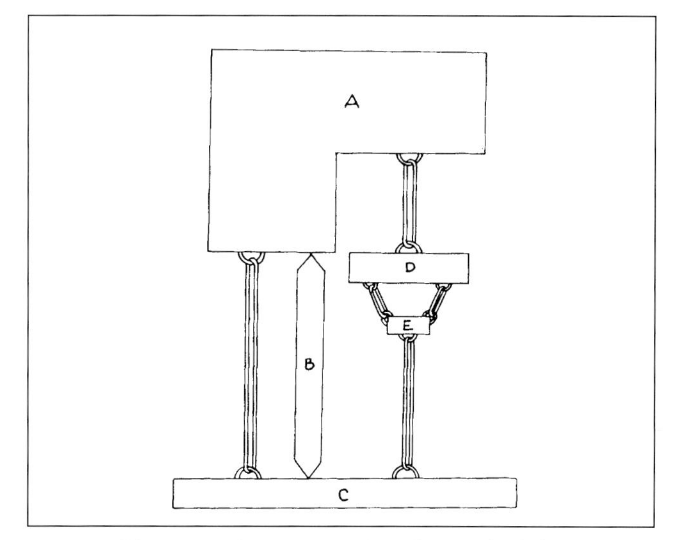

Figure 1. Diagrammatic representation of muscular balance of head and neck region. A: Head (minus upper face). B: Vertebral column. C: Shoulder girdle. D: Mandible F: Hyoid bone.

Fonder and others described the effect that occlusion has on posture.[41-43] Guzay[44] evaluated the function of the mandible from an engineering perspective and reported that the center of mandibular rotation was not at the temporomandibular joint but instead at the level of the second cervical vertebra *(Figure 2)*.

Rocabado described that, as the vertical dimension of occlusion is altered, there is a significant change in the cervical posture.[45] He described that the stability of the cranium over the cervical spine is extremely

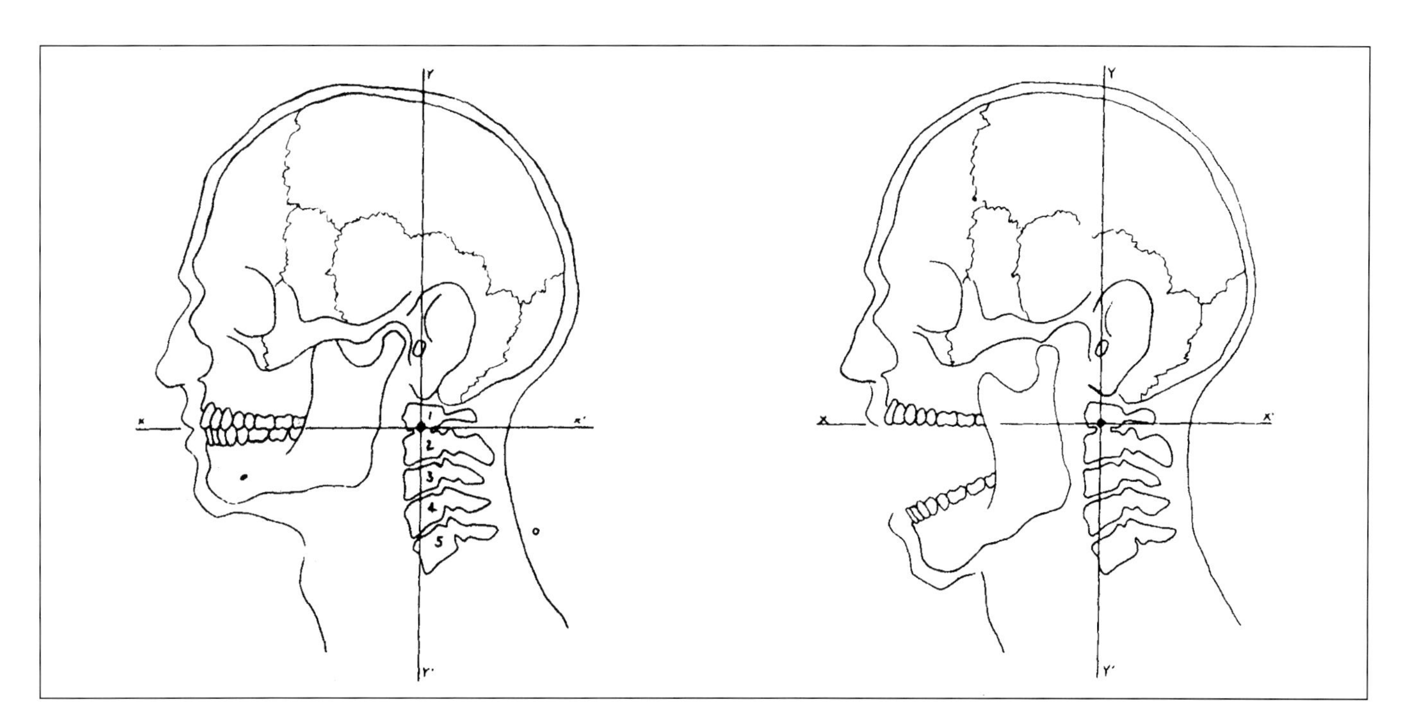

Figure 2. The apex of the combined muscular control of the mandible to all functioning movements is located at the dens between the atlas and axis of the cervical vertebrae. The condyle translates forward and downward as the mouth opens.

important in diagnosis and treatment of head, neck, and face pain.

Posture and alterations of posture are unique. Alteration of posture within the upper quarter, as with the mandible, occurs in three dimensions. A very typical scenario is seen in the patient who presents with a head forward posture, which is frequently seen with the temporomandibular disorder (TMD) or CMD patient. As a head forward posture develops, it must involve the neck, shoulder, and mandible. Kraus described changes that could be expected with increasing severity of postural alterations as described below.[46]

Forward Head Posture

1. Adaptive shortening of suboccipital muscles
2. Irritation of the greater and lesser occipital nerves
3. Facet strains of occiput-atlas and the atlas-axis articulations
4. Soft tissue tension, especially the periosteum
5. Potential involvement of the vertebral artery
6. Altered firing of mechanoreceptors
7. Lost rest position for the tongue
8. Increased activity of supramandibular muscles.

Decrease in Cervical Lordosis

1. Shortening of suprahyoid and stretching of infrahyoid muscles
2. Elevation of hyoid bone
3. Imbalance between anterior/posterior cervical musculature
4. Mid-cervical facet joint strain
5. Altered firing of mechanoreceptors
6. Loss of side bending motion and rotation of the head
7. A change in the resting vertical dimension of the mandible
8. Changes in the habitual closure pattern of the mandible
9. Alteration of a normal swallowing sequence
10. Clenching is more likely to occur.

Increase in Kyphosis of the Upper Thoracic Spine

1. Thoracic outlet syndrome
2. Increase disc pressure in the lower cervical and upper thoracic area
3. Flattening of mid-thoracic area
4. Hypomobile thoracic joints
5. Hypermobile cervical thoracic junction
6. Alteration of nasal-diaphramatic breathing
7. A change of the resting vertical dimension of the mandible.

Protraction and Elevation of the Shoulder Girdle and Internal Rotation of the Glenohumeral Joint

1. Increase tension in the trapezius and levator scapulae
2. Sternocleidomastoid (SCM) and scalene muscles have a greater mechanical advantage
3. Latissimus dorsi shorten leading to lower back pain
4. Compression of the sterno-clavicular joints and acromio-clavicular joints
5. Shoulder girdle muscle imbalance
6. A change in the resting vertical dimension of the mandible.

Anatomy and Function of the Spine

Anatomy of the Cervical Spine

The head sits atop the cervical spine and weighs approximately 15 pounds with its center of gravity at the sella turcica. The center of gravity is anterior to the occipitoatlantal (OA) articulation in the normal, healthy state placing more weight anterior to the OA joints. The resultant force vectors created by gravity tend to tip the head forward. If the center of gravity moves forward, as with a patient in a head forward posture, the cervical spine and its musculature are subjected to greater forces as the fulcrum (spine) is being moved further from the load. Every inch that the head is moved anterior from its neutral position will increase the effective "weight" of the head by approximately 15 pounds, assuming an average head weighs 15 pounds. Thus, one inch of a forward head posture results in an effective weight of 30 pounds, while two inches of forward head posture results in an effective weight of 45 pounds. The overall posture is altered as the central nervous system attempts to maintain the optic, otic, and occlusal planes level with the surroundings.[47] These planes are maintained at the expense of the musculoskeletal system. Lower body orthopedic conditions can, in turn, alter head posture. For example, a leg length discrepancy resulting in a pelvic tilt must be compensated for by upper quarter accommodation. The head and cervical spine must accommodate while maintaining the optic, otic, and occlusal planes.[45]

Function of the Cervical Spine

The cervical spine is made up of seven vertebrae. Due to its function and anatomy, it can be divided into an upper cervical or craniovertebral region [occiput-atlas, atlas-axis (AA)] and the lower cervical spine, C3–C7. The principal motion in the first articulation, occiput-atlas, is principally a nodding motion (flexion-extension) of about 15–20 degrees. Side flexion is about 10 degrees, and rotation is negligible. The atlas unlike the other vertebrae has no vertebral body and no spinous process. The axis is anatomically similar to the other cervical vertebrae in shape, with the exception of the odontoid process or dens. The dens projects into vertebral canal of the atlas and forms the most mobile articulation within the spine. Flexion-extension is about ten degrees and side bending only five degrees, but approximately 50% of rotation occurs between atlas-axis prior to other cervical vertebrae being activated. Talking and chewing would be all but impossible without movement at C1–C2.

Articulation between the vertebrae occur at seven pairs of highly innervated synovial facet joints called zygapophyseal joints from the occiput to C7. Vertebrae from C3 to T1 also have additional saddle shaped articulations known as uncovertebral joints of Loachka, which act as guides in flexion and extension. The greatest movement in flexion-extension occurs at C5–C6 and as a result we find that the intervetebral discs are easily damaged in this area. Inter-vertebral discs are located between each vertebra, giving the spine approximately one half of its height, as well as its characteristic curvatures. The discs are composed of an outer cartilaginous anulus fibrosis and the internal nucleus pulposis. Their function is to absorb stress and allow motion to occur. The musculature of the area and its interrelation to the craniomandibular complex is very evident, yet its relationship to the entire upper quarter is seldom considered nor understood.[48,49]

Thoracic Spine

In order to understand the complex interrelationship involved in upper quarter function, we must also consider the thoracic spine. The thoracic spine acts completely or not at all; however, for our understanding, we will consider it only from the cervical-thoracic junction (C7–T1) to T3, which is the most significant area from a functional perspective. The upper thoracic spine articulates with the sternum via the ribs. The first two ribs and sternum ultimately articulate with the mandible through the infrahyoid attachments to the hyoid bone. This is attached to the mandible via the suprahyoid muscles. The first two ribs attach to the upper and lower cervical spine through the scalene muscles. The sternum and clavicle are attached to the occiput by the sternocleidomastoid muscles (SCM). The shoulder girdle (scapula, humerus, acromioclavicular joint, clavicle, and sternoclavicular joint) is related to all other structure of the upper quarter either directly through joints or through cervical attachments to the scapula.

The muscles of the scapula attach it to the occiput (upper trapezius muscle), upper cervical spine (levator scapula), lower cervical spine (upper trapezius), upper thoracic spine (middle trapezius and rhomboids), ribs (serratus anterior and pectoralis minor), mandible (omohyoid), and to the sternum, directly through the acromioclavicular and sternoclavicular joints. The humerus attaches to the ribs and sternum (pectoralis major and latissimus dorsi) and to the scapula (supraspinatus and infraspinatus, teres major and minor, coracobrachialis, and deltoid muscles).[49-52]

As can be clearly seen, the structural and biomechanical interrelationship of the upper quarter is quite involved. This area of the upper quarter must be prime concern to the dentist treating orofacial pain and TMD.

Forward Head Posture

Forward head posture can be the result of many things such as a flexion-extension injury, shoulder injury, temporomandibular joint (TMJ) pathology, mandibular overclosure, airway obstruction, dysphagia, and other chronic conditions. This may result in the cervical spine being held in an extreme extended position, producing a "closed-packed" joint position.[45] Such positioning results in overstretching of capsular and intervertebral ligaments of the vertebral joints. The range of motion will be decreased and joints can become compressed, encouraging degeneration within the joints and discs. Such postural distortion results in what is termed a "crossed syndrome," where postural muscles (pectoralis major and minor, upper trapezius, levator scapula, and SCM) shorten and tighten while the phasic muscles (serratus anterior, rhomboids, middle and lower trapezius) are stretched and weakened.[53] This is confirmed by Davis' Law which states that "if muscle ends are brought closer together, muscle tonus is increased which shortens the muscle causing hypertrophy. If muscle ends are separated beyond normal, tonus is lessened or lost causing the muscle to become weak."[54] With continued collapse in forward head posture, the scapulae protract, elevate, and internally rotate causing rolled and elevated shoulders. In order for the head to maintain its three horizontal reference planes, the cranium rotates posteriorly on the atlas, causing the lower cervical spine to flex, losing its normal lordotic curve. In order to maintain the body's center of gravity, the thoracic spine loses its normal kyphotic curve, flattening the upper back. This results in a stretching of the supra and infrahyoid musculature causing a posterior-inferior pull upon the mandible, producing the tendency for an open mouth posture. To close the mouth, the masseter and temporalis muscles must contract. As a result, the mandible and its condyles are retracted posteriorly and superiorly into a "closed-pack" position, thus reducing the mandible's resting vertical dimension. The constant hyperactivity of the musculature can produce musculoskeletal dysfunction, trigger points, degenerative changes due to compression, compression syndromes, vascular dysfunction, and peripheral nerve entrapment. Each of these disorders can lead to local and/or referred pain.[30,31,53]

Another frequent occurrence with forward head posture is an extension of the cranium on the upper cervical spine. This often results in a mechanical impingement of the occipital nerves, creating pain that may extend from the suboccipital region to the supraorbital area. Supraorbital pain may result from communications between upper cervical nerves and the supraorbital branch of the trigeminal nerve.[4] Convergence between the trigeminal and cervical nerves C1–C3 frequently occurs and is well documented. Convergence occurs within the spinal tract nucleus of the trigeminal nerve, or the spinal trigemino-cervical complex. This area is a prime center for transmission of nociceptive and mechanoreceptor impulses, as well as having an influence on the sympathetic nervous system. Neurons from cranial nerves V, VII, IX, X, XI, and XII also interact within this complex.[46,47,55-62] This may explain the referred pain patterns commonly seen in patients suffering from head, neck, and face pain. Because of this complex neuroanatomical and neurophysiologic relationship, a cranial nerve exam should be performed on all craniomandibular patients.

Forward head posture significantly alters the position of the hyoid bone. The hyoid is the only non-articulate bone in the body, yet serves as the insertion for muscles, ligaments, and fascia from the cranium, cervical spine, and shoulder girdle. The position of the hyoid bone tends to remain at a vertical height between C3–C4. Reduction in the cervical spine lordosis results in an elevation of the hyoid and affects all attached structures. Normal tongue posture and swallowing may also be adversely affected.[46] Treatment of temporomandibular disorders while ignoring the forward head posture will doom any treatment to ultimate failure.[18,47]

A total of 31 segmental pairs of spinal nerves exit the vertebrae via the intervertebral foraminae. Involvement of these nerve roots can produce symptoms which are specifically diagnostic for the nerve roots involved. Differential diagnoses can be made by evaluating dermatomes, myotomes, and sclerotomes innervated by each nerve *(Figure 3).*

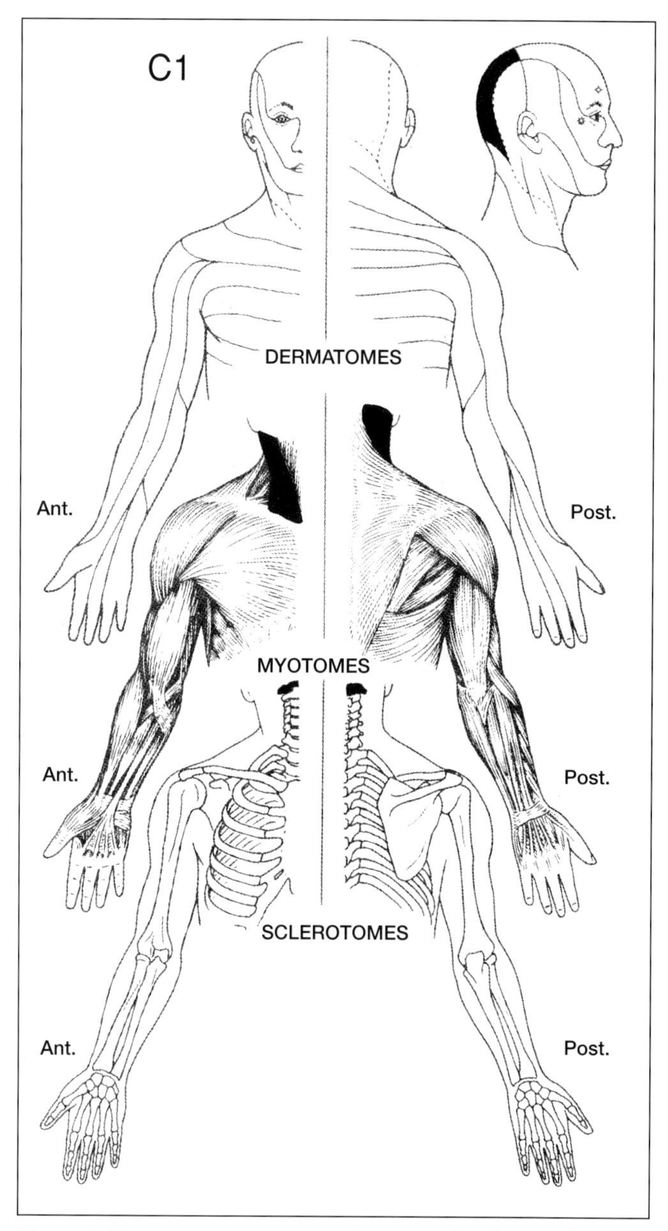

Figure 3. Dermatome, myotome, sclerotome distribution for C1.

Developmental Relationships

A dermatome represents a spinal nerve that supplies a specific strip of skin that extends from the posterior midline to the anterior midline. A myotome represents a group of muscles innervated from a single spinal segment. Sclerotome represents the area of bone innervated from a single spinal segment. These can be clinically evaluated by examining the motor function and reflexes associated with a particular nerve.[49,63] Time and space do not permit a review of each cervical nerve; however, we will consider evaluation of C1 as an example since our focus has been on this area *(Figure 3).*

C1—Dermatome
Skin: Posterior scalp
Forehead } perceived pain
Retro-orbital

C1—Myotome
Nerves: Cranial XI (spinal accessory)
Suboccipital nerve
Muscles: Sternocleidomastoid (C1–C4)
Longus Capitis (C1–C4)
Rectus Capitis anterior (C1–C2)
Rectus Capitis laterals (C1)
Rectus Capitis posterior (C1)
Obliqis capitis inferior (C1)
Obliqis capitis superior (C1)
Splenius capitis (C1–C4)
Splenius cervicis (C1–C4)

C1—Sclerotome
Bones: Vertebra and periosteum
Atlas
Occiput
Ligaments: Atlanto-occipital
Medial atlanto-occipital
Alar
Apical dental
Cruciform
Accessory atlantoaxial
Articular capsule
Nuchal
Anterior atlanto-occipital membrane
Posterior atlanto-occiptal membrane

Neurologic Assessment
Motor Function: Head flexion
Head rotation
Fixation and steadying of neck
Extension
Reflexes: Jaw jerk
Head retraction
Sensory: Posterior scalp
Forehead skin

Evaluating and treating upper quarter disorders can be quite complex. Dentistry should take the lead in the management of upper quarter disorders in an interdisciplinary effort. Without correction of a patient's craniomandibular disorder, as well as normalization of the cervical spine and shoulder girdle, treatment of forward head posture will most often be only transitory. The reverse is also true. A CMD condition cannot be successfully treated if the upper quarter is ignored. Despite the need for dental involvement, many will choose not to actively treat upper quarter problems. Good communication and interdisciplinary relationships must be developed with other health care providers to bring maximum benefit for these conditions. For this to occur, it is necessary for the dentist to screen for upper quarter dysfunction. This can readily be carried out through clinical and radiological evaluation.

Clinical Evaluation
The patient should be viewed from the frontal, lateral and posterior. A plumb line or visual grid is helpful in identifying body asymmetry. The following observations should be made with ideal alignment :

Frontal:
- Facial symmetry (optic, otic and occlusal planes should be parallel and perpendicular to floor)
- Ear height level
- Chin in midline
- Sternocleidomastoid muscles should be of equal size and angulation
- Suprascapular sulcus should be of equal depth
- Shoulder height should be equal without anterior rolling
- Arms should hang the same distance from the torso and be of equal lengths, and hands should point in the same direction (palms toward the body)
- Height of the anterior-superior iliac crest should be level
- Knees should be level
- Middle malleolus' level
- Arch height of feet equal
- Foot angulation should be the same
- Check for long second metatarsal (Morton's foot)

Rear (refer to Illustration 1):
- Ear height level
- Mastoids level
- Shoulder height should be level
- Scapulae should be level and not "winged," protracted, retracted or elevated
- Iliac crest and posterior superior iliac spine should be level
- Inferior buttock folds should be level

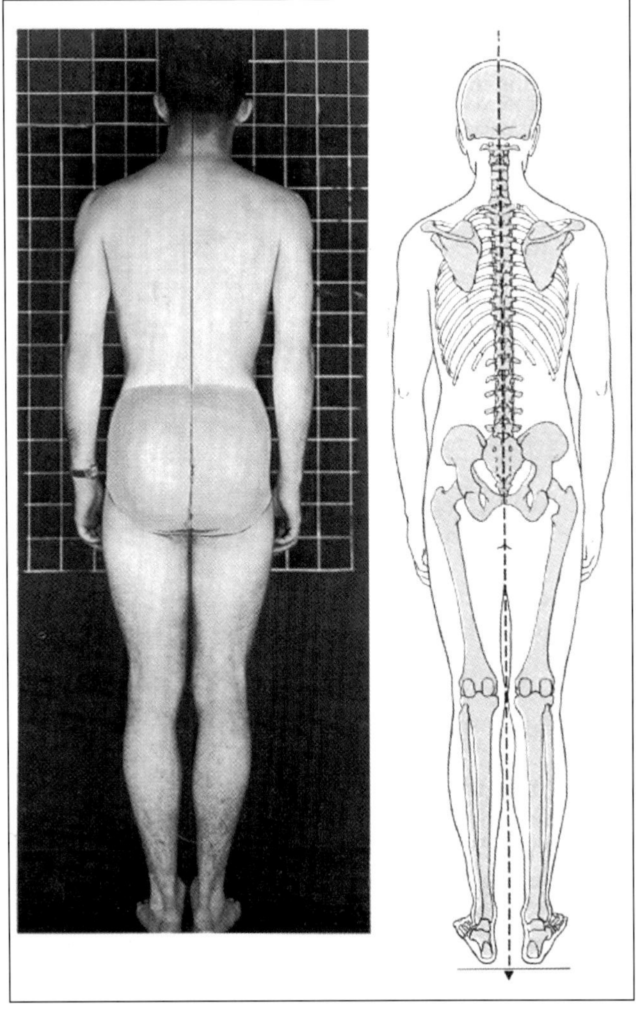

Illustration 1. Ideal alignment: posterior view.

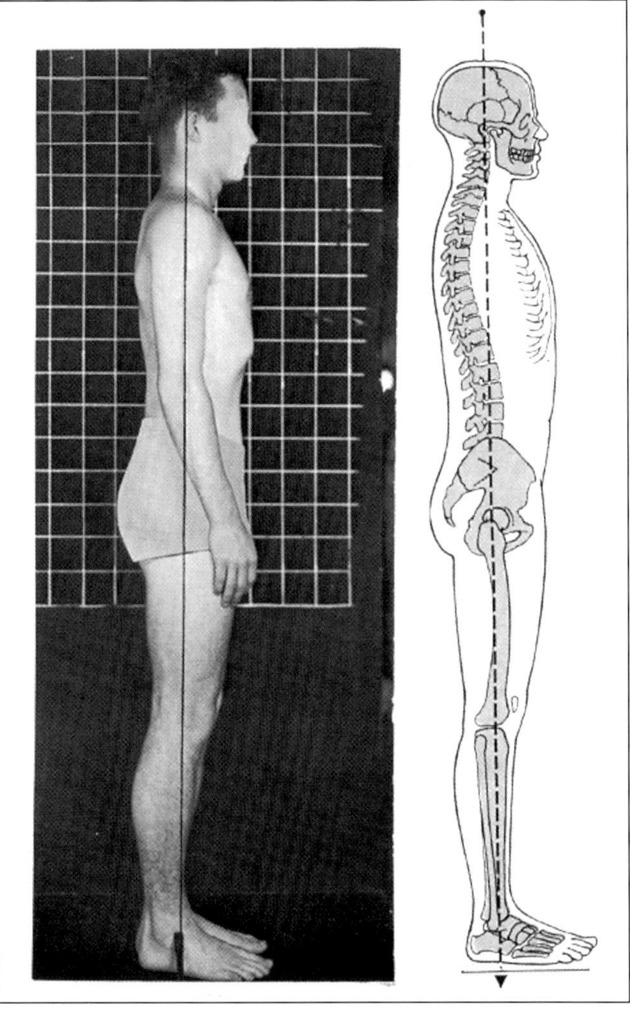

Illustration 2. Ideal segmental alignment: side view.

From a lateral view, a plumb line should fall through the external auditory meatus (EAM) with the odontoid process lying just behind the cervical vertebral bodies, the glenohumeral joint and lumbar vertebral bodies. The plumb line should fall slightly behind the center of the hip joint, slightly anterior to the center of the knee joint, through the calcaneous-cubudal joint and anterior to the lateral malleolus *(Illustration 2)*.

Lateral:

- EAM should be positioned over cervical spine
- Malar process should be in line with the sterno-clavicular junction
- SCM angulation should be 45–60 degrees
- Occiput should not be tipped back at OA
- Normal cervical lordotic curve of lower cervical with a slight kyphotic curve of upper cervical
- Depth of cervical curve from a vertical tangent through occiput and the apex of the thoracic spine should not be greater than 6 cm
- Shoulder should not be rolled forward or elevated
- Normal kyphotic thoracic curve and normal lordotic lumbar curve
- Anterior and posterior superior iliac spine should be evaluated with the angle being level for males and 5–10 degrees for females
- Knees should not be locked

  Reference [63]

Cervical Screening Evaluation

Active Motion

Normal cervical neck flexion should allow 80–90 degrees forward bending with the chin touching the chest. Initial flexion is nodding and occurs mostly between OA and AA joints. Extension should allow the forehead to be nearly horizontal or parallel to the floor (70–90 degrees). Normal side flexion should be approximately 45 degrees from the sagittal plane, with most movement taking place between OA and AA joints. Rotation should allow 70–90 degrees of movement with the chin being in line with the shoulder. Rotation and side flexion always occur together; 50% of rotation occurs at AA joints while the remaining 50% is evenly distributed throughout the cervical spine.[48]

Passive Motion

Any previously noted restricted range of motion (ROM) should be evaluated with passive motion. This is a more accurate evaluation of joint movement without muscle action. "End feel" is a valuable observation in passive motion. It is defined as the "feel" at the end of a patient's ROM. Normal end feel, when it is bone to bone, will produce a hard, unyielding and painless end point similar to that felt when fully extending the elbow. Normal soft tissue approximation will produce a yielding compression preventing further movement as can be felt in knee flexion. Normal tissue stretch produces a hard yet springy feel as is felt when bending the fingers back toward the dorsal surface of the hand. Occasionally pain will prevent any determination of end feel. Within the cervical spine, capsular pathology is said to exist if there is pain and/or limitation with passive movement with no limitation of flexion, equal limitation of lateral flexion and rotation, and a marked limitation in extension. A non-capsular pattern is said to exist with minimal limitation or with a full ROM and pain. Pain would indicate ligament or tendinous inflammation, fibrosis, or adhesions. Pain produced by all passive movement except flexion is often indicative of a disc lesion.[49]

Resisted Isometric Movements

Isometric contraction within the ROM of the cervical spine against resistance is an effective way to assess pain and muscle weakness. Muscle weakness without pain is often associated with either a ruptured tendon or a neurologic lesion. Myotome and reflex testing can be done to indicate the specific nerve root involved.

C1–C2—Neck flexion
C3—neck side flexion
C4—shoulder elevation
C5—shoulder abduction
C6—elbow flexion and/or wrist extension
C7—elbow extension and/or wrist flexion
C8—thumb extension and/or ulnar deviation
T1—adduction of the thumb and/or abduction of the little finger[49]

Cervical Gliding

With the patient in a supine position, the operator should cradle the occiput in the hands. Assure the patient that you are not going to jerk or twist the head and instruct him or her to relax and not to assist in the movements. The operator lifts the head in a gliding fashion keeping the face up and avoiding flexion or extension. Such a movement will engage the vertebrae as they glide to their maximum range followed by succeeding facets being engaged. The effect is a ratcheting movement as each facet is engaged. If you feel binding, you should consider a potential facet disorder at that level. Lateral gliding should also be evaluated for freedom of movement.[48]

Occipitoatlantal (OA) Evaluation

While holding the patient's head in the hands, place the index finger on the transverse process of C1 (just inferior and anterior to the mastoid). When the head is rotated, the transverse process on the side to which the head is rotated will rotate away from the palpating finger. If it remains prominent, there is a restriction at OA. Another technique to evaluate OA is to have the patient tuck the chin back and nod the head in forward side bending which moves this articulation. Rotation of AA can be evaluated by flexing the head fully, thus locking the facets, and evaluating rotation at C1–C2.[48]

Forminal Compression Test (Spurling Test)

With the palms of the operators' hands on the parietal area, the head is compressed caudally. The head is then side flexed to each side while compressing the cervical spine. If the procedure is painful and pain radiates into the arm on the side to which the head is flexed, there is the possibility for foraminal nerve root compression.[49]

Distraction Test

With fingers under the occiput, lift the patient's head to decompress the cervical spine. While distracting the spine, the patient should lift their shoulders, thus further decompressing the vertebra. If pain is relieved or decreased, a reduction of nerve root compression has occurred.[49]

Shoulder Decompression Test

The patient's head is flexed sideways while applying downward pressure on the opposite shoulder. Increased pain may indicate nerve root irritation or compression, foraminal stenosis, or adhesions around the dural sleeve of the nerve.[48]

Lower Cervical Nerve Root Test
In this test the patient's head is extended and flexed to the side. The neck is then rotated to the same side and held for 30 seconds. Pain will be felt on the side to which the head is rotated if nerve root compression exists.[48]

Vertebral Artery Test
The movement for this test is the same as the lower cervical nerve root test with the exception that the chin is retruded before movements are begun. If dizziness or nystagmus occur, the vertebral artery may be compressed.[64]

Shoulder Abduction Test
The patient places his or her hands on top of the head while keeping the elbows back and holding the position for 30 seconds. Relief or a decrease of symptoms indicates a cervical extradural compression, such as a nerve root compression or a herniated disc.[49]

Valsalva Maneuver
The patient takes a deep breath and, while holding it, bears down as when having a bowel movement. An increase in pain indicates the possibility of a herniated disc, tumor, or osteophyte.[48]

Dizziness Test
Hot and cold is alternated behind the patient's ear one side at a time. If dizziness is experienced, it is indicative of an inner ear problem.

The patient's head is actively rotated as far as possible to the right and left. Next, while keeping the patient's head straight and the eyes fixed on an object, the shoulders are rotated right and left as far as possible. If dizziness occurs with both movements, the vertebral artery may be involved. If dizziness occurs only when the head is rotated, the problem is likely related to the inner ear.[49]

Brachial Plexus Tension Test (Adson's Test)
While monitoring the radial pulse, have the patient raise the arm beside the head, flex the elbow by placing the palm of the hand behind the back, and externally rotate the elbow. While the patient takes a deep breath, the head is rotated toward the side being tested. If there is a compression of the subclavian artery, the pulse will be reduced. Symptoms of tingling, paresthesia, pain, or a sensation of heat or cold may occur if the brachial plexus is compressed.[48]

Scanning Palpation
With the patient sitting or standing, cradle the forehead with one hand while standing beside the patient. Palpate the facet joints of each vertebra from C1–T2 using the tip of the middle finger from the opposite side and the thumb from the near side of the spine. This will produce compression of neurologic structures. The pressure should be perpendicular to the facet which will produce a more vertical angulation as you palpate the vertebra.[65]

Springing Test
With the patient supine and the forehead resting on a support, palpate the spinous processes of C1–T1 with the thumbs, feeling for "springiness." Then move the thumbs laterally to the side of the spinous process and, by using alternating pressure, move the spinous process from side to side rocking the vertebra. Next, move the thumbs further laterally to rest on the distal aspect of the transverse process. Press anteriorly in an alternating right to left fashion to rotate the vertebra. Move further laterally to the transverse process and glide the vertebra laterally back and forth. All of these movements should produce a "springy" feel. A "hard" feel or lack of springiness may indicate a vertebral condition at that level.[49]

Radiographic Evaluation
Radiologic evaluation of the cervical spine is another valuable tool in differential diagnosis of the orofacial pain patient. Tomography, nuclear magnetic resonance imaging (MRI), and myelograms may be helpful in many cases, yet standard films can be of great value. These films should be taken without the ear rods from the head positioner in place so that a more normal cervical posture can be observed. The standard views include anteroposterior (AP), Odontoid (AP through an open mouth), lateral (neutral, flexion, and full extension), and a 45 degree oblique view, right and left.

Craniometrics
Craniometrics is the measurement of bony landmarks, angles, and relationships which can be very valuable in assisting in the identification of craniomandibular-cervical relationships. These measurements are most useful when paired with other historical, physical, and radiologic data.

Radiographic Views

Anteroposterior
In the anterior view, C1–C2 is obscured by the mandible, thus it is used to view C3–C7. The examiner should evaluate the shape of the vertebrae, look for lateral wedging (disc space narrowing) and cervical scoliosis, and rule out the presence of a cervical rib *(Figure 4)*.[66-68]

Odontoid View
The odontoid view is an AP view at the upper cervical region taken with the mouth open and the head tilted

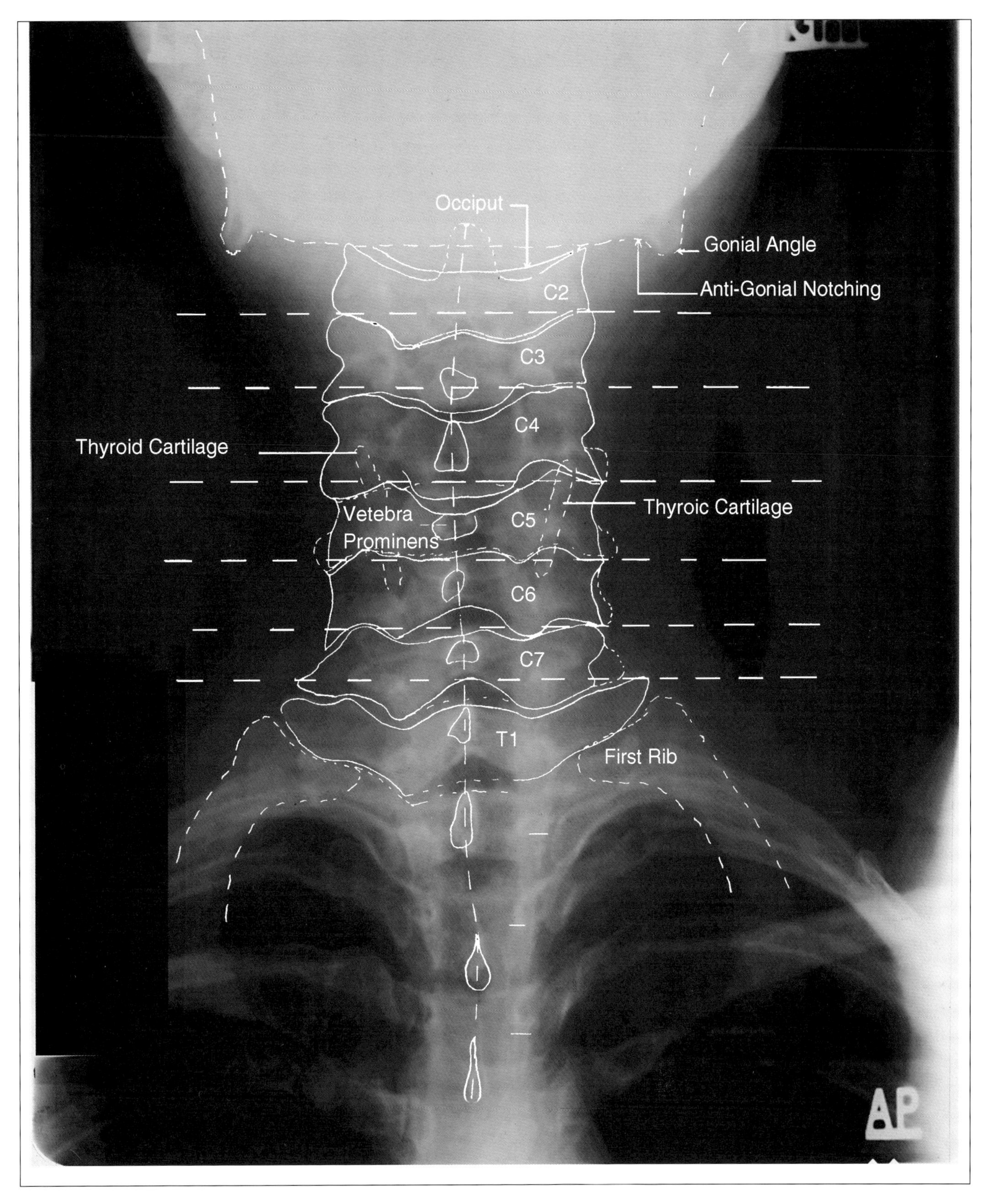

Figure 4. Anteroposterior cervical spine radiograph. Note that C3 through C7–T1 can be easily visualized.

slightly into extension. The spacing between the atlas and axis should be equal with the odontoid process centered *(Figure 5)*.[66-68]

Lateral Oblique

Lateral oblique radiographs are important when nerve or vertebral artery entrapment are suspected. They reveal the intervertebral foraminae, as well as the joints of luschka and the zygapophyseal joints. The most important area to evaluate is the intervertebral foramina. Other pathology to be considered is lipping at the joints of luschka and the facet joints *(Figures 6 and 7)*.[66-68]

Lateral

The lateral cervical radiograph is probably the most diagnostic of the cervical spine series. Much can be learned from this view, including overall curvature of the cervical spine, shape of the vertebrae including fusions, collapse, or wedging, disc space (normally 4–6 mm), lipping; osteophytes, displacement, soft tissue width (2.6–4.8 mm at anterior inferior boarder of C3), instability (more than 3.5 mm of horizontal displacement of one vertebra compared to its adjacent vertebra), atlanto-dental interval (no greater than 3 mm); OA relationship, and the hyoid relationship *(Figure 8)*.[66-68]

Lateral Flexion and Extension

Lateral flexion and extension views reveal the results of these two movements on the vertebrae. Flexion will reveal the articular facets and the integrity of the posterior ligaments. The space between the posterior border of the atlas and the anterior border of the odontoid process should not increase significantly, and a smooth curve of the vertebral bodies should exist. Extension will stretch the anterior longitudinal ligament and changes along the anterior aspect of the vertebral body should be noted. A smooth curve of the vertebral bodies should be observed *(Figures 9 and 10)*.[66-68]

Pillar View

Another cervical view which is sometimes used is the AP Pillar radiograph. The spine is placed into extension, and the beam will come from a 50–70 degree cephalad angulation in order to be parallel with the facet joints and articular processes. It is used to evaluate the superior and inferior articular facets, alignment of the lateral margins of the articular processes, the laminae, and the spinous processes.[66-68]

Analysis of Radiographic Views

Cervical Gravity Line

A vertical line extending from the distal apex of the odontoid process to the distal edge of the body of C7 is referred to as the cervical gravity line. The vertebral bodies should remain anterior to this line. In an ideal cervical curve, the centers of the bodies of the vertebra to the gravity line are 7–10 mm *(Figure 11)*.[69]

Atlanto Dental Space

The atlanto dental space is a measurement of the space between the posterior surface of the anterior arch of the atlas and the anterior border of the odontoid process. This space should not exceed 3 mm in adults and should not increase with flexion or extension. Steele suggests the canal distance be divided into thirds with one-third being the dens, one-third the spinal cord, and the remaining one-third space should be divided with one-half being dorsal to the spinal cord and one-half ventral to the cord.[70]

George's Line (diagnostic line or posterior vertebral line)

George's line is a line drawn along the posterior border of the vertebral bodies that delineates the anterior wall of the spinal canal. This line should be a smooth line connecting the superior and inferior borders of the vertebral bodies. Normal cervical lordosis produces an arc approximately 17 cm in length. The posterior canal line (PCL) is drawn at the spinolamina, which is the bony cortex line in each vertebra produced by the union of the right and left vertebral lamina and the spinous process. This line indicates the posterior aspect of the spinal column. The anterior vertebral line (AVL) is a line drawn between the superior and inferior anterior borders of the vertebra. Even with the loss of normal cervical lordosis, this should remain a smooth line. An irregularity of this line indicates an anterior or posterior lysthesis (slippage) of the vertebra. The spinal canal measured between the posterior vertebral line (PVL) and PCL should range from 16–30 mm at C1 (21.4 mm average) decreasing to 13–24 mm at C7 (17.5 mm average). Any widening or stenosis of less than 12 mm should be noted *(Figure 11)*.[48,49]

Spinal Canal Diameters for Adults

	Range	Average
C1	16–30 mm	21.4
C2	16–28 mm	19.2
C3	14–25 mm	19.1
C5	14–25 mm	18.5
C7	13–24 mm	17.5

Reference[48]

Stress Lines

Jackson suggested that the intersection of a line drawn parallel to the posterior surface of the body at C2 and a second line drawn parallel to the posterior surface of C7 should intersect at the point of most stress on the cervical spine. The normal location for maximum stress is C4–C6.[71]

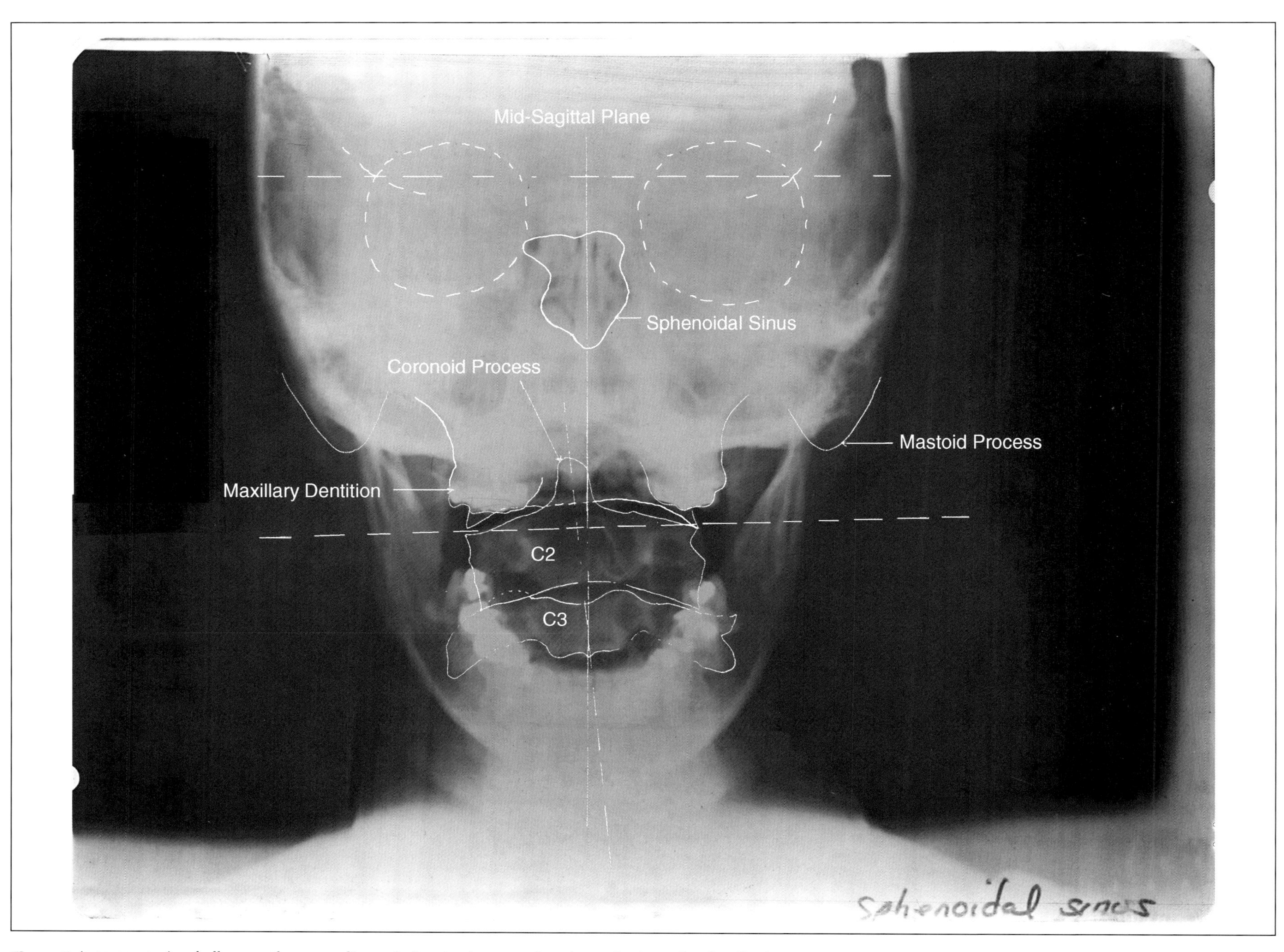

Figure 5. Anteroposterior skull—mouth open radiograph. Spacing between the atlas and axis can be visualized.

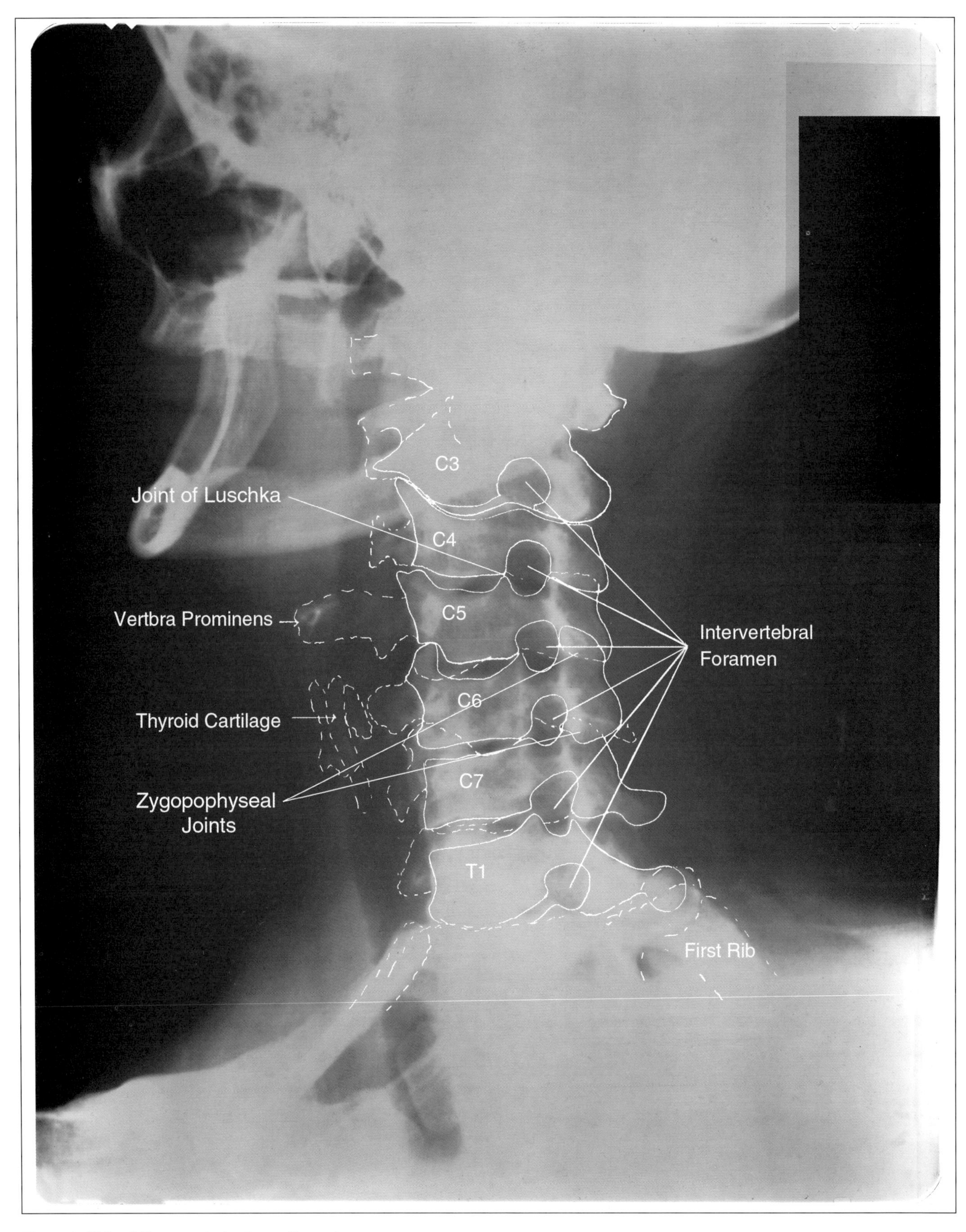

Figure 6. Right oblique cervical spine radiograph.

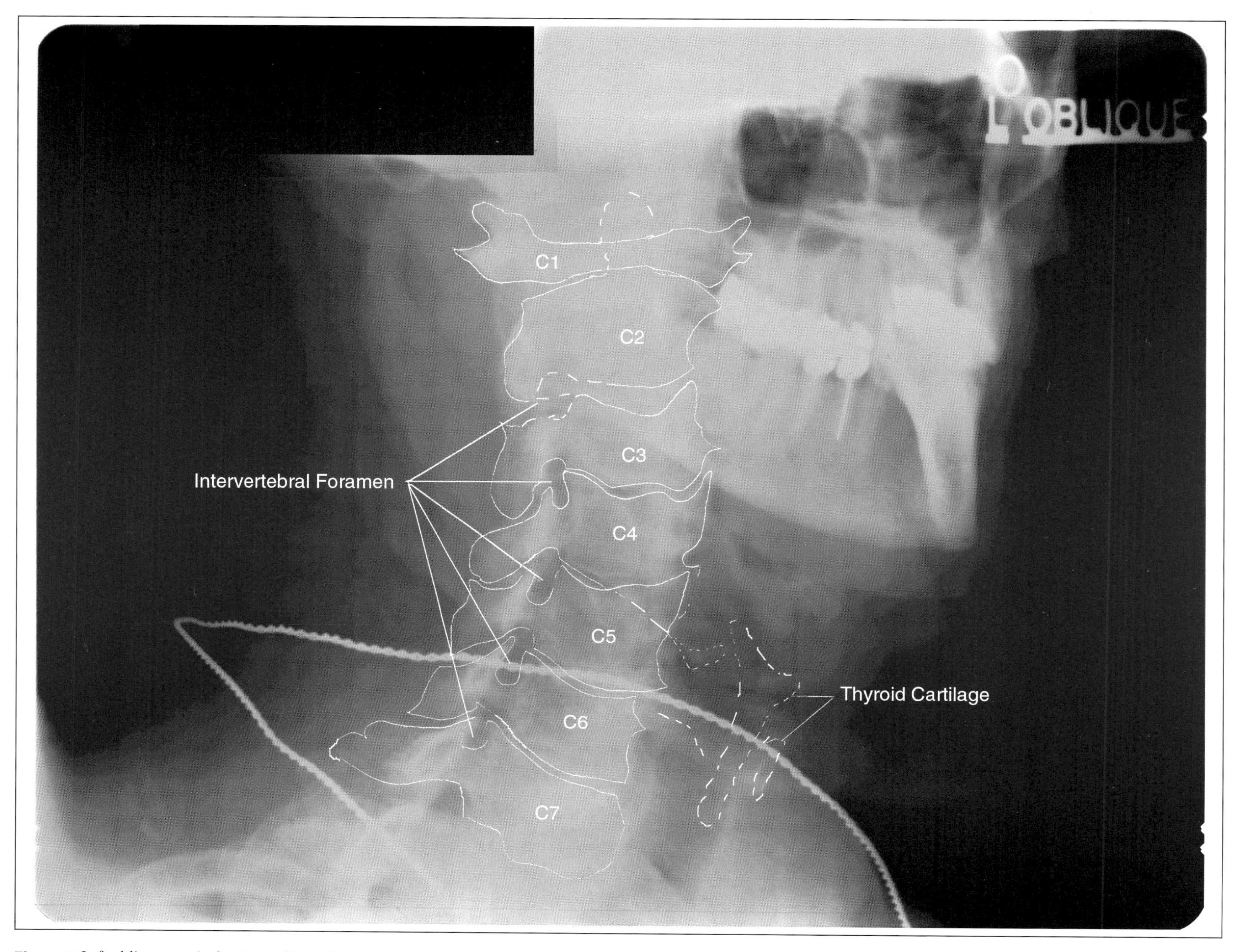

Figure 7. Left oblique cervical spine radiograph.

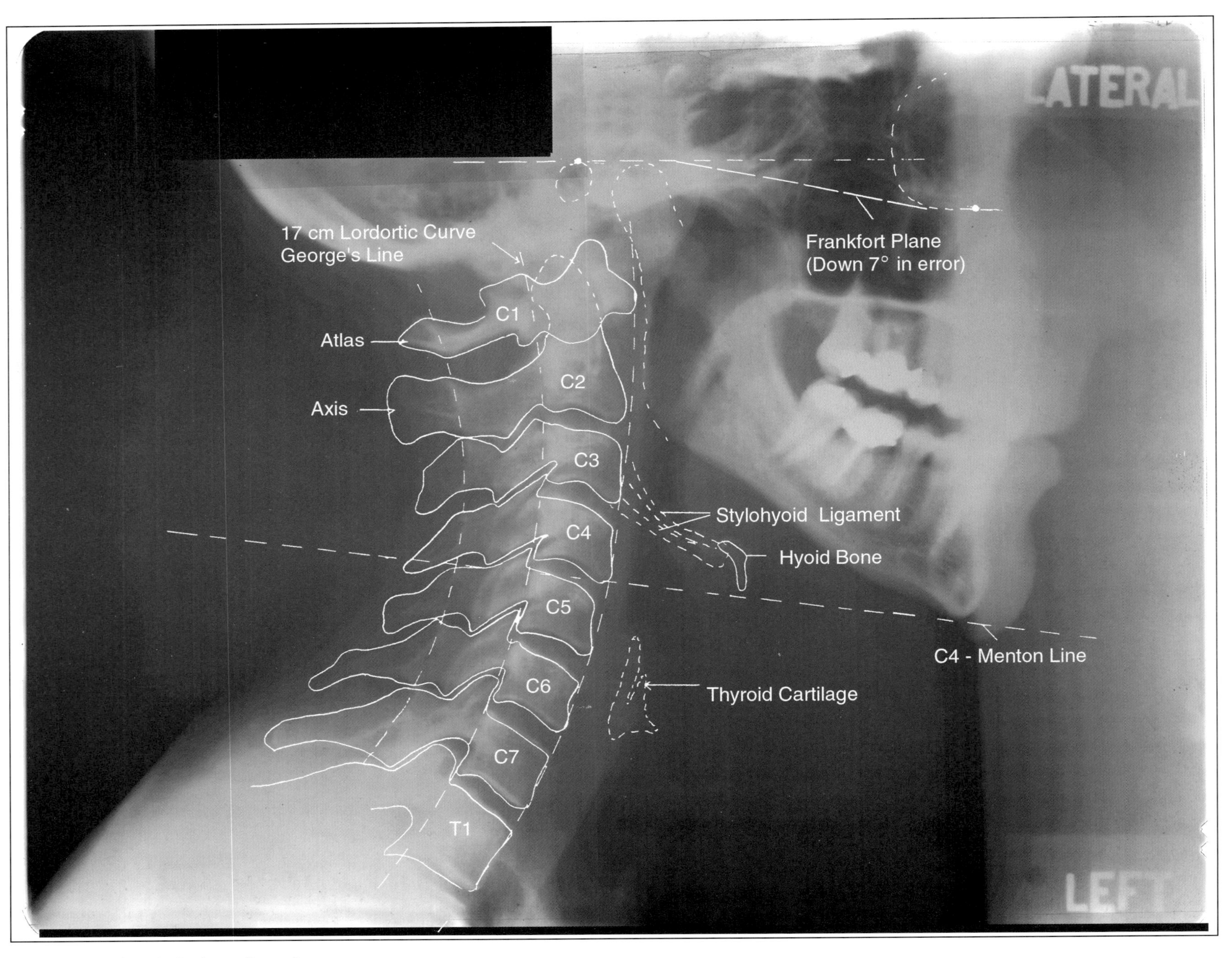

Figure 8. Lateral cervical spine radiograph.

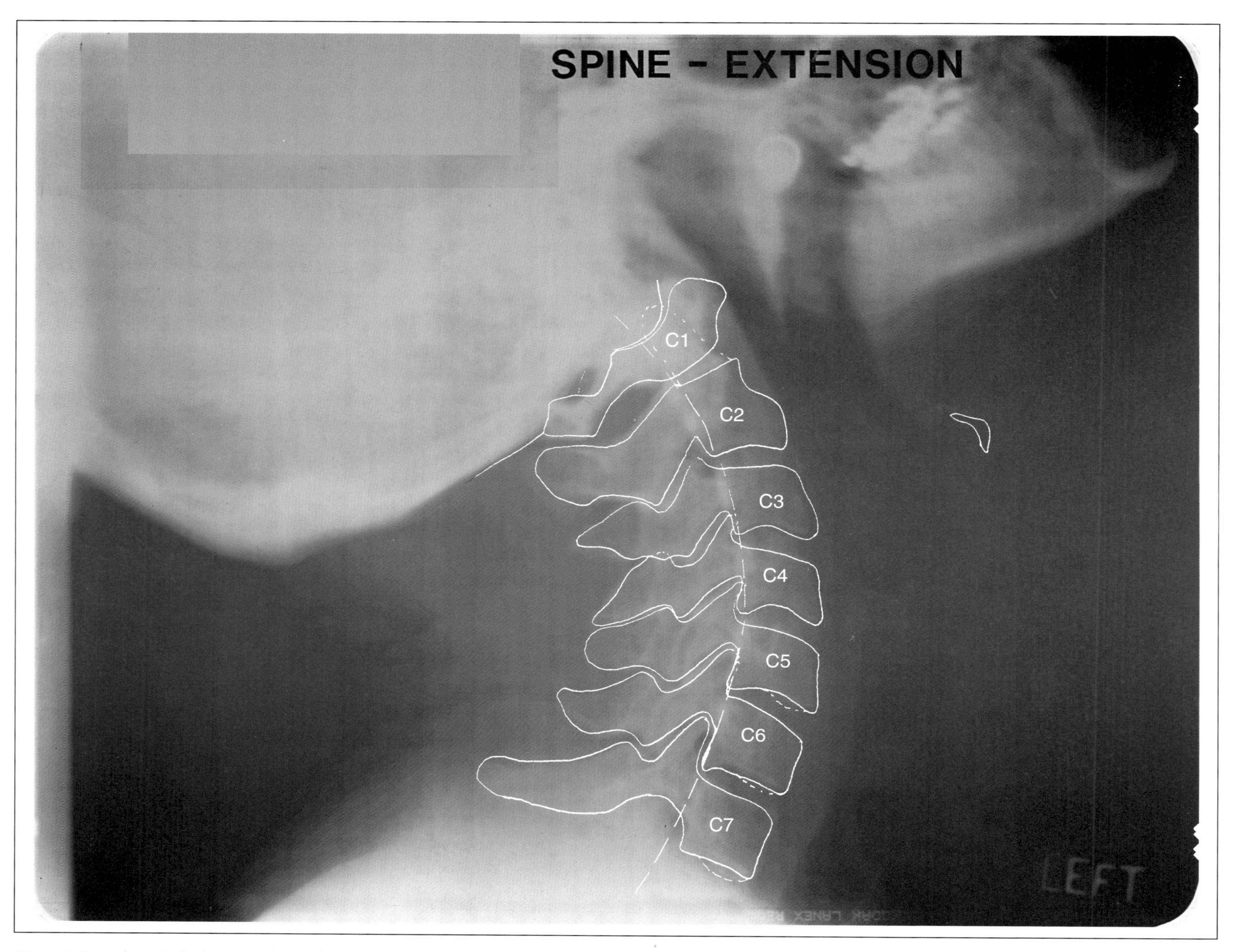

Figure 9. Lateral cervical spine extension radiograph.

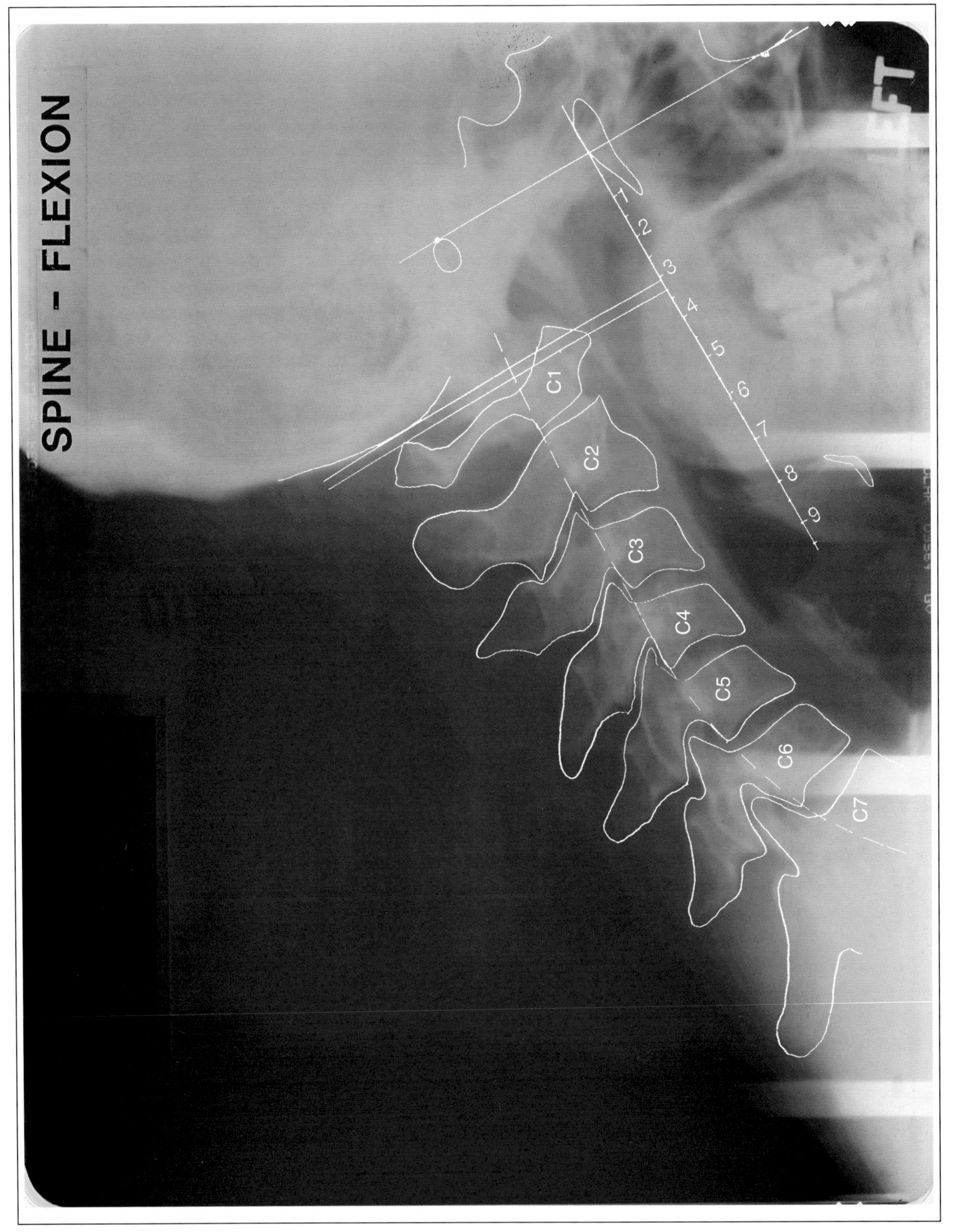

Figure 10. Lateral cervical spine flexion radiograph.

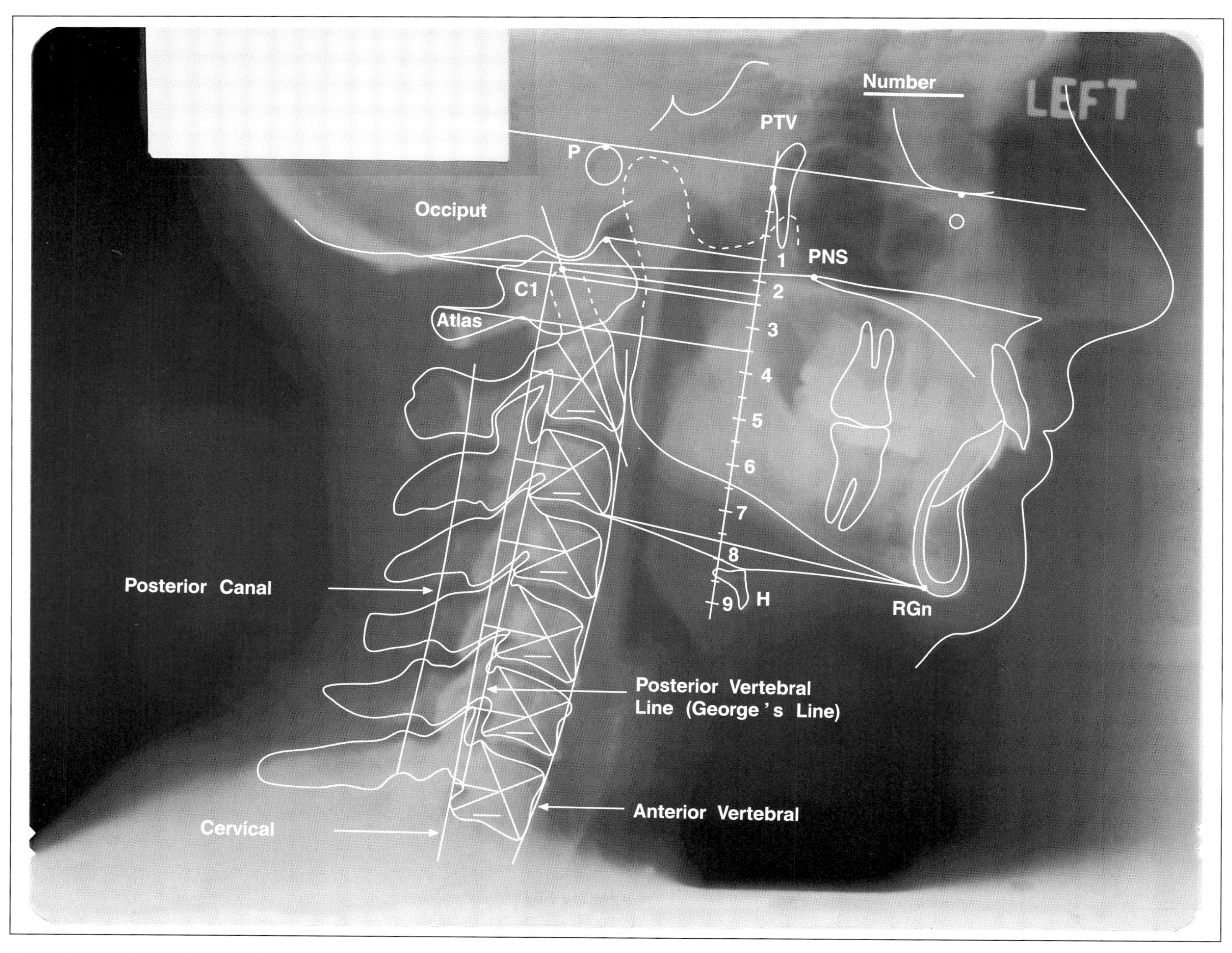

Figure 11. Lateral cervical spine radiograph.

Prevertebral Soft Tissue Measurement
Measurements from the body of the cervical vertebrae can be made to the retrolaryngeal and retrotracheal soft tissue at C4–C7. Retropharyngeal space should be between 1 and 7 mm with an average of 3.4 mm. Retrotracheal space ranges from 9–22 mm with an average of 14 mm.[48]

Airway
Tracing the anterior aspect of adenoid tissue at the rear of the nasopharynx and the distal border of the tongue gives a good indication of pharyngeal airway. This measurement should be approximately 11.6 mm with a range of 10–15 mm.[72]

Rocabado's Evaluation
The most well known craniometric analysis of the cervical spine has been previously published by Rocabado.[73] Biomechanical relationships are extremely important when treating upper quadrant disorders. Rocabado presented:

1) a detailed analysis for completing cephalometric studies of craniovertebral relationships
2) the relationship of the hyoid apparatus to the cervical spine
3) the determination of normal or abnormal architecture of the cervical spine.

Definitions and Cephalometric Points

- Retrognathion (RGN) is the most inferior posterior point of the mandibular symphysis.
- Hyoidale (H) is the most superior anterior point of the body of the hyoid bone.
- McGregor's plane (MGP) is a line that connects the posterior nasal spine to the basi-occiput.
- The odontoid plane (OP) is a line that extends from the anterior inferior angle of the odontoid to its apex.
- A normal measure of the posterior-inferior angle at the intersection of MGP and OP is 101 degrees +/- 5 degrees.
- The measurement for the distance between the basi-occiput to the posterior arch of the atlas is 4–9 mm (less than 4 mm indicates craniovertebral compression).
- Normal cervical lordosis and a normal craniovertebral relationship will show a normal hyoid bone below a C3-RGN plane *(Figure 12)*. With a straight cervical curvature and a normal craniovertebral relationship or with an extension of the occiput where MGP to OP angle is less than 96 degrees, the hyoid bone should lie on the line from C3-RGN *(Figure 13)*.
- When a reversed cervical curvature (kyphosis) is present and either a normal craniovertebral relationship or an extension of the occiput where MGP to OP angle is less than 96 degrees, the hyoid bone will be above the line of C3-RGN forming a negative triangle (C3-RGN-H) *(Figure 14 and 15)*.[68] A negative triangle indicates that the hyoid lies superior to C3-RGN.

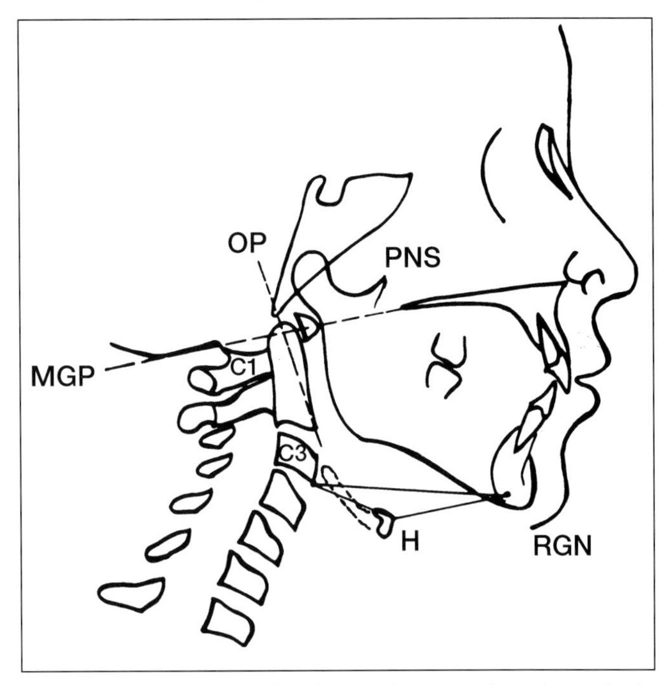

Figure 12. Normal cervical lordosis with a normal craniovertebral relationship.

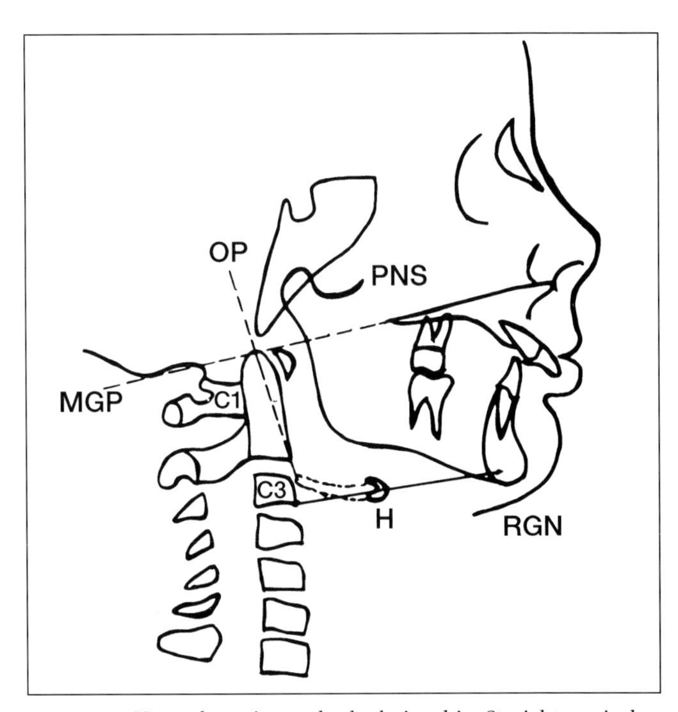

Figure 13. Normal craniovertebral relationship. Straight cervical spine.

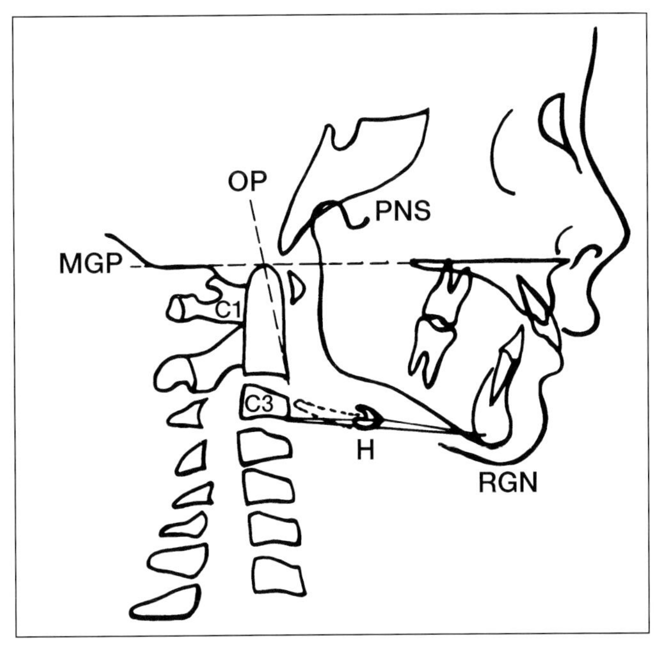

Figure 14. Normal craniovertebral relationship. Inverted cervical curvature.

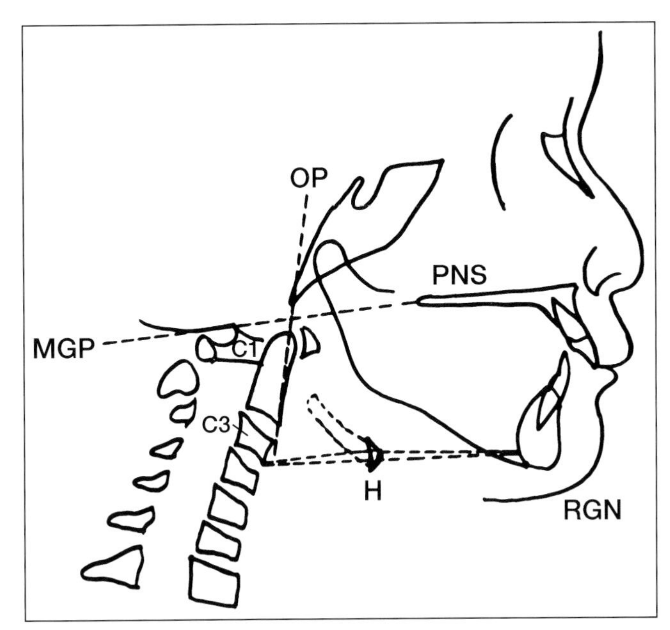

Figure 15. Extension of craniovertebral joints. Reversed cervical curvature.

By relating the cranium, cervical spine, mandible, and hyoid bone into a functional biomechanical unit, the clinician is able to identify a normal versus an abnormal architecture of the cervical spine, as well as relationships of craniomandibular and craniocervical structures. Manual orthopedic techniques directed to the upper quarter and mandibular orthopedic repositioning appliances may modify these relationships, making it imperative that the physical medicine specialist and/or physical therapist work concurrently with the dentist in treating these conditions. Evaluating these relationships at the initiation of treatment alerts the practitioner to potential cervical spine, craniomandibular, or craniovertebral disorders, and establishes a baseline for outcomes evaluation.

Conclusion

It has not been unusual in craniomandibular practice for a patient's signs and symptoms to be intensified following placement of an intraoral orthosis or to have symptoms continue despite good ROM and comfort of the masticatory musculature. Head, neck, and shoulder pathology may be either a contributing factor or the primary etiology. Due to this intimate relationship, a complete upper quarter evaluation is necessary with every orofacial pain or TMD patient. Actual treatment of upper quarter abnormalities may be referred to an appropriate health care provider. However, it is critical for the dentist to be involved in the diagnosis and treatment of such patients to properly evaluate this region for possible concomitant pathology and/or dysfunction. The techniques presented will allow the practitioner to perform a comprehensive screening exam of the cervical spine. In the differential diagnosis of orofacial pain and TMD, it is imperative that an upper quarter evaluation be performed, otherwise significant etiologic factors may be potentially overlooked, which will ultimately compromise treatment rendered.

References

1. Jankelson RR: *Neuromuscular Dental Diagnosis and Treatment.* St. Louis: Ishiyaku EuroAmerica, Inc., 1990.
2. Ash MM, Ramfjord SP: Anatomy, physiology, and pathophysiology of occlusion. In: Ash MM and Ramfjord SP, eds. *Occlusion, 4th Ed.* Philadelphia: W.B. Saunders; 1995;1-29.
3. Gelb M: Diagnostic tests. In: Kaplan AS and Assael LA, eds. *Temporomandibular Disorders Diagnosis and Treatment.* Philadelphia: W.B. Saunders; 1991; 371-385.
4. Cooper BC: Craniomandibular disorders. In: Cooper BC and Lucente FE, eds. *Management of Facial, Head and Neck Pain.* Philadelphia: W.B. Saunders; 1989;153-254.
5. Guyton AC: Membrane physiology, nerve, and muscle. In: Guyton AC, ed. *Textbook of Medical Physiology.* Philadelphia: W.B. Saunders Co.; 1986;87-148.
6. Sheikholeslam A, Moller E, Loos J: Pain, tenderness and strength of human elevator muscles. *Scand J Dent Res* 1980;88:60-66.

7. Garry JF: Early iatrogenic, orofacial muscle, skeletal, and TMJ dysfunction. In: Morgan D, ed. *Diseases of the Temporomandibular Apparatus—A Multidisciplinary Approach.* St. Louis: C.V. Mosby Co., 1982;35-69.

8. Marks MB: Allergy in relation to orofacial dental deformities in children. *J Allergy* 1965;36:293-302.

9. Bushy RS: *Alterations in Certain Anatomical Relations Accompanying the Change From Oral to Nasal Breathing.* M.S. Thesis, University of Illinois, Chicago: 1965.

10. Harvold EP, et al.: Primate experiments on oral respiration. *Am J Orthod* 1981;79:359-372.

11. Quinn GW: Airway interference and its affect upon growth and development of the face, jaw, dentition, and associated parts. *N C Dent J* 1978; 60:28-31.

12. Rubin RM: Mode of respiration and facial growth. *Am J Orthod* 1980;78:504-510.

13. McNamara JA: Influence of respiratory pattern on craniofacial growth. *Angle Orthod* 1981;51:269-299.

14. Hannuksela A: The effect of moderate to severe atrophy on the facial skeleton. *Eur J Orthod* 1981;3:187-193.

15. Marks MB: *Stigmata of Respiratory Tract Allergies.* A Scope Publication. Kalamazoo, NJ: Upjohn Co., 1977.

16. Meredith GM: The airway and dentofacial development. *Ear Nose Throat J* 1987;66:190-195.

17. Rubin RM: Effects of nasal airway obstruction on facial growth. *Ear Nose Throat J* 1987;66:212-219.

18. Kaplan AS, Assael LA: *Temporomandibular Disorders—Diagnosis and Treatment.* Philadelphia: W.B. Saunders, 1991.

19. Ozbec MM: Natural head posture, upper airway morphology and obstructive sleep apnea severity in adults. *Eur J Orthod* 1998;20(2):133-143.

20. Dunn J: Physical therapy. In: Kaplan AS and Assael LA, eds. *Temporomandibular Disorders—Diagnosis and Treatment.* Philadelphia: W.B. Saunders; 1991;455-460

21. Kraus S: Cervical spine influences on the craniomandibular region. In: Kraus S, ed. *Clinics in Physical Therapy. TMJ Disorders—Management of the Craniomandibular Complex Vol. 18.* New York: Churchill Livingstone; 1988;367-404.

22. Higbie EJ, Seidel-Cobb D, Taylor LF, Cummings GS: Effect of head position on vertical mandibular opening. *J Orthop Sports Phys Ther* 1999;29:127-130.

23. Shankland WE: Craniofacial pain syndromes that mimic temporomandibular joint disorders. *Ann Acad Med Singapore* 1995;24:83-84.

24. Bonica JJ: Regional pains. In Bonica JJ, ed. *The Management of Pain, 2nd Ed.* Philadelphia: Lea and Febriger; 1990; 651:858.

25. Bricker SL, Langlais RP, Miller CS: *Oral Diagnosis, Oral Medicine and Treatment Planning (ed 2nd).* Philadelphia, Lea and Febriger, 1994.

26. Adams GL, Boies LR, Hilger PA: *Fundamentals of Otolaryngology.* Philadelphia: W.B. Saunders, 1989.

27. Cummings CW, Krause CW: *Otolaryngology-Head and Neck Surgery Vol. 1.* St. Louis: Mosby, 1993.

28. Cummings CW, Schuller DE: *Otolaryngology-Head and Neck Surgery Vol. 2.* St. Louis: Mosby, 1993.

29. Anthony M: The role of the occipital nerve in unilateral headache. In: Rose CF, ed. *Advancement in headache research proceeding of the 6th International Migraine Society.* London: John Libbey; 198; 257:262.

30. Travell JG, Simons DG: *Myofascial Pain and Dysfunction—The Trigger Point Manual.* Baltimore: Williams and Wilkins; 1984;1-164.

31. Rachlin ES: *Myofascial Pain and Fibromyalgia—Trigger Point Manual.* St. Louis: Mosby, 1994.

32. Ernest EA: Temporal tendinitis: A painful disorder that mimics migraine headache. *J Neurol Orthopaed Med Surg* 1987;8:159-167.

33. Wilk SJ: Surgical management of refractory craniomandibular pain using radiofrequency thermolysis: A report of thirty patients. *J Craniomand Pract* 1994;12:93-99.

34. Shankland WE: Ernest Syndrome as a consequence of stylomandibular ligament injury: Report of 68 cases. *J Pros Dent* 1987;57:501-506.

35. Shankland WE: Ernest Syndrome (insertion tendinosis of the stylomandibular ligament) as a cause of craniomandibular pain: Diagnosis, treatment and report of two cases. *J Neurol Orthop Med Surg* 1987;8:253-257.

36. Ernest EA: The Ernest Syndrome: An insertion tendinosis of the stylomandibular ligament. *J Neuro Orthop Med Surg* 1986;7:427-438.

37. De Araujo Lucas G, Laundana A, Chopard RP, Raffaelli E: Anatomy of the lesser occipital nerve in relation to cervicogenic headache. *Clin Anat* 1994;7:90-96.

38. Gelb H: *New Concepts in Craniomandibular and Chronic Pain Management.* London: Mosby-Wolf, 1994.

39. Travell J, Simons D: *Myofascial Pain and Dysfunction—The Trigger Point Manual Vol. 2.* Baltimore: Williams and Wilkins, 1992.

40. Tilley L: Atlanta Craniomandibular Society's Framework Philosophy. *J Craniomandib Pract* 1987;(5)2:163-164.

41. Fonder A: *The Dental Physician.* Rock Falls: Medical-Dental Inc., 1985.

42. Miralles R, et al.: Increase of the vertical occlusal dimension by means of a removable orthodontic appliance and its effect on craniocervical relationships and position of the cervical spine in children. *J Craniomandib Pract* 1997;15(3):221-228.

43. Vig PS, Showfety KJ, Phillips C: Experimental manipulation of head posture. *Am J Orthod* 1980;77:258-268.

44. Guzay C: Quadrant Thearom. *Basal Facts* 1978;(2)1:187-190.

45. Rocabado M: *Dentistry I.* Rocabado Institute for Craniomandibular and Vertebral Therapeutics, Atlanta: Institute of Graduate Health Sciences, 1984.

46. Kraus S: *TMJ Disorders—Management of the Craniomandibular Complex.* New York: Churchill-Livingston, 1988.

47. Saunders H: *Evaluation, Treatment and Prevention of Musculoskeletal Disorders.* Edina, MN: Educational Opportunities, 1985.

48. Bland JH: *Disorders of the Cervical Spine—Diagnosis and Medical Management.* Philadelphia: W. B. Saunders, 1988.

49. Magee DJ: *Orthopedic Physical Assessment, 3rd Ed.* Philadelphia: W. B. Saunders, 1997.

50. Moore KL: *Clinically Oriented Anatomy, 3rd Ed.* Baltimore: Williams and Wilkins, 1992.

51. Rohen JW, Yokochi C: *Color Atlas of Anatomy.* New York: Igaku-Shoin, 1988.

52. Williams PL, Warwick R: *Gray's Anatomy, 36th Ed.* Philadelphia: W. B. Saunders, 1986.

53. Chaitow L: *Modern Neuromuscular Techniques.* New York: Churchill-Livingston, 1996.

54. Walker-Delaney J: *Neuromuscular Techniques.* Tampa: Neuoromuscular Research Group, 1988.

55. Mannheimer JS, Dunn J: Cervical spine. In: Kaplan AS and Assael LA, eds. *Temporomandibular Disorders Diagnosis and Treatment.* Philadelphia: W.B. Saunders; 1991;50-94.

56. Hardebo, JE: On pain mechanisms in cluster headache. *Headache* 1991;31:91-106.

57. Anthony M: The role of the occipital nerve in unilateral headache. In Rose CF, ed; *Advancement in headache research proceeding of the 6th International Migraine Society.* London: John Libbey; 1986;257:262.

58. Kerr FLW: Structural relations of trigeminal spinal tract to upper cervical roots and solitary nucleus in cats. *Exp Neurol* 1961;4:134-138.

59. Kerr FLW: Mechanism, diagnosis and management of some cranial and facial syndromes. *Surg Clin North Am* 1963;43:951-961.

60. Kerr FLW: The ultrastructure of the spinal tract of the trigeminal nerve and the substantia gelatinosa. *Exp Neurol.*

61. Pfaller K, Adrvidsson J: Cervical distribution of trigeminal and upper cervical primary afferents in the rat studied by antigrade transport of horseradish peroxidase conjugated to wheat germ agglutinin. *J Comp Neurol* 1988;268:91-108.

62. Oleson J: Clinical and pathophysiological observations in migraine and tension-type headache explained by integration of vascular, supraspinal and myofascial imputs. *Neurol Clin* 1990; 46:135-132.

63. Kendall FP, McCreary EK: *Muscle Testing and Function.* Baltimore: Williams and Wilkins, 1983.

64. Vernon, H: *Upper Cervical Syndrome.* Baltimore: Williams and Wilkins, 1988.

65. Sweat R, Robinson K: Scanning Palpation of the Cervical Spine. *Inter-Examiner Reliability Study.* Atlanta: Joint Motion Conference, 1987.

66. Greenan D: *A Practical Atlas of TMJ and Cephalometric Radiology.* Atlanta: Imaging Systems, Inc, 1990.

67. Grossman RI, Yousem DM: *Neuroradiology.* St. Louis: Mosby, 1994.

68. Backus A: Radiographic anatomy and positioning of the thoracic and cervical spine. In: Bontrager KL, ed. *Textbook of Radiographic Positioning and Related Anatomy 3rd Ed.* St. Louis: Mosby Yearbook; 1993;271-312.

69. Rocabado M: Radiographic study of the craniocervical relation in patients under orthodontic treatment and the incidence with related symptoms. *J Craniomandib Pract* 1987;(5)1:36-42.

70. Dvorak J, Dvorak V: *Manuel Medicine: Diagnostics.* New York: Thieme-Stratton Inc., 1984.

71. Jackson R: *The Cervical Syndrome.* Springfield: Charles C. Thomas, 1978.

72. Riley R, Guilleminault C, Powell, Simons FB: Palatopharyngoplasty failure, cephalometric roentgenograms, and obstructive sleep apnea. *Ortholaryngol Head Neck Surg* 1985;93(2):240-244.

73. Rocabado M: Biomechanical relationship of the cranial, cervical, and hyoid regions. *J Craniomandib Pract* 1983(1)3:61-66.

Illustrations 1 and 2 are reprinted, with permission, from *Muscle Testing and Function* by F. P. Kendall and E. K. McCreary (Williams and Wilkins, 1983). Figure 1 is reprinted, with permission, from *Disorders of the Cervical Spine* by J. H. Bland, MD (Saunders, 1987). Figure 2 is reprinted, with permission, from "The Dental Distress Syndrome Quantified" by A. C. Fonder (*Basal Facts* 1987;9[4]:141-167). Figure 3 is reprinted, with permission, from *Diseases of the Temporomandibular Apparatus* by D. H. Morgan, DDS (Mosby, 1982). Figures 12, 13, 14, and 15 are reprinted, with permission, from "Biomechanical Relationship of the Cranial, Cervical, and Hyoid Regions" by M. Rocabado, RPT (*Cranio,* Vol. 1, No. 3, p. 64).

DIFFERENTIAL DIAGNOSIS

A New Perspective on Temporomandibular Disorders and the Differential Diagnosis of Head, Neck, & Face Pain, and Dysfunction

David M. Hickman, Michael W. Mazzocco, Robert W. Graves, and Bryan D. Weaver

Overview

For over 60 years, medicine and dentistry have equated head, neck, and facial pain, and dysfunction with a nebulous syndrome called temporomandibular disorders (TMD). Attention was first given to Costen, an otolaryngologist, in 1934.[1] Costen described this syndrome of the stomatognathic system which bears his name as a condition resulting from the loss of vertical dimension of occlusion. This disorder was later diagnosed as temporomandibular syndrome. This syndrome was first defined in the medical dictionary as a dysfunction of the temporomandibular joint caused by deforming arthritis as a result of mandibular overclosure or displacement.[2] During the 1950s, Harry Sicher became the dominant figure who established functional anatomy as a basis for treatment.[3] The importance of muscle physiology came into focus through the use of electromyographs by Moyers,[4] Prozansky,[5] MacDougall,[6] and Perry.[7] Radiography began to evolve through transcranial imaging,[8] arthrography,[9] the development of tomography,[10] and cinefluorography.[11] Kraus,[12] Travell,[13] Sicher,[14] and Schwartz[15] focused on the treatment of masticatory musculature.

Schwartz became the principal figure of the decade of the 1960s. He introduced the term temporomandibular pain-dysfunction syndrome.[15] Thilander,[16] Kawamura,[17] and Storey[18] provided advances in neurophysiology relative to the temporomandibular apparatus. In this decade, muscle and emotional components were thought to be the significant etiologic factors in the development of this disorder. Biomechanics of the temporomandibular joint and internal derangements were, for the most part, ignored.

It was during the 1970s that myofascial pain dysfunction syndrome (MPD) was introduced and muscle therapy was emphasized by Laskin.[19] Etiology and treatment continued to be directed toward the musculature throughout much of this decade. William Farrar rapidly became the dominate influence of the 1970s. He redeveloped and reemphasized the concept of occlusal factors being significant etiologic factors for development of internal derangements of the temporomandibular joint. This philosophy continued into the 1980s.[20]

Within this most recent decade, controversy over the definition of temporomandibular disorders continues; terminology and etiologies remain vague and nebulous. A recent National Institute of Health/National Institute of Dental Research (NIH/NIDR) position statement on TMD concludes: "Given the lack of epidemiological information and the collection of as yet undefined etiologies to be described as TMD, a conventional disease classification system would be difficult to describe, possibly misleading and unlikely to receive broad acceptance."[21] These conclusions relegate TMD to a specific category of conditions having no defined common etiology or biologic explanation. The apparent difficulty lies in the management of those signs and symptoms, which are present and overlap other medical conditions.

The term "TMD" has been used to characterize the generalized, nonspecific complex of headache, neckache, earache, face pain, tenderness of muscles to palpation, sensation of bite change, difficulty chewing and/or swallowing, gross temporomandibular joint sounds, and limited range of motion. The above mentioned report goes on to relate: "Nonetheless, there is consensus that initiation of treatment should be based on patient history and physical examination and may include laboratory analysis, imaging and consideration of psychosocial factors. Patient history should include medical, dental and social data, as well as quantification of pain and dysfunction. The physical examination should encompass orofacial tissues, musculature and neurologic function. Particular attention should be paid to determination of functional range of motion, occlusal status, existence of parafunctional conditions and the presence of joint or muscle tenderness and cutaneous hyperalgesia. Psychosocial assessments should determine the extent to which pain and dysfunction interfere with or diminish the patient's quality of life and, when used, must be administered by skilled professionals using validated instruments. The consideration of psychosocial factors has the potential for inappropriate use."[21] Thus, despite numerous efforts to define and differentiate TMD, most clinicians are perplexed and frustrated when attempting to determine a clinical diagnosis and treatment plan when confronted with signs and symptoms of head, neck, and face pain, and dysfunction.

Model Synthesis

Selye's entire General Adaptation Syndrome (GAS) paradigm reinforces this foundation concept of limited body responses to multiple etiologies. He defined stress as the state manifested by a specific syndrome, which consists of all the nonspecifically induced changes within a biologic system. Briefly, Selye summarizes stress as the nonspecific response of the body to any demand. Early in his medical training, Selye observed that a certain nonspecific symptom complex was common to infectious diseases. Each patient felt and looked ill, experienced diffuse aches and pains in the joints, intestinal problems, loss of appetite, fever, and enlarged tonsils. Thus, the presence of generalized infectious disease could be determined by a few specific signs, which could be followed by a further differential diagnosis that led to a specific remedy. It is the presence of these nonspecific symptoms and the body's limited response to multiple etiologies that has thwarted efforts to accurately distinguish TMDs from other causes of head, neck, and facial pain, and dysfunction.[22] The dental profession is currently capable of moving beyond the utilization of nonspecific signs and symptoms to develop a diagnosis of TMD, as determined by the National Institute of Health/National Institute of Dental Research, and formulate a specific diagnosis for the specific disease process as illustrated in *Figure 1.*

Earlier efforts by the NIDR to define TMD based their research on several operative definitions. First, disease was defined as an "objective biologic event involving disruption of specific body structures or organ systems caused by pathologic, anatomic or physiologic changes." Second, illness was defined as "a subjective experience or self attribution that a disease is present, yielding physical discomfort, emotional distress, behavioral limitation and psychosocial disruptions." Claims were made that progressive pathologic changes cannot be reliably diagnosed in TMDs and concluded that this condition is more usefully considered to be an illness. This was the creation of Dworkin's psychosocial model of TMD.[23] Previous paradigms to differentiate TMD have hinged upon only the nonspecific symptom complex. By ignoring the progressive pathologic changes which to date cannot be reliably diagnosed in TMDs, treatment is inherently limited to the nonspecific components. The persistent question remains: Is it possible to further differentiate clinical signs and symptoms?

Literature analyses and syntheses are becoming increasingly important as a means of periodically bringing coherence to a research area, contributing new knowledge revealed by integrating single studies, and quickly informing scientists of the state of the field. As a result, there is a need for approaches that can provide replicable, reliable, and trustworthy results. Over the last decade, many researchers have begun using the statistical meta-analysis approach to integrate studies. However, the single studies conducted in many areas are not of the type amenable to statistical meta-analysis but are more appropriate for descriptive analysis and synthesis. Reports of diagnostic accuracy often differ. The authors utilized an existing method to summarize disparate reports that use a logistic transformation and linear regression to produce a summary receiver operating characteristic curve. The curve is useful for summarizing a body of diagnostic literature accuracy, comparing technologies, detecting outliers, and finding the optimum operating point of the test. Summary Receiver Operating Characteristic Curves took into account possible test threshold differences between studies.

Several methods are also available for analyzing multicategory and continuous test data. The usefulness of applying these methods is constrained by publication bias and the generally poor quality of primary studies of diagnostic test accuracy. By extending the logic of meta-analysis to diagnostic testing, the method provides a new tool for technology assessment.[24-27]

Applications of meta-analysis have begun to appear with some regularity in the dental research literature. Careful consideration of the principles involved in the meta-analytic process provide a basis of understanding upon which controversies may be resolved. This process reaffirms the need for close collaboration between statisticians and other scientists in the performance of a meta-analysis, and the value of such close collaboration in the evaluation and interpretation of a meta-analysis performed by others.[28-30]

The authors conducted a descriptive meta-analysis of the related literature to determine a disease based model of head, neck, and facial pain, and dysfunction.[31-48] The results are represented in *Figure 1.*

Foundation Concepts

Differential diagnosis of head, neck, and face pain, and dysfunction can be a tremendous challenge for the clinician. This challenge primarily arises duc to the anatomical complexity of the region. Neurophysiology reveals the vast area of the somatosensory cortex dedicated to the head, neck, and face. The overlapping neural pathways of cranial nerves V, VII, IX, and X and cervical nerves C1–C3 are well referenced in the literature, especially the association between the trigeminal nerve and upper cervical nerves. The numerous nociceptive and proprioceptive receptors of joint capsules, coordination of the musculature, and the biomechanics of intracapsular temporomandibular structures are only now being truly understood. The central nervous system is bombarded with somatosensory and autonomic input from fibers supplying these areas. This particularly becomes apparent in individuals suffering head and neck pain, and orthopedic discrepancies of the mandible as it relates to the cranial base, as well as other pathologic processes affecting these areas. Within this intricate neurophysiology, one is able to see the apparent interrelationship of pain mechanisms and autonomic involvement of several different but interrelated areas.[49-58]

In health, individual homeostatic mechanisms maintain a stable internal environment necessary for survival. Homeostasis is dynamic, not static, and the physiologic processes are variable, maintaining the internal environment within a narrow range. Adaptation is the ability of an organism to adapt to stressors which are defined as any stimuli affecting an organism. Stressors may have desirable or undesirable effects depending on the organism's response to the particular stressor. As stressors (microtraumas, macrotrauma, etc.) are applied, disease may result if the stressor is sufficient to inhibit normal physiologic functioning, surpassing the organism's ability to adapt. The thrust of the paradigm presented in *Figure 1* revolves around the organism's inability to adapt to stressors, resulting in disease.[59] Through proper medical and dental history, examination, imaging, laboratory studies, differential diagnostic injections, electrophysiologic studies, etc., it is possible to develop a differential diagnosis. If health professionals are to properly differentiate the conditions causing head, neck, and face pain, and dysfunction, a differential diagnosis from at least 135 disorders must be considered. Approximately 20 of these conditions might be considered to be within the realm of musculoskeletal disorders traditionally known as "temporomandibular disorders."[60] Weldon Bell has taught that a diagnosis should do the following: properly differentiate and classify the disorder, establish the etiology of pain and dysfunction, if possible, and provide a basis for prognosis when effective treatment is rendered. He, of course, advocated that the treatment

Figure 1
Differential Diagnosis of Head, Neck, and Facial Pain, and Dysfunction

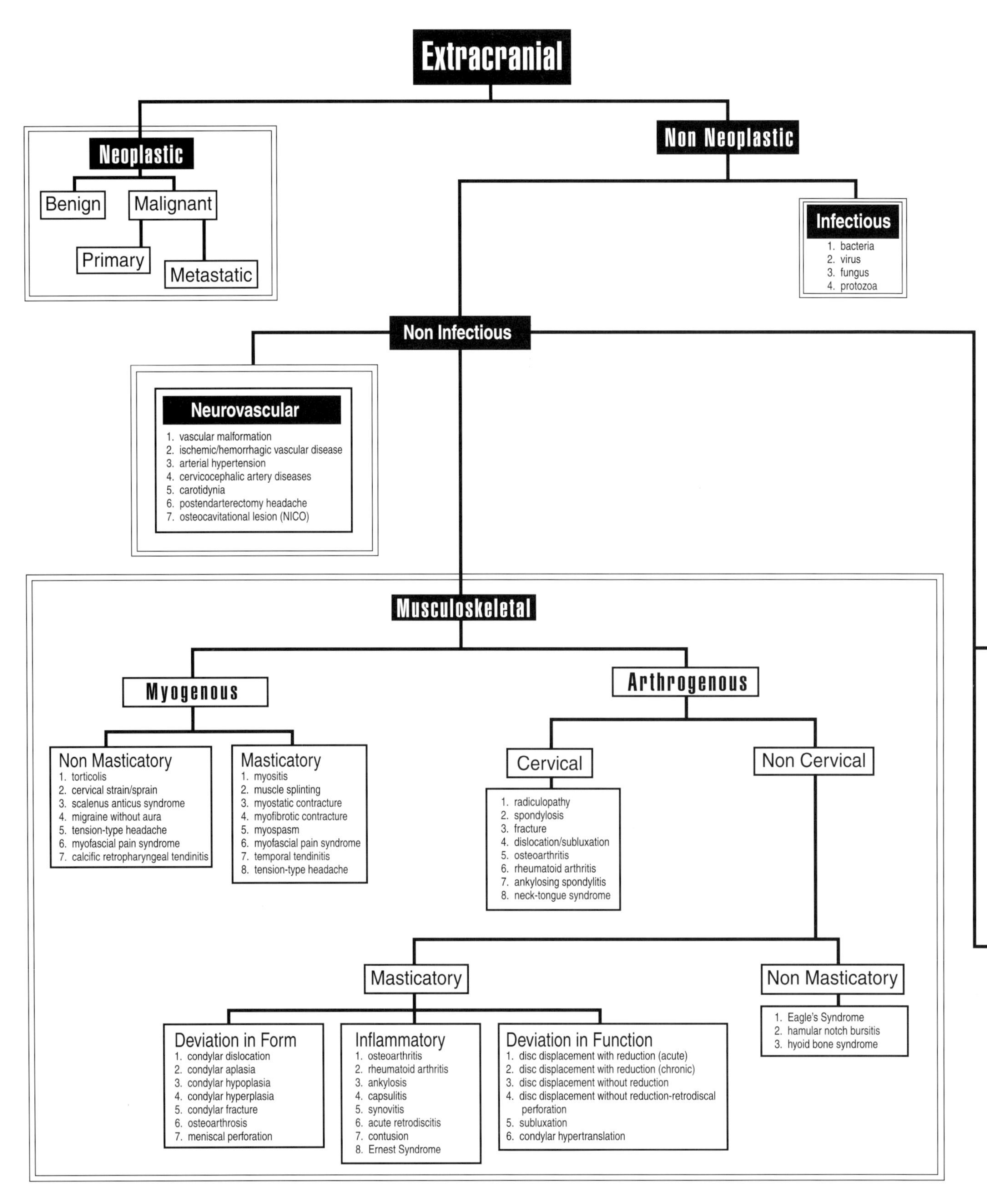

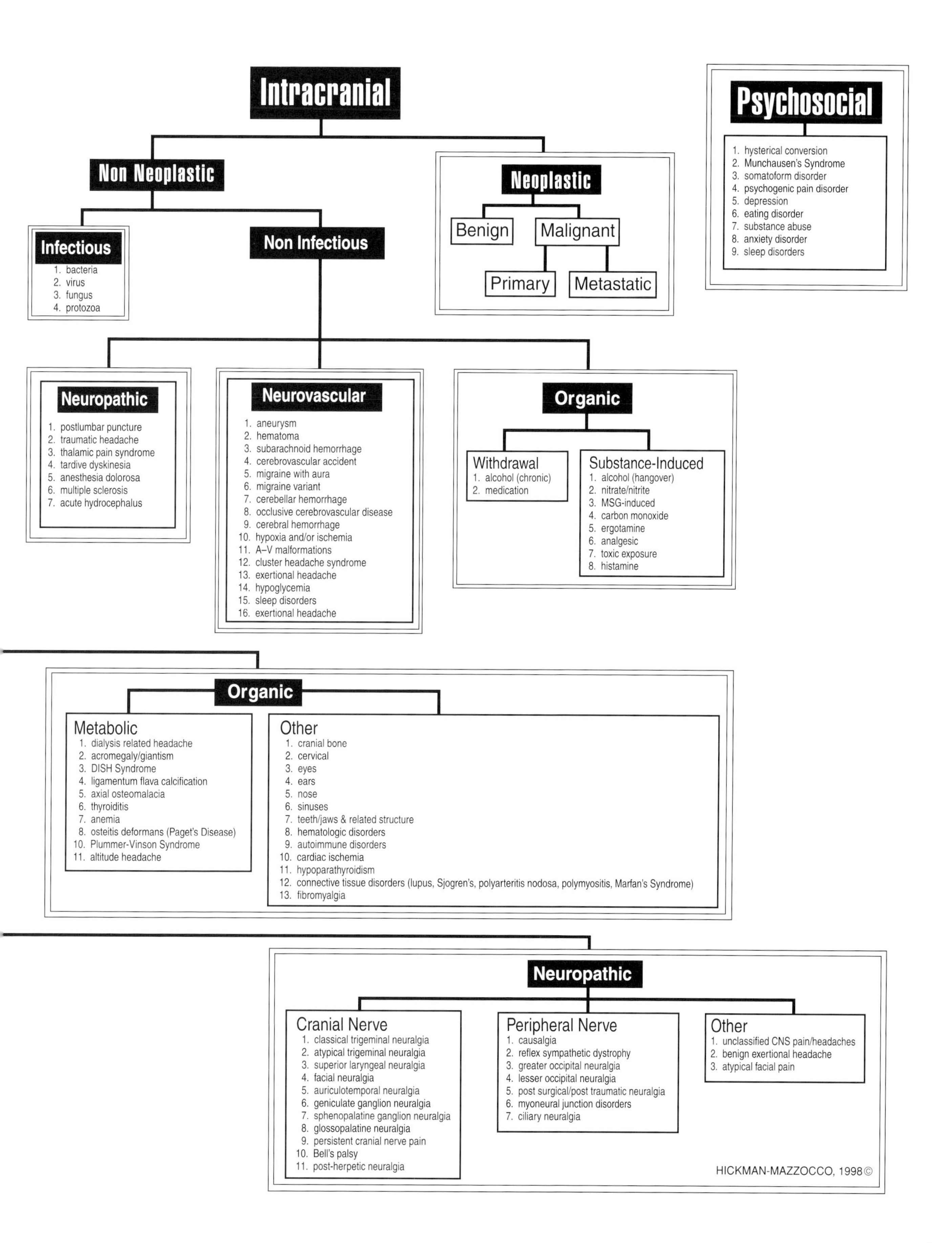
Intracranial
Non Neoplastic
Infectious
1. bacteria
2. virus
3. fungus
4. protozoa
Non Infectious
Neoplastic
Benign
Malignant
Primary
Metastatic
Psychosocial
1. hysterical conversion
2. Munchausen's Syndrome
3. somatoform disorder
4. psychogenic pain disorder
5. depression
6. eating disorder
7. substance abuse
8. anxiety disorder
9. sleep disorders
Neuropathic
1. postlumbar puncture
2. traumatic headache
3. thalamic pain syndrome
4. tardive dyskinesia
5. anesthesia dolorosa
6. multiple sclerosis
7. acute hydrocephalus
Neurovascular
1. aneurysm
2. hematoma
3. subarachnoid hemorrhage
4. cerebrovascular accident
5. migraine with aura
6. migraine variant
7. cerebellar hemorrhage
8. occlusive cerebrovascular disease
9. cerebral hemorrhage
10. hypoxia and/or ischemia
11. A–V malformations
12. cluster headache syndrome
13. exertional headache
14. hypoglycemia
15. sleep disorders
16. exertional headache
Organic
Withdrawal
1. alcohol (chronic)
2. medication
Substance-Induced
1. alcohol (hangover)
2. nitrate/nitrite
3. MSG-induced
4. carbon monoxide
5. ergotamine
6. analgesic
7. toxic exposure
8. histamine
Organic
Metabolic
1. dialysis related headache
2. acromegaly/giantism
3. DISH Syndrome
4. ligamentum flava calcification
5. axial osteomalacia
6. thyroiditis
7. anemia
8. osteitis deformans (Paget's Disease)
10. Plummer-Vinson Syndrome
11. altitude headache
Other
1. cranial bone
2. cervical
3. eyes
4. ears
5. nose
6. sinuses
7. teeth/jaws & related structure
8. hematologic disorders
9. autoimmune disorders
10. cardiac ischemia
11. hypoparathyroidism
12. connective tissue disorders (lupus, Sjogren's, polyarteritis nodosa, polymyositis, Marfan's Syndrome)
13. fibromyalgia
Neuropathic
Cranial Nerve
1. classical trigeminal neuralgia
2. atypical trigeminal neuralgia
3. superior laryngeal neuralgia
4. facial neuralgia
5. auriculotemporal neuralgia
6. geniculate ganglion neuralgia
7. sphenopalatine ganglion neuralgia
8. glossopalatine neuralgia
9. persistent cranial nerve pain
10. Bell's palsy
11. post-herpetic neuralgia
Peripheral Nerve
1. causalgia
2. reflex sympathetic dystrophy
3. greater occipital neuralgia
4. lesser occipital neuralgia
5. post surgical/post traumatic neuralgia
6. myoneural junction disorders
7. ciliary neuralgia
Other
1. unclassified CNS pain/headaches
2. benign exertional headache
3. atypical facial pain
HICKMAN-MAZZOCCO, 1998©

should specifically and appropriately relate to the diagnosis.[61] In the differential diagnostic paradigm which is illustrated in *Figure 1*, TMDs cannot be included because they do not meet the specific criteria of diseases as stated previously.

When formulating a differential diagnosis of head, neck, and face pain, and dysfunction, one would logically begin by determining whether the disorder is intracranial or extracranial *(Figure 1)*. This would be investigated and determined through standard medical-neurologic evaluation, imaging, blood chemistry, etc. Following the differentiation between intracranial or extracranial pathology, one would begin to formulate a differential diagnosis by beginning at a molecular level, where all pathologic processes begin. Tissue injury is initiated at this level or results from structural alteration within the cell. The normal cell constantly modifies its structure and function in response to changing demands and stresses. The body will attempt to maintain normal homeostasis; however, if the cell encounters excessive physiologic stressors or certain stimuli, it may undergo adaptation. The cell will attempt to achieve a steady but altered state while maintaining the usual functions, regardless of the continued stress. Atrophy, hypertrophy, and hyperplasia are the cell's principal means of adaptation. If the adaptive capacity of the cell is exceeded, cell injury or even death may occur.[62]

Realizing that all forms of tissue injury begin with molecular or structural alteration within the cell, it is necessary to continue our examination of pathology by examining disease at the cellular or subcellular levels. Neoplasia is literally defined as "new growth." It progresses as an uncontrolled growth of cells with no relation to physiologic needs. Hypertrophy, hyperplasia, metaplasia, and dysplasia are disturbances of cell growth and differentiation. Once the offending stimulus is removed, tissue will return to its normal state. However, neoplasia proceeds uncontrolled, and escapes the normal homeostatic controls of cell division.[63]

Progression toward a differential diagnosis would logically flow from neoplasia/nonneoplasia to infectious/noninfectious. Microorganisms create infection by invading and multiplying within tissue to produce a host response. Infection may be caused by a variety of microorganisms: bacteria, viruses, fungi, and protozoa.

Infections commonly occur within the head, face, and neck. Bacterial infections may invade fascial planes leading to a cellulitis which may ultimately coalesce into an abscess. The temporomandibular joint may become involved by the direct extension from infection resulting in pain and/or ankylosis. Pain may occur within the temporomandibular joint or any of its associated structures.[64] These pain patterns are extensive and result from the pathology, altered biomechanics, or pain referral patterns mediated by the central nervous system.[61,62] A careful and specific differential diagnosis is obviously a necessity to properly initiate and guide treatment.

Disease processes commonly creating head, neck, and face pain, and dysfunction may be further differentiated into musculoskeletal, neurovascular, neuropathic, and organic pathology as illustrated in *Figure 1*. Tension headache, cerebral vascular accident, trigeminal neuralgia, and hematologic disorders, respectively, are examples within these categories causing head, neck, and facial pain, and dysfunction.[31-48] However, careful study enables the health care practitioner to further subdivide extracranial, musculoskeletal conditions into a specific or differential diagnosis. Inspection of the algorithm reveals several areas which will necessitate subcharts, such as diseases of the eyes, ears, and sinus pathology. Further differentiation within these categories is currently under consideration, but beyond the scope of this paper. Also, it is not the purpose of this paper to explain each pathway within the illustrated paradigm shown in *Figure 1*. A complete definition of this diagnostic flow-chart would require an entire text to be written. However, the majority of the so-called "TMDs" will fall within the extracranial, musculoskeletal portion of the presented paradigm.

Use of the Algorithm

When studying head and neck disorders, the broad category of extracranial, musculoskeletal may be contrasted by further subdivision into myogenous and arthrogenous disorders. Pain and dysfunction of myogenous or arthrogenous origin would obviously emanate from cervical, noncervical, masticatory, or nonmasticatory structures as illustrated within the algorithm *(Figure 1)*.[35,36,42,56,57,64-66] Specific masticatory disorders are defined within the arthrogenous, noncervical or myogenous, masticatory categories. It must be realized that many of the traditional TMD types of pain and dysfunction should be categorized only within the myogenous or arthrogenous, noncervical, masticatory categories. With a careful and thorough history, examination, imaging, laboratory measurements, and electrophysiologic evaluation, the astute clinician is capable of formulating a differential diagnosis specific to the pathologic process.

The biomechanical and neurologic relationships between cervical and head and neck structures are complex and extensive. Many of the clinical situations evaluated on a daily basis may present with one or multiple conditions occurring concomitantly, requiring a specific or differential diagnosis. Typically seen in the pain clinic is the patient with head, neck, and face pain. As illustrated in *Figure 1*, this pain may frequently be the result of musculoskeletal, myogenous, nonmasticatory pathology (e.g., myofascial pain of the superior trapezius) or musculoskeletal, myogenous, masticatory pathology (e.g., temporal tendinitis) or two conditions occurring concomitantly with overlapping pain patterns. The convergence of the trigeminal nerve and upper cervical root fibers on the same sensory neurons within the subnucleus caudalis is one anatomic and physiologic basis for the referral of pain between trigeminal and cervical territories.[49-58]

The patient with longstanding pain is often referred for evaluation of temporomandibular joint pain. This pain may result from a chronic capsulitis, or a rheumatoid arthritis[64] [musculoskeletal, arthrogenous, noncervical, masticatory, inflammatory, *(Figure 1)*]. More frequently, in patients with longstanding pain, this perceived or referred pain is often the result of myofascial pain,[64-66] a tendinitis of the short and/or long head of the temporalis muscle, possibly an inflammatory response of the stylomandibular ligament,[58,68,70] or a lesser occipital neuralgia.[58,72,73] Myofascial trigger points of the medial pterygoid, lateral pterygoid, masseter, and sternocleidomastoid muscles frequently refer pain into the area of the temporomandibular joint.[64,65] A tendinitis of the insertions of the short or long heads of the temporalis tendons may refer pain into the area of the temporomandibular joint,[56,67,68] as well as pathology at the insertion of the stylomandibular ligament (Ernest Syndrome).[58,69-71] A lesser occipital neuralgia frequently refers pain into the parietal, temporal, retroorbital areas and/or the ear.[31,58,72,73] These conditions may occur concomitantly with or without intracapsular pathology of the temporomandibular joint. Each of these diseases may display localized or referred pain into the temporomandibular joint.[58,67-71] The health care practitioner needs to specifically differentiate these conditions into primary and secondary diagnoses with or without any anatomic or physiologic relationships. This requirement is necessary to identify the condition(s), as well as guide the treatment required.

Further consideration of a diagnostic process requires that acute versus chronic pain be considered. This is an issue as complicated as the development of a differential diagnostic paradigm, and no consensus exists. In a disease based model, pain is a symptom usually resulting from an underlying peripheral injury. When does peripheral or acute pain become centrally mediated, or is all pain a continuum with central effects? Psychological factors are involved in all pain but tend to play a much greater role with persistent, chronic pain. Further, longstanding pain must be differentiated from persistent acute, recurrent (arthritic pain, migraine headaches, trigeminal neuralgia, or cancer) or chronic pain. Chronic pain may be accompanied by central manifestations such as depression or anxiety. These psychological effects may precede or follow the conscious awareness of pain. Chronic pain research is not definitive. Based on current information, chronic pain may be either a disease or an illness. Chronic pain would be appropriately categorized within the intracranial, nonneoplastic, noninfectious, neuropathic section or the psychosocial section of the algorithm *(Figure 1)*, depending on whether the psychologic behavior was the cause or the result of the pain.[74-76]

Conclusion

As in any discipline of dentistry or medicine, evolution of the art and science must occur if our profession is to flourish and keep pace with evolving knowledge and technology. A paradigm has been developed and presented for a diagnostic algorithm from a review of the dental and medical literature. Today's knowledge of functional anatomy, neurophysiology, pathophysiology, and diagnostic techniques, combined with advancements in technology, have given the health care provider the ability to specifically differentiate head, neck, and face pain, and dysfunction.

The NIH/NIDR position paper on temporomandibular disorders has stated that a classification system would be difficult to develop because there is no defined etiologic or biologic explanation for the condition. As previously stated, the term "TMD" has been used to characterize the generalized, nonspecific complex of headache, neckache, earache, face pain, tenderness of muscles to palpation, sensation of bite change, difficulty chewing and/or swallowing, gross temporomandibular joint sounds, and limited range of motion. There is common agreement that the term "TMD" is misused, misunderstood and has been overused as an all-encompassing diagnosis for these nonspecific signs and symptoms, thus the use of TMDs as a diagnosis may be inappropriate. Much of the confusion has stemmed from the lack of understanding of the neuroanatomical and biomechanical relationships within the head and neck, as well as the interrelationships between these structures. Most of science regarding these neuroanatomic and pathophysiologic relationships have only recently evolved in the scientific and clinical areas.

Disease classifications systems are developed hierarchically within the realm of biologic categorization. It must be remembered that within this paradigm there are multiple systems interacting. As dental, medical, and basic sciences evolve, it is hoped that this classification system will allow dynamic change to occur. The proposed paradigm is a combined effort by the authors to develop a diagnostic flow-chart enabling the health practitioner to logically develop a differential diagnosis that is specific for a particular disease or diseases.

References

1. Costen JB: Syndrome of ear and sinus symptoms dependent upon disturbed function of the temporomandibular joint. *Ann Otol Rhinol Laryngol* 1934;43:1.
2. *Dorland's Illustrated Medical Dictionary (ed 26).* Philadelphia: W.B. Saunders Co., 1981.
3. Sicher H. *Oral Anatomy.* St. Louis: C.V. Mosby Co., 1949.
4. Moyers RE: An electromyographic analysis of certain muscles involved in temporomandibular movement. *Am J Orthod* 1950;36:481.
5. Prozansky S: The application of electromyography in dental research. *J Am Dent Assoc* 1950;44:49.
6. MacDougall JDB, Andrew BL: An electromyographic study of the temporalis and masseter muscles. *J Anat* 1953;87:37.
7. Perry HT: Implications of myographic research. *Angle Orthod* 1955;25:179.
8. Updegrave WJ: An evaluation of temporomandibular joint roentgenography. *J Am Dent Assoc* 1953;46:408-419.
9. Norgaard F: *Temporomandibular Arthography.* Copenhagen: Munkgaerd.
10. Ricketts RM: Laminography in the diagnosis of temporomandibular joint disorders. *J Am Dent Assoc* 1953;46:620.
11. Berry HM, Hoffman FA: Cinefluorography with image intensification for observing temporomandibular movement. *J Am Dent Assoc* 1956;53:577.
12. Kraus H: *Principles and practice of therapeutic exercises.* Springfield, IL.: Charles C. Thomas, 1950.
13. Travell J, Rinzler SH: The myofascial genesis of pain. *Postgrad Med* 1952;11:425.
14. Sicher H: Problems of pain in dentistry. *Oral Surg Oral Med Oral Pathol* 1954;7:149-160.
15. Schwartz LL: A temporomandibular pain-dysfunction syndrome. *J Chronic Dis* 1956;3:284.
16. Thilander B: Innervation of the temporomandibular joint capsule in man. *Trans R School Dent* 1961;7:1.
17. Kawamura Y, Majima T: Temporomandibular joint sensory mechanisms controlling activities. *J Dent Res* 1964;43:150.
18. Storey AT: Sensory function of the temporomandibular joint. *Can Dent Assoc J* 1968;34:294.
19. Laskin DM: Etiology of pain-dysfunction syndrome. *J Am Dent Assoc* 1969;79:147.
20. Farrar WV: Diagnosis and treatment of anterior dislocation of the articular disc. *NY J Dent* 1971;41:348.
21. National Institute of Health Technology Assessment Conference Statement on Management of Temporomandibular Joint Disorders. Draft May 2, 1996, MD.
22. Selye H: *The Stress of Life.* New York: McGraw Hill Book Co., 1980.
23. Dworkin SF: Perspectives on the interaction of biologic, psychologic and social factors in TMD. *J Am Dent Assoc* 1994;125:856-863.
24. Littenberg B, Moses LE: Estimating diagnostic accuracy from multiple conflicting reports: a new meta-analytic method. *Med Decis Making* 1993;13(4):313-321.
25. Bland CJ, Meurer LN, Maldonado GA: Systematic approach to conducting a non-statistical meta-analysis of research literature. *Acad Med* 1995;70(7):642-653.
26. Irwig L, Macaskill P, Glasziou P, Fahey M: Meta-analytic methods for diagnostic test accuracy. *J Clin Epidemiol.* 1995;48:119-132.
27. Yach D: Meta-analysis in epidemiology. *S Afr Med J* 1990;78:94-97.
28. Oakes M: The logic and role of meta-analysis in clinical research. *Sta Methods Med Res* 1993;2:147-160.
29. Proskin HM, Volpe AR: Meta-analysis in dental research: a paradigm for performance and interpretation. *J Clin Dent* 1994;5:19-26.
30. Reynolds NR, Timmerman G, Anderson J, Stevenson JS: Meta-analysis for descriptive research. *Res Nurs Health* 1992;15:467-475.
31. Adams RD, Victor M: Pain and other disorders of somatic sensation, headache and backache. In: Adams RD, ed. *Principles of Neurology, 6th Ed.* New York: McGraw Hill; 1997;125-224.
32. Andreoli TE, Bennett JC, Carpenter CCJ, Plum F, Smith LH: *Essentials of Medicine, 2nd Ed.* Philadelphia: W.B. Saunders, 1990.
33. Aronoff GM: *Evaluation and treatment of chronic pain.* Baltimore: Williams & Wilkins, 1992.
34. Bell WE: *Orofacial Pains: Classification, Diagnosis, Management, 4th Ed.* Chicago: Year Book Medical Publishers, Inc., 1989.

35. Bonica JJ: Regional pains. In: Bonica JJ, editor. *The Management of Pain, 2nd Ed.* Philadelphia: Lea and Febiger; 1990;651-858.

36. Bricker SL, Langlais RP, Miller CS: *Oral Diagnosis, Oral Medicine and Treatment Planning, 2nd Ed.* Philadelphia: Lea and Febriger, 1994.

37. Cummings CW, Krause CW: *Otolaryngology—Head and Neck Surgery Vol. 1.* St. Louis: Mosby, 1993.

38. Cummings CW, Schuller DE: *Otolaryngology—Head and Neck Surgery Vol. 2.* St. Louis: Mosby, 1993.

39. Fricton JR, Kroening RJ, Hathaway KM: *TMJ and Craniofacial Pain: Diagnosis and Management.* St. Louis: Ishiyaku EuroAmerica, 1988.

40. Fonder AC: *The Dental Physician.* Univeristy Publications: Blacksburg, VA, 1997.

41. Kaplan AS, Assael LA: *Temporomandibular Disorders—Diagnosis and Treatment.* Philadelphia: W.B. Saunders Co.; 1991;105-515.

42. Kelley WM, et al:. *Textbook of Internal Medicine.* Philadelphia: Lippencott-Raven, 1997.

43. Orban SL: *Orban's Oral Histology and Embryology.* St. Louis: Mosby Year Book, 1991.

44. Rocabado ML, Iglarsh ZA: *Musculoskeletal Approach to Maxillofacial Pain.* Philadelphia: J.B. Lippencott Co., 1991.

45. Rosenberg RN: *Comprehensive Neurology.* New York: Raven Press, 1991.

46. Saper JR, Silberstein S, Gordon CD, Hamel RL: *Handbook of Headache Management.* Baltimore: Williams and Wilkins, 1993.

47. Schottenfeld D, Fraumeni JF: *Cancer Epidemiology and Prevention, 2nd Ed.* New York: Oxford University Press; 1996;587-1370.

48. Merskey H, Bogduk N: *Classification of Chronic Pain—Descriptions of Chronic Pain Syndromes and Definitions of Pain Terms.* Seattle: International Association for the Study of Pain, 1994.

49. Hardebo JE: On pain mechanisms in cluster headache. *Headache* 1991;31:91-106.

50. Anthony M: The role of the occipital nerve in unilateral headache. *Advancement in headache research proceeding of the 6th International Migraine Society.* London: John Libbey; 1986;257:262.

51. Kerr FLW: Structural relations of trigeminal spinal tract to upper cervical roots and solitary nucleus in cats. *Exp Neurol* 1961;4:134-138.

52. Kerr FLW: Mechanism, diagnosis and management of some cranial and facial syndromes. *Surg Clin North Am* 1963;43:951-961.

53. Kerr FLW: A mechanism to account for frontal headache in posterior-fossa tumors. *J Neurosurg* 1961;18:605-609.

54. Kerr FLW: The ultrastructure of the spinal tract of the trigeminal nerve and the substantia gelatinosa. *Exp Neurol* 1966;16:359-376.

55. Pfaller K, Adrvidsson J: Cervical distribution of trigeminal and upper cervical primary afferents in the rat studied by antigrade transport of horseradish peroxidase conjugated to wheat germ agglutinin. *J Comp Neurol* 1988;268:91-108.

56. Kraus SL: *TMJ disorders—Management of the Craniomandibular Complex.* New York: Churchill Livingston, 1988.

57. Oleson J: Clinical and pathophysiological observations in migraine and tension-type headache explained by integration of vascular, supraspinal and myofascial imputs. *Neurol Clin* 1990;46:135-132.

58. Shankland WE: Craniofacial pain syndromes that mimic temporomandibular joint disorders. *Ann Acad Med Singaphone* 1995;24:83-84.

59. Muir BL: Homeostasis and adaptation. In: Muir BL, ed. *Pathophysiology—An Introduction to the Mechanisms of Disease.* New York: John Wiley and Sons; 1988;3-18.

60. Moses AJ: *Controversy in Temporomandibular Disorders: Clinician's Guide to Critical Thinking.* Chicago: Futa Book Publishers, 1997.

61. Bell WE: *Temporomandibular Disorders: Classification, Diagnosis and Management.* Chicago: Year Book Medical Publishers, Inc., 1986.

62. Kumar V, Cotran RS, Robbins SL: Cell injury, death and adaptation. In: Kumar V, ed. *Basic Pathology, 5th Ed.* Philadelphia: W.B. Saunders Co.; 1992;3-25.

63. Sheldon H: Neoplasia. In: Sheldon H, ed. *Boyd's Introduction to the Study of Disease (ed 11).* Philadelphia: Lea and Febringer; 1992;244-251.

64. Bell WE: *Temporomandibular Disorders: Classification, Diagnosis, Management.* Chicago: Year Book Medical Publishers Inc., 1990.

65. Travell JG, Simons DG: *Myofascial Pain and Dysfunction—The Trigger Point Manual.* Baltimore: Williams and Wilkins, 1984.

66. Rachlin ES: *Myofascial Pain and Fibromyalgia—Trigger Point Manual.* St. Louis: Mosby, 1994.

67. Ernest EA: Temporal tendinitis: A painful disorder that mimics migraine headache. *J Neurol Orthop Med Surg* 1987;8:159-167.

68. Wilk SJ: Surgical management of refractory craniomandibular pain using radiofrequency thermolysis: A report of thirty patients. *J Craniomandib Pract* 1994;12:93-99.

69. Shankland WE: Ernest Syndrome as a consequence of stylomandibular ligament injury: Report of 68 cases. *J Pros Dent* 1987;57:501-506.

70. Shankland WE: Ernest Syndrome (insertion tendinosis of the stylomandibular ligament) as a cause of craniomandibular pain: Diagnosis, treatment and report of two cases. *J Neurol Orthop Med Surg* 1987;8:253-257.

71. Ernest EA: The Ernest Syndrome: An insertion tendinosis of the stylomandibular ligament. *J Neuro Orthop Med Surg* 1986;7:427-438.

72. De Araujo Lucas G, Laundana A, Chopard RP, Raffaelli E: Anatomy of the lesser occipital nerve in relation to cervicogenic headache. *Clin Anat* 1994;7:90-96.

73. Plaffenrath V, Dankekar R, Pollmann W: Cervicogenic headache—The clinical picture, radiological findings and hypotheses on its pathophysiology. *Headache* 1987:27:495-499.

74. Hanson RW, Gerber KE: *Coping with Chronic Pain—A Guide to Patient Self-Management.* New York: The Guilford Press, 1990.

75. Cailliet R: Chronic pain. In: Cailliet R, ed. *Pain Mechanisms and Management.* Philadelphia: F. A. Davis Co., 1993;246-261.

76. Gatchel RJ, Turk DC: *Psychological Approaches to the Pain Management—A Practitioner's Handbook.* New York: The Guilford Press, 1996.

Fibromyalgia and Myofascial Pain Dysfunction Affecting the Head and Neck: Update and Differential Diagnosis

M. Bergamini, S. Prayer Galletti, and C. Bergamini

Introduction

Neuromuscular dentistry and craniomandibular orthopedics are based upon the fundamental concept that myofascial pain syndrome (MPS) is often the cause of the symptomatic manifestations related to masticatory dysfunctions. Myofascial pain syndrome involved in such manifestations predominantly affects the head and neck musculature.[1] The capability to investigate masticatory muscular function by means of modern sophisticated electronic measurement devices was pioneered by B. Jankelson.[2] The work of Travell and Simons,[3] collected in their famous "Myofascial Pain and Dysfunction—The Trigger Point Manual," is also an essential contribution to our science. An eminent colleague has wittily called this text "the Bible of the craniomandibular orthopedist!" These authors have emphasized the role of masticatory muscles in the pathogenesis of craniomandibular dysfunction and symptoms. The misleading concept concerning the role of the temporomandibular joint (TMJ) as the origin of masticatory dysfunctions can now be considered under a new light. It is becoming clear that muscular disorders are the etiologic source of the clinical manifestations. The TMJ is often secondarily involved, only after muscular hypertonicity interferes with normal disc/condyle dynamics.[4]

Craniomandibular orthopedists must be knowledgeable regarding MPS, but also aware of chronic muscle disorders whose signs and symptoms mimic myofascial manifestations. The author's investigation was initiated by the need to understand the reason for the lack of treatment response in certain patients with apparent myofascial syndrome.

Recently, the medical literature[5-7] has focused upon two syndromes: the fibromyalgia syndrome (FS) and the chronic fatigue syndrome (CFS). MPS, even though frequently reported, has been generally considered a minor subject of concern to chiropractors, physiotherapists, and occasionally dentists. The symptoms of MPS are often inappropriately referred to as temporomandibular disorders (TMD) by many dentists. The misunderstanding still goes on!

A comparison among MPS, FS, and CFS requires a concise report of each and an analysis of any clinical and/or humoral parameters which could be helpful in developing a correct differential diagnosis. The lack of a definite distinction among these syndromes has been noted by several authors. Merskey[8] has stated that "FS and MPS require a better understanding" and Tunks[9] has recently concluded that "... there is need for more clinical studies comparing fibromyalgia with myofascial pain and with control groups to develop diagnostic criteria with adequate specificity, sensitivity and inter-rater reliability."

Very recently, it has been observed that patients affected by chronic facial pain show a high co-morbidity with other stress-associated syndromes, based on a possible malfunction of the hypothalamic-pituitary-adrenal stress hormonal axis.[10] Similar implications were observed also regarding CFS.[11]

Myofascial Pain Syndrome (MPS)

MPS appears to be the most frequent cause of muscular pain and of chronic nonspecific pain. Even if its pathogenesis has not yet been completely clarified, clinical aspects characterizing the syndrome are now very well known.

MPS has been defined by Travell and Simons[3] as "pain and/or autonomic phenomena referred from active myofascial trigger points (TrPs) with associated dysfunction." The myofascial trigger point is defined by the same authors as "an hyperirritable spot, usually within a taut band of skeletal muscle or in a muscle's fascia, that is painful on compression and that gives rise to characteristic referred pain, tenderness and autonomic phenomena."

Although MPS can occur in any part of the body, it is more likely to be found in the head and neck. There is wide evidence that the masticatory apparatus is one of the most involved, thus provoking a major cause of craniomandibular pain.[1] The reasons the masticatory apparatus is so affected by MPS can be detected in its peculiar structure, mainly related to the dentition, which is something quite different from any other body apparatus. In fact, either during or subsequent to growth, and due to multiple pathologic events on dental structures, the relationship between the dental arches happens to undergo complex alterations. The consequence of such phenomena is a modification of dental occlusion requiring continuous muscular compensation which may lead to the onset of a myofascial condition. Clinical manifestations of MPS of head and neck can be either of a "localized" or of a "spread" type with more extensive signs and symptoms.[7] This distinction is very relevant in craniomandibular orthopedic practice.

The dental occlusion often requires accommodative muscle adaptation which can cause "localized" MPS of both primary masticatory muscles, as well as other associated muscles influenced by postural mechanisms through neural and biochemical involvement. While the clinical symptomatology can be extremely variable, the pattern is generally similar. Pain may be the only relevant symptom or it can be associated with dysfunctional signs, involving the head and neck and influencing chewing ability. Headache is the most common manifestation of myogenous dysfunction.[12] Neck pain and/or stiffness and temporomandibular joint involvement may also result from muscle over-accommodation to a noncompatible intercuspation of the teeth. Puzzling pain distribution may be present, especially when teeth and alveolar regions are affected or nerve entrapment phenomena contribute to generate painful complex syndromes like atypical neuralgias.[13] One should remember that pain is not always the most relevant symptom. Autonomic and/or proprioceptive disorders, such as vertigo, nausea, fatigue, sensorial alterations, etc., described by Bergamini and Prayer Galletti,[14] may contribute to the clinical condition, creating difficulty formulating diagnosis and treatment.

The "spread" type of MPS has multiple origins involving skeletal muscle structures of various areas. Diffuse dysfunctional and postural problems may lead to a vicious cycle in which a craniomandibular malrelationship may exist, but a single therapeutic approach cannot resolve the clinical puzzle.

MPS affects people of all ages, of both sexes, but appears to be more common in females. Even children are not immune, since quite often infantile headaches are due to musculature contraction, caused by dental malocclusion.[15,16]

According to Simons,[17] the myofascial pain diagnosis requires the presence of all of the five major criteria and at least one of the four minor criteria reported in *Table I*. These criteria are well suited for the masticatory apparatus, as well as the head and neck area. Nevertheless, we would like to add another practical criterion derived from the specific experience gathered in treating MPS patients, which will be described when discussing differential diagnosis. At present it is worthwhile to consider that in the past ten years we utilized both surface electromyography (EMG) and low frequency, high intensity transcutaneous electrical nerve stimulation (TENS) of branches of cranial nerves V and VII for testing and reducing muscular hypertonicity, characteristic of MPS. Basmajian and De Luca[18] have proposed the rationale for employing surface EMG: 1) surface EMG is a noninvasive technique and can provide suitable data on muscular activity if properly utilized, and 2) muscular tonus and hypertonicity have an exact correlation with the EMG signal which gives a great deal of information when developing a differential diagnosis.[19] However, it must be remarked that surface EMG has not been widely utilized by other health care specialists involved in myofascial diagnosis.

Table I
Clinical criteria for the diagnosis of myofascial pain syndrome

Major criteria

1. Regional pain complaint
2. Pain complaint or altered sensation in the expected distribution of referred pain from a myofascial trigger point
3. Taut band palpable in an accessible muscle
4. Exquisite spot tenderness at one point along the length of the taut band
5. Some degree of restricted range of motion when measurable

Minor criteria

a. Reproduction of clinical pain complaint or altered sensation by pressure on the tender spot
b. Elicitation of a local twitch by transverse snapping palpation at the tender spot or by needle insertion into the tender spot in the taut band
c. Pain alleviated by elongation (stretching) of the muscle or by injecting the tender spot
d. Improvement of symptoms after low-frequency TENS on myofascial TrPs*

From McCain, modified.[15]

*Criterion derived from clinical experiences in treating MPS by means of neuromuscular modalities

The value of low frequency TENS for reduction of muscle hypertonicity is well documented.[2,4] MPS in most cases is a well defined musculoskeletal disorder which can be easily diagnosed following the above mentioned criteria. However, the clinical behavior of patients, as well as the response to therapies,[20] can create difficulties in determining the existing pathological condition. In these specific cases, a differential diagnosis can be rather problematic, as will be later clarified.

Fibromyalgia (FS)

The term fibromyalgia was first introduced by Hench.[21] Moldofsky's research[22] followed, demonstrating EEG alterations observed in patients with chronic pain and fatigue syndromes. The most typical aspects will be described later by Yunus.[23] A classification of fibromyalgia has been validated by the Multicenter Criteria Study based on appropriate pain controls and blinded observations.[24] According to Yunus and Masi,[6] fibromyalgia can be defined as "a form of non articular rheumatism characterized by musculoskeletal aching and tenderness on palpation of tendino-musculoskeletal sites called tender points" (TePs). They have classified FS as primary, secondary, concomitant, and localized. However, FS is no longer considered a rheumatic disease because of the lack of typical humoral findings. The above mentioned classification is no longer accepted and FS is now considered as a primary manifestation, sometimes isolated or associated with other diseases. Moreover, the syndrome previously called "localized" fibromyalgia is characterized by pain in a few contiguous anatomic sites and often due to traumatic etiologic factors. As reported by Yunus and Masi,[6] this is in contrast with the fundamental concepts concerning FS and, in the author's opinion, it rather suits MPS.

Fibromyalgia syndrome affects mainly females (70–90%) in their fifth decade and shows a chronic development since symptoms can last more than 5 years.[15] Fibromyalgia syndrome is a frequent pain disorder in which a reproducible physical finding, the presence of palpable fibrositic TePs, is found. This is associated with characteristic symptoms of generalized muscular aching, stiffness, fatigue, and non-restorative sleep. Fibromyalgia syndrome can be viewed as consisting of a central set of core features, which are essential for diagnosis, superimposed on a variable number of ancillary manifestations, often seen in association with, but not integral to, the final diagnosis of the condition.[15] The core features are generalized pain and widespread tenderness over discrete anatomical areas already described as "fibrositic tender points." Ancillary features are of two types:

1) Fatigue, non-restorative sleep, and morning stiffness can be considered almost characteristic since they occur in over 75% of individuals.

2) Irritable bowel syndrome, Raynaud's phenomenon, headache, subjective swelling, non-dermatomal paraesthesiae, psychological distress, and marked functional disability are less common, occurring in perhaps 25% of cases.

Pain, best described as "chronic muscular aching," is the central dominating feature of FS and is considered essential to diagnosis. The typical historical findings are chronicity, persistence, and the absence of a migratory pattern of symptomatology. The preponderance of chronic muscular aching is shown by a study of Yunus[25] in which all of the clinical features of FS were compared with those of patients with rheumatoid arthritis, as well as with normal controls *(Table II)*. Fibromyalgia patients have lower pain thresholds not only over TePs, but also over control points, which are not generally tender in rheumatoid arthritis patients and normal controls.[26,27] The body distribution of pain in a large FS population is shown in *Table III*. This reports data from four different clinical trials.[23,28,29]

Table II
Percentage frequency of symptoms in patients with fibromyalgia and rheumatoid arthritis compared with healthy controls

Symptoms	Fibromyalgia	Rheumatoid arthritis	Healthy controls
Pain	94	79	0
Fatigue	85	62	10
Stiffness	76	66	0
Anxiety	72	47	31
Poor sleep	62	32	9
Generalised aching	60	40	0
Mental stress	60	33	25
Swelling	40	56	5
Depression	37	26	9
Paraesthesia	36	9	2

From McCain.[15]

Table III
Pain in different part of the body of FS patients reported by different authors

	Wolfe (1985)	Leavitt (1986)	Yunus (1981)	McCain Scudds (1988)
Low back	95	80	65	66
Neck	90	65	35	34
Shoulders	90	75	55	54
Hips	80	70	35	38
Hands	75	65	55	52
Knees	70	70	68	66
Chest wall	70	30	—	—
Feet	70	50	18	18
Elbows	65	52	22	24
Ankles	55	55	20	22
Wrists	55	55	15	14

From McCain.[15]

Fibrositic TePs are areas of mild tenderness in normal individuals, but palpation of these sites in fibromyalgia patients often causes extreme pain and withdrawal. The American College of Rheumatology (ACR) Classification Criteria for sensitivity and specificity of diagnosis established nine paired sites.[24] When 11 of 18 tender points can be elicited together with the criterion of widespread muscular aching, FS must be suspected *(Table IV)*.

Table IV
Topographical location of the 18 most recurrent TePs

Sites	Features
Occiput	Bilaterally at the suboccipital muscle insertion
Low cervical	Bilaterally at the anterior aspect of the intertransverse spaces at C5-C7
Trapezius	Bilaterally at the midpoint of the upper border
Supraspinatus	Bilaterally at the origin above the medial border of the scapular spine
Second rib	Bilaterally upper surfaces just lateral to the costochondral junctions
Lateral epicondyle	Bilaterally, 2 cm distal to the epicondyles
Gluteal	Bilaterally, in upper outer quadrants of buttocks in anterior fold of muscle
Greater trochanter	Bilaterally, posterior to the trochanteric prominence
Knee	Bilaterally, at the medial fat pad proximal to the joint line

From McCain.[15]

TePs must be carefully distinguished from TrPs. Palpation of tender points causes pain localized to the area of palpation. Pain does not radiate to adjacent areas and no muscle hardness or induration can be appreciated. Active trigger points, on the contrary, do refer pain to distant areas usually in a typical pattern[3] and can be felt on palpation as hard nodules in the muscular belly. These differences have led to the clinical axiom: "TePs are to fibromyalgia as TrPs are to myofascial pain.[15]

Many non-specific ancillary features occur frequently enough to be considered as adjunctive characteristics. Most frequently reported are morning stiffness, sleep disturbance, and fatigue occurring in over 75% of cases.[30] These symptoms may also be seen in rheumatic diseases such as rheumatoid arthritis, but their frequency is less significant. Other symptoms which are present in 25% of FS patients are non-dermatomal paraesthesiae, subjective joint and interjoint swelling, headache, irritable bowel syndrome and Raynaud's phenomenon. [23,24,30,31]

The coincidence of FS with certain autoimmune and rheumatic diseases has been noted. Many researches have shown that the most frequently associated pathologies are rheumatoid arthritis (RA), systemic lupus erythematosus (SLE), Raynaud's phenomenon, and Sjogren syndrome.[32] Some authors emphasize that many painful and disabling symptoms, typical of autoimmune syndromes, could depend on the presence of FS. Another typical sign is livedo reticularis, which also might be associated to FS as demonstrated by cutaneous biopsies.[33] Surprisingly, there has been no apparent research performed regarding the relationship between autoimmune diseases and MPS.

Psychological disturbances are frequently present in fibromyalgia patients. However, studies report that only a minority of patients have true major psychiatric disorders. It is a common opinion that psychological distress is likely to be the result of rather than the cause of chronic pain.[34,35] Researchers do not agree on anxiety and depression levels in FS compared to those in rheumatoid patients.[36-38] As a consequence, it may be reasonable to consider psychological disturbances as an epiphenomenon of fibromyalgia, rather than a marker of the syndrome. Nevertheless, recent studies[39] have shown that a mind body intervention, including patient education, meditation techniques and movement therapy, appear to be an adjunctive treatment for patients with fibromyalgia. The most current treatment modalities are those utilizing anti-depressive drugs such as amitriptyline and cyclobenzaprine. The use of such drugs is based upon the pathogenetic observations about the role of neurohormonal involvement, as will be later described.

Chronic Fatigue Syndrome (CFS)

Even if medical literature has dealt at length with CFS in the last few years, it is hard to define this syndrome properly because of its poor clinical features. According to the criteria established by Sharpe,[40] CFS consistently occurs with the following signs and symptoms:

1) Severe physical and mental fatigue induced by physical or mental effort.
2) Associated symptoms including myalgia, headache, depression, poor concentration, and others.
3) Absence of abnormalities on conventional medical investigation.
4) Functional disability.
5) Duration of illness longer than six months.

A consistent anamnestic feature in CFS patients is a previous viral infection within a period of six months before its onset. This has been reported to occur in 72% of patients.[41] Nevertheless, a viral infection is not pathognomonic because a unique agent has not yet been detected.

An important clinical feature is related to the psychiatric condition of CFS patients, mainly represented by depression, as well as psychic instability. These observations have suggested a possible link with a viral brain infection, so that Wessely has called CFS "benign encephalomyelitis."[42]

However, current authorities now emphasize similarities rather than differences between CFS and FS.[43,44] Yunus and Masi[25] consider CFS as a subgroup of fibromyalgia characterized by severe fatigue as a predominant symptom.

Pathogenetic Hypothesis

The pathogenesis of chronic myalgias is still far from being completely understood. A rational analysis of the subject requires a careful description of all the factors potentially involved in causing such myalgias.

Infectious Factors

A great deal of viral, microbial and also parasitic agents have been implicated, in MPS,[3] FS, and CFS. Epstein-Barr virus, as well as Borrellia Burgdoferi, are the most investigated.[45] The former may produce a chronic infection which mimics CFS , while the latter is supposed to be the etiologic agent of Lyme disease which can mimic FS.[46,47] Relationships between retroviruses and CFS,[48] and between parvovirus B19 and FS[49] have been suggested, but this has not been confirmed.

Research on muscular biopsies, using molecular techniques, has shown enteroviral genic sequences in 50% of a group of FS patients who were, however, free from enteroviral infections.[50] Moreover, very interesting data from clinical observations confirm that up to 70% of FS and CFS patients have been affected by a "flu-like" syndrome as the initiating element of the myalgic syndrome.[51]

All these controversial data lead to the conclusion that an infectious pathogenesis of chronic myalgia must be taken into consideration but with caution.

Hormonal and Neurohormonal Factors

Recent research has focused attention on the influence of neurohormonal dysfunctions, including either functional deficiencies of the inhibitory neurotransmitters at the spinal or supraspinal levels (e.g., serotonin, norepinephrine, enkephaline, GABA, and somatostatin) or an overactivity of excitatory neurotransmitters (e.g., substance P, cholecystokinin, and other peptides) or both.[52] These disorders could depend, to some extent, on a genetic predisposition[53] and could be triggered by stressor agents such as viral infections (see above) and traumatic events.

Serotonin, a pain inhibitor and a sleep mediator, appears to be deficient in FS. This fact has been suggested by the low serum or plasma tryptophan levels,[52,54] decreased transport of tryptophan,[52] decreased cerebrospinal fluid[55] and low serum serotonin levels.[56] Obviously, a simple serotonin deficiency cannot cause FS, since not all patients show this defect. An abnormal hypothalamic-pituitary adrenal axis may also play a significant role in FS pathogenesis.[57] Such a disorder is tested by low neuropeptide Y levels found in FS patients' plasma. These substances are normally present in a high rate in the central nervous system (CNS) and particularly in the hypothalamus, hippocampus, and cerebral cortex, while they show low plasma levels in FS patients. This fact is very significant due to the involvement of these neuropeptides in the regulation of food intake, and cardiovascular and neuroendocrine function.[58] Moreover, low levels of neuropeptides Y could induce an abnormal response to stress due to an alteration of ACTH production by the adrenal cortex.[57]

Russell reported high levels of substance P in cerebrospinal fluid in FS patients.[58] Substance P is an 11-aminoacid peptide which has a role in the neurotransmission of pain from the periphery to the CNS. Its physiologic functions are influenced by serotonin,[59] while the combination of low serotonin levels and high substance P levels may be responsible for the lower than normal pain threshold in FS.[54]

Remarkably, in FS an abnormal production of somatomedine C has been detected.[60] This substance is closely related to growth hormone secretion and plays a critical role in muscle homeostasis and repair;[61,62] similar data have been confirmed by Bagge.[63] An interesting issue comes from the observation that about 80% of the total daily production of growth hormone is secreted during the stage-4 of sleep. Since stage-4 is the most disturbed in FS[64] and since FS patients also show low somatomedine C levels it appears that any disturbance in this hormone production may be a predisposing factor in muscle microtrauma and/or impairs the normal healing of muscle microtrauma. Such a hypothesis is in accord with Jacobsen's[65] findings of lower levels of serum type III procollagen in FS patients due to inadequate growth hormone production.

The crucial issue from all these studies is that an unknown substance might be responsible for the alteration in pain perception at a central level according to the fundamental algometric research by Granges and Littlejohn.[66] They demonstrated the threshold of pain to be significantly lower in FS patients compared to MPS patients and pain free controls *(Table V)*. Following Russell's more recent research,[67] several chemical pain factors such as serotonin, substance P, nerve growth factor, and dinorphin A appear to be implicated in the pathogenesis of fibromyalgia, shedding new light on the development of innovative therapies.

Table V
Comparison of various algometric parameters response between a study group of fibromyalgia patients, myofascial pain patients, and pain-free controls

	Fibromyalgia Syndrome	Myofascial Pain Syndrome	Pain-free Controls	Statistical Significance
Sum of pressure pain threshold at all 18 tender/trigger points (kg/cm^2) and at all 4 control points	51.5 (±9.5)	79.7 (±18.3)	113.0 (±31.8)	.0001
Sum of pressure pain threshold values over control points only (kg/cm^2)	19.3 (±6.8)	26.0 (±7.6)	33.9 (±9.1)	.0001
Mean pain threshold at 1 tender/trigger point site (kg/cm2)	1.7 (±0.5)	2.9 (±0.8)	4.3 (±0.3)	.0001
Mean pain threshold at 1 control point site (kg/cm2)	4.8 (±1.7)	6.5 (±1.9)	8.4 (±2.0)	
Total number of tender/trigger points (mean number)	15.2 (±2.3)	7.2 (±3.9)	2.7 (±3.3)	.0001

From Granges and Littlejohn.[66]

Immunological Factors

Several studies confirm that FS commonly accompanies autoimmune, rheumatic and non-rheumatic diseases like rheumatoid arthritis, Sjogren's syndrome, Raynaud's phenomenon, and hypothyroidism. This suggests a possible connection with immune system alterations.[68] Livedo reticularis, which is a typical feature of an immuno-mediated vascular condition, is commonly seen in FS patients. Skin biopsies have revealed abnormal serum immunoglobulin deposits at the dermal-epidermal junction in fibromyalgia.[33,69] Alterations in T cells and natural killer cells have been investigated but results are not consistent.[54,70]

Studies conducted by Goldenberg and Komaroff[71] described abnormalities of immune function such as elevated serum antibodies to some viruses, abnormal levels of circulating immune complexes, Epstein-Barr virus–related T lymphocyte dysfunction, and monocyte alterations. Another possible link between immunological disturbances and FS is revealed from the research on the influence of sleep-wake cycles on the immune system.[72] Jacobsen[73] has performed the screening for autoantibodies in patients with FS compared to healthy people. In a high percentage they found anti-smooth muscles and even anti-striated muscle autoantibodies. Such antibodies were not present in healthy controls. However, these findings have not been confirmed in subsequent studies.

Advanced research on immunological abnormalities in patients with CFS have shown an imbalance between different NK lymphocyte subsets and an increase of some NK CD4 and B CD19 lymphocyte subsets.[74] These observations, however, need subsequent controlled studies to compare to clinical observations.

Finally, alterations of the cytochemical network, including α interferon, IL2, IL6 production, etc., have been taken into account, with controversial results.[70] *Table VI* reports a synthesis of the major immunological issues of FS and CFS.

Psychological Factors

Recent literature regarding connections between the psychological profile and chronic pain does not clarify whether psychological disorders, so common in FS patients, represent the cause rather than the effect of this myalgic syndrome. Furthermore, it has not been confirmed that psychological factors can predispose one to chronic myalgias. The most diffuse and effective personality evaluation test is the Minnesota Multiphasic Personality Inventory (MMPI).[75] So tested chronic myalgic patients have shown a psychological profile related to the neurotic triad (hypochondria, depression, and hysteria). Studies[76] conducted on FS patients utilizing the MMPI established no direct connections between FS fundamental features (number of TePs, fatigue, and sleep disturbances) and the degree of psychological disorders. Instead pain severity seems to be directly related to the psychological disorder.

According to another study on a rather large group of FS and MPS patients,[77] 60% of FS patients showed an MMPI profile classified as psychosomatic, 28% depressed, and the remaining group were affected by a specific psychological disorder. In MPS patients, on the contrary, the percentages were respectively 15%, 25%, and 0%, with 60% of patients presenting no psychological disorders. Psychological pathology is not relevant in the pathogenesis of localized chronic pain, but it becomes more significant in conditioning the

Table VI
Immunological assessment in fibromyalgia and chronic fatigue syndrome

Measure	Fibromyalgia	Chronic fatigue syndrome
Mitogen stimulation	Normal	Normal or ↓ Natural killer activity
Lymphocyte enumeration	Usually normal ⅓ have ↑ CD4/CD8 ratio	Normal Slight ↑ CD4 ↓ CD4/CD8 ratio
Cytokine	Normal	↑ IFN-α Normal IFN Slight ↑ IFN production Normal IFN-γ production Normal IL-1 production
Circulating immune complexes	Normal	↑ in 60–67%
IgG subclasses	Normal (no subclass ↓)	↓ IgG subclasses

From Fricton.[20]

symptomatology of diffuse syndromes. An hypothesis has been put forward: psychological alterations might act as predisposing factors in some MPS patients for a more systemic syndrome, but further research on this issue is required.[78] Two additional studies using a different type of evaluation test (SCL 90R) established significant abnormal scores for depression and anxiety scales in FS patients.[34,15] Recently, the medical literature has referred to the relationships between a previously experienced sexual harassment and delayed development of a FS syndrome.[79]

Peripheral Factors

In MPS genesis the essential factor is trauma which acts through two different patterns, either separate or combined. A single traumatic event is often the cause resulting from an automobile accident (whiplash), sport injuries, domestic accidents, or potentially from iatrogenic causes.[4] This kind of trauma leads to acute MPS, certainly the most well known and accepted, but often improperly described as a "sprained muscle." It can affect one or several healthy muscle groups, as well as muscles already affected by chronic MPS. The forced stretching of a previously contracted muscle is the typical mechanism of action. Acute MPS generally improves with spraying and stretching techniques, specifically in the case of sport injuries. Repetitive microtrauma elicited by improper body posture, work habits, improperly fitting shoes, etc. (all producing an effect on posture) may be a major influence leading to chronic MPS. Very often a skeletal deformity acts as an essential cofactor. As a consequence, the muscles that are most involved in postural maintenance are those which must compensate for the skeletal disorder through excessive accommodation, and thus these muscles are the most frequently affected by myofascial involvement.

According to Simons,[3,80] microtrauma can produce damage to the sarcolemmal membrane which creates an excess of Ca^{++} ions transported from extracellular fluid into the muscle fiber, thus provoking a muscular sustained contraction. This activates the ATP dependent pump to eliminate the excess Ca^{++} and depletes ATP stores as has been verified from muscular taut bands. Actin and myosin filaments are not able to return to their physiologic resting length as a result of these depleted ATP stores. Eventually TrPs can degenerate into granular structures localized in areas of muscular fibrosis.[15]

In FS, peripheral factors are likely to be less important than central factors.[81] Nevertheless, the fact that they can contribute pathogenically to some extent is suggested by the decrease of peripheral pain and tenderness in FS patients when injected epidurally with opioid drugs,[82] or following regional sympathetic blockade.[83] It is still unknown if these findings might be secondary to central related reflex mechanisms, or instead represent an epiphenomenon.

Trauma is probably an important peripheral factor in initiating or aggravating FS in some patients who are neurohormonally susceptible to this condition.[84] Also, environmental stimuli such as weather alterations, and physical and mental stress need to be considered as peripheral factors.[85]

To summarize, theories on the pathogenesis refer to two basic mechanisms: the first of central origin, represented by neurohormonal alterations, or by immunological modifications with a possible infectious origin and psychological disturbances of various degrees. The second mechanism has a peripheral origin involving mechanical factors with postural modifications. These two mechanisms could interact in diagnosing chronic myalgic syndromes.

A critical evaluation of currently available data suggests that the primary defect in fibromyalgia is most likely of central origin, i.e., a complex network of neurohormonal dysfunctions leading to aberrant central pain mechanisms, which alone can cause FS. In other patients, interactions of additional factors, including peripheral influences (e.g., trauma, mechanical stress) may increase and produce a vicious cycle. Thus, for any given situation the patient complains of more pain than would be expected and the pain fluctuates according to the external environmental factors, such as weather change, posture, and stress. Therefore, FS can be defined as an "aberrant central pain mechanism with peripheral modulation."[81]

In the case of MPS, peripheral factors are likely to be the more active. It is well known from the experience collected following treatment results of masticatory dysfunctions that the removal of mechanical/postural alteration often leads to clinical improvement. Nevertheless, the possible action of central mechanisms should not be underestimated since these influences promote and affect the perception and spread of symptoms. In this event, a true FS should be suspected.

How does a localized problem become more generalized and meet American College of Rheumatology (ACR) criteria that defines diffuse fibromyalgia? There is evidence that vertebral dysfunction at one level may induce changes at other levels, with subsequent activation of segmental reflex arcs. When central pain-modulating factors are operating and when such reflex arcs occur in a number of segments rather than in just one, the spread of changes to the dorsal horns may occur. Thus, sensitization of dorsal horn neurons may take place over a wide area of the spinal cord and hence the syndrome becomes diffuse.[27] Pathogenetic relationships between FS and MPS, according to the author's referred opinions, are illustrated in *Figure 1.*

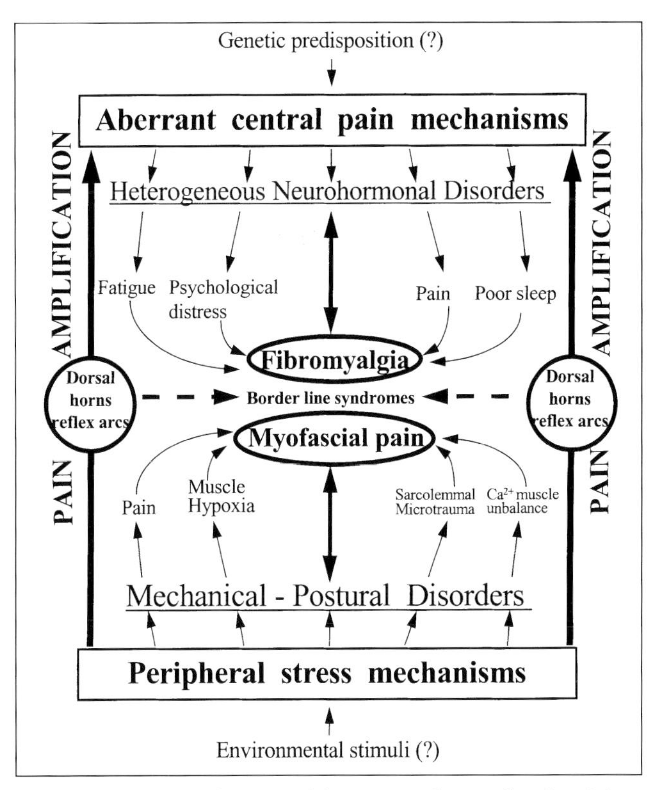

Figure 1. Schematic diagram of the proposed central and peripheral mechanisms interactingly operating in FS and MPS.

Differential Diagnosis

The topic of differential diagnosis of chronic myalgias related to the head and neck area will be discussed following this sequence:

1) Differential diagnosis between "localized" MPS, mostly of occlusal origin, and "spread" MPS.
2) Differential diagnosis between MPS and FS or CFS.

The distinction between "localized" and "spread" MPS is fundamental for a craniomandibular practice because spread MPS treatment requires a multidisciplinary approach. Besides the previously described diagnostic criteria, craniomandibular orthopedic procedures require the combined use of surface EMG of masticatory muscles and low frequency, high intensity transcutaneous electrical neural stimulation (TENS) applied to branches of cranial nerves V and VII. The use of surface EMG to record patient response to low frequency acupuncture-like TENS facilitates a differential diagnosis. Experience acquired through clinical observation of a large number of patients, confirms that a diffuse muscular imbalance almost always gives typical EMG data.[19] Commonly, masticatory muscles tested before and after TENS application show a noticeable improvement in values, thus confirming that TENS application has positively influenced all the tested muscles. On the contrary, when the posterior temporalis and anterior digastric muscles, which are closely related to cervical posture, maintain signs of hypertonicity following TENS and when the modification of the existing occlusion into a myocentric occlusion does not modify the muscular imbalance, there is a strong implication that upper quarter postural problems exist, concurrently.[19]

A differential diagnosis between MPS and FS or CFS is a complex clinical problem. Chronic myalgic syndromes are characterized by specific features and distinctive diagnostic parameters; nevertheless, a high percentage of FS patients show symptoms of the head and neck region which are similar to craniomandibular MPS. This creates problems when attempting to develop a diagnosis. This subject has been thoroughly investigated in a worldwide literature search; however, our personal clinical experience allowed us to achieve some additionally valuable data. We shall first discuss data collected from the medical literature and compare it with findings obtained in the authors' clinical practices.

The authors agree that MPS frequently shows a more acute onset, a more regional localization, an objective trigger point phenomenon, and a better response to treatment.[86] Fibromyalgia syndrome instead tends to be more insidious at the onset, more widespread, characterized by subjective TePs, and it is more unpredictable in its prognosis (differential characteristic between TePs, and myofascial TrPs have been described above). Following these criteria, FS and MPS should be easily distinguished and categorized *(Table VII)*. Unfortunately, there are many borderline conditions in which clinical features create diagnostic confusion. Active TrPs may spread via activation of satellite or secondary TrPs resulting in the gradual transformation from a regional myofascial presentation to a subsequent global fibromyalgic picture. The mechanism for creation or activation of secondary TrPs involves excessive compensation for the previous lack of use of muscle groups related to the area where the myofascial problem began.

Table VII
Comparison between clinical features of fibromyalgia and myofascial pain syndrome

	Fibromyalgia	Myofascial pain
Sex	Female/male 10:1	Female/male 2:1
Age	40–60 years primarily	All ages
Duration of the symptoms	Chronic	Acute or chronic
Tender/trigger point pain	Local, non-radiating	Referred to distinct reference zones
Tender/ trigger point distribution	Widespread	Regional
Tender/trigger point anatomy	Muscle-tendon junction	Muscle belly
Stiffness	Widespread	Regional
Fatigue	Debilitating	Usually absent
Twitch response	Absent	Present
Treatment	Drugs	Local injection. Stretch and spray therapy. Orthopedic realignment
Prognosis	Seldom cured	Usually good

From McCain,[15] modified.

Other borderline situations have been reported. Patients with FS who did not satisfy all the fibromyalgic criteria have been described,[87] while other authors[35,88] theorized that these disorders may coexist or could be a continuum of development from one phase to the other. Littlejohn[89] described an epidemic Australian pain syndrome which started with a localized pattern and developed into a generalized syndrome. There are also conflicting results concerning TrP count, palpation-induced pain, and referred pain, which suggest more clinical studies are needed to compare FS and MPS, and to develop specific, sensitive, and reliable diagnostic criteria.[24,25,66,90]

Many comparative studies on FS and MPS symptomatology reported no relevant differences in anamnestic symptoms.[8,73,91,92] Sleep disturbances, fatigue, and paraesthesias are present in different percentages in both syndromes. Several ancillary disorders found in FS may possibly be linked to referred pain due to myofascial pain: i.e., irritable bowel syndrome might occur with myofascial TrPs in the abdominal wall, dysmenorrhea and dyspareunia may be caused by TrPs in the pyriformis muscle, and headaches by TrPs in the upper neck and jaws muscles.[3]

It is evident from our review of the general medical literature that a suitable differential diagnostic criteria between FS and MPS has not been established; thus it is worthwhile to evaluate the diagnostic criteria and modalities previously mentioned. In our experience FS should be suspected when several anamnestic results and objective measurements are observed. Long lasting and severe symptoms coupled with previous multiple therapeutic failures can be considered diagnostically relevant. Sleep disturbances, persistent pain during the night and morning, anxiety, and depression contribute to FS suspicion. We have observed that MPS patients often get relief from sleeplessness while symptoms worsen during waking hours. Of paramount importance will be a clinical examination directed at detecting palpation tenderness in the typical tender sites of masticatory and cervical muscles, their bilateral distribution, and the lack of coincidence between muscular soreness and evidence of taut bands within the tested muscles. When muscular and non-muscular soreness (e.g., cutaneous, articular, etc.) is determined for the head and neck, the clinician should extend palpatory maneuvers below the cervical area towards the chest, hips, and legs, following the multicenter criteria study rules that were previously mentioned.

When FS is suspected, it may be difficult to decide whether to submit such patients to functional exams of the masticatory apparatus or to refer to an appropriate FS therapist. If FS symptoms are very evident, it may be judicious to immediately refer to an FS therapist since FS patients who are psychologically disturbed do not respond well to modalities used for functional analysis. However, this fact caused us to submit suspected FS patients to TENS to determine if there is a difference in the response in these patients.

It has been the experience of the authors that low frequency, high amplitude TENS is easily accepted by MPS patients with single or multiple applications; however, almost unfailingly, we have observed that patients who are affected by FS generally respond adversely to TENS stimulation. It has been the authors' experience to observe that patients exclusively affected by FS show normal or even low resting EMG activity when compared to MPD/TMD patients. The authors acknowledge that it is very rare to find people affected only by FS. Simons stated that up to 72% of patients affected by FS also have active TrPs. Simons' impression about surface EMG in MPS diagnosis is very similar to the authors'. Moreover, one should be aware that low EMG values do not always mean healthy muscles. Several recent studies seem to give more credit to EMG frequency analysis as reported by Thomas.[93]

Conclusions

Dealing with the present research, the authors' principal aims were:

1) To determine a proper connection between MPS and those myalgic syndromes which have been investigated during the last ten years in the domain of musculoskeletal and rheumatic diseases.
2) To determine if any biochemical or biophysical issue creates the initial onset of musculoskeletal pain in subjects undergoing chronic muscle stress.
3) To establish suitable diagnostic criteria for the differential diagnosis between MPS and FS.

Since the three syndromes present similar characteristics which often overlap but which may have quite different clinical outcomes, our purpose has been that of investigating the pathogenetic mechanisms they may have in common.

Many studies suggest that MPS may evolve into FS when other pathogenic factors are superimposed.[91,92] As a consequence, it is possible to find borderline situations creating various clinical features. Due to the lack of personal experience, the authors can only accept the evidence in the medical/dental literature that considers chronic fatigue syndrome as a special kind of FS, where fatigue is likely to be the most significant symptom. The authors feel assured that MPS is principally determined by peripheral mechanisms acting on posture, while FS is probably determined by central acting factors. However, in MPS, the reason similar morphological and functional situations may or may not develop muscular pain in different patients has not been ascertained. Researchers have a clearer understanding regarding pathogenic circuits that are activated and that can affect proprioceptive and nociceptive systems. Neurohormonal connections that lower pain threshold at the CNS level are also found to be involved. In the authors' opinion, this should be a major area for future research, potentially resulting in additional therapeutic solutions.

It must be observed that all clinical suggestions for diagnosis found in the general literature are only dealing with anamnestic data and the clinical examination of patients. Special attention has been placed on algometric parameters. No laboratory tests have been performed to identify one or more of the mentioned syndromes. Instead, the authors' proposal of verifying the response of patients to low frequency, high amplitude TENS and the capacity of this stimulation to affect pain can be considered an objective approach. A careful search of the literature covering many years revealed that Arroyo and Cohen[94] had achieved similar results. A brief description of their study, entitled "Abnormal responses to electrocutaneous stimulation in fibromyalgia," can be useful to better understand the consistency of the phenomenon. They used an electronic stimulator (Dynex III, Medtronic Ltd.,

Minneapolis, USA) where the frequency was adjustable from 1 to 100 Hz, the current output was adjustable in increments of 1 mA from 0 to 60 mA, and the pulse width was adjustable in increments of 15 microseconds from 40 to 250 microseconds. Ten FS patients and ten controls were studied; a fixed stimulation frequency of 100 Hz was utilized, and electrodes were applied on five points of the hand not corresponding to habitual tender point sites. Perception threshold resulted to be similar to controls, while pain tolerance was markedly reduced in all FS patients, inducing an intensification of pain. A persistent sensation of burning lasting from 20 seconds to several minutes following stimulation was observed in all patients. The conclusion of the authors was that such phenomena confirm the central origin of pain in FS patients which could interfere with the antinociceptive system (e.g., endogenous peptides action). The authors' conclusions confirm their previous studies on mediation and control of pain.[95]

It is the impression of the authors that low frequency, high amplitude TENS may be used as a tool for differential diagnosis of FS versus MPD; however, more controlled studies must be carried out to confirm these clinical impressions. Our findings are similar to Arroyo and Cohen's research, who showed that individuals suffering from FS respond poorly to high frequency TENS.

Moreover, one should consider some other topics regarding the contents of this paper. It is fundamental to possess adequate understanding of musculoskeletal pain. This will enable one to achieve a more accurate differential diagnosis and, if feasible, a more effective treatment. However, the utility of existing modalities as aids in developing a precise diagnosis is poorly recognized by general health care specialists. Due to this lack of knowledge, opinions regarding MPS have been controversial, and treatment is not well defined. The fundamental advantages reached by means of surface EMG are not sufficiently appreciated in diagnosis by other health care specialists. Moreover, the orthopedic realignment of skeletal structures to eliminate perpetuating factors of muscular impairment is considered by the majority of muscle pain specialists as adjunctive treatment following the physical maneuvers to eliminate TrPs.

The practice of orthopedic realignment is the fundamental basis of any craniomandibular treatment whenever the occlusal malrelationship plays a major role in modifying masticatory muscles' equilibrium. Data collected through clinical experience confirm that TMJ pain is often a referred pain from myofascial TrPs within cervical, as well as masticatory, muscles. Temporomandibular joint referred pain must be distinguished from arthrogenic TMJ pain by means of differential diagnostic data. On the basis of such experience, one can presume that MPS affecting other areas should be treated following the same criteria.

Another concept that should be considered is that in many cases MPS should be regarded as the primary etiologic factor in the development of pain. This may occur concomitantly with other chronic autoimmune diseases, not just in combination with FS as has been commonly reported. This fact could assist ancillary management of patients affected by chronic diseases such as systemic lupus erithematosus, rheumatoid arthritis, etc.

In conclusion, the subject of chronic muscular disorders is still uncertain. Advancements have given health care practioners an improved ability to diagnose MPS while a definitive diagnosis of FS as well as CFS, remain undefined. The only certainty derived from clinical experience and review of the literature is that muscular pain syndromes such as FS, are in fact a reality and may exist with or without other conditions occurring simultaneously. It is rarely localized, and it is most often associated with either MPS or systemic immune diseases. It is also evident that FS is very difficult to treat due to its uncertain origin and pathogenesis. When FS and MPS of the head and neck area overlap, craniomandibular treatment modalities may become ineffective. However, we can assume that our proposed diagnostic procedures, even if not "the gold standard," are the most suitable means at our disposal currently.

The pharmacological treatment of musculoskeletal disorders must finally be considered. We have mentioned above that some central analgesic drugs such as tramadol could be even more effective than antidepressive drugs in treating fibromyalgia. Pharmacologic management of MPS has not been investigated by researchers and has had little emphasis. Nevertheless, it is interesting to consider that in the last few years several studies have been conducted regarding the effects of magnesium in reducing muscle irritability.[96,97] The authors believe that any effort to find a truly effective pharmacological aid in treating musculoskeletal disorders will be a helpful means to support the orthopedic therapies for masticatory disorders.

The possibility that FS might be the result of an improperly treated MPS in patients showing specific disposition toward the onset of the syndrome such as age, central sensitization, neurohormonal alterations, etc., should be also taken into consideration. If such a hypothesis can be validated, proper diagnosis and treatment of any myofascial disorder could represent a valuable protective means against the onset of a secondary FS.

References

1. Fricton J, Kroening R, Haley D: Myofascial Pain and Dysfunction of the Head and Neck: a revue of the clinical characteristics of 164 patients. *Oral Surg Oral Med Oral Pathol* 1985:60;615-623.
2. Jankelson B: Neuromuscular aspects of occlusion. *Dent Clin North Am* 1979:23;157.
3. Simons DG, Travell JG, Simons LS: *Myofascial Pain and Dysfunction—The Trigger Point Manual, 2nd Ed.* Baltimore: William and Wilkins, 1999.
4. Jankelson RR: *Neuromuscular Dental Diagnosis and Treatment.* St. Louis: Ishiyaku EuroAmerica, 1989.
5. Goldenberg DL: Fibromyalgia, chronic fatigue syndrome, and myofascial pain syndrome *Curr Opin Rheumat* 1994:6;223-233.
6. Yunus MB, Masi TA: Fibromyalgia, restless legs syndrome, periodic limb movement disorder, and psychogenic pain. In: McCarty DJ, Koopman WJ, eds. *Arthritis and Allied Conditions Vol. II.* Philadelphia: Lea and Febiger, 1993.
7. Goldenberg DL: Fibromyalgia, chronic fatigue syndrome and myofascial pain syndrome. *Curr Opin Rheumat* 1993:5;199-208.
8. Merskey H: The classification of fibromyalgia and myofascial pain. In: Vaeroy H, Merskey H, eds. *Progress in Fibromyalgia and Myofascial Pain.* Amsterdam: Elsevier Science, 1993.
9. Tunks E: Clinical experimental investigations in fibromyalgia and myofascial pain. In: Vaeroy H, Merskey H, eds. *Progress in Fibromyalgia and Myofascial Pain.* Amsterdam: Elsevier Science, 1993.
10. Korszun A, Papadopoulos E, Demitrack M, Engleberg C, Crofford L: The relationship between temporomandibular disorders and stress-associated syndromes. *Oral Surg Oral Med Oral Pathol Oral Radiol Endod* 1998, 86 (4):416-420.
11. Demitrack MA, Crofford LJ: Evidence for and pathophysiologic implications of hypothalamic-pituitary adrenal axis dysregulation in fibromyalgia and chronic fatigue syndrome. *Ann NY Acad Sci* 1998:840;684-697.
12. Vargo CP, Hickman DM: Cluster-like signs and symptoms respond to myofascial/craniomandibular treatment: a report of two cases. *J Craniomandib Pract* 1997:15;89-93.
13. Bergamini M, Prayer Galletti S, Tonelli P: A classification of musculoskeletal disorders of the stomatognatic apparatus. In: Bergamini M, Prayer Galletti S, eds. *Pathophysiology of Head and Neck Musculoskeletal Disorders, Frontiers of Oral Physiology Vol. 7.* Basel: Karger, 1990.
14. Bergamini M, Prayer Galletti S: Systematic manifestations of musculoskeletal disorders related to masticatory dysfunctions. In: Coy R, ed. *Anthology of Craniomandibular Orthopedics Vol. II.* Collinsville, Illinois: Buchanan Pub., 1992.
15. McCain GA: Fibromyalgia and myofascial pain syndromes. In: Wall PD, Melzack R, eds. *Textbook of Pain, 3rd Ed.* Churchill and Livingstone, 1994.
16. Fricton JR: Myofascial pain syndrome. Characteristics and epidemiology. In: Fricton JR, Awad E, eds. *Advances in Pain Research and Therapy Vol. 17.* New York: Raven Press Ltd., 1990.
17. Simons D: Muscular pain syndromes. In: Fricton JR, Awad E, eds. *Advances in Pain Research and Therapy Vol. 17.* New York: Raven Press Ltd., 1990.
18. Basmajian JV, De Luca CJ: *Muscles Alive, 5th Ed.* Baltimore: Williams and Wilkins, 1985.
19. Cooper BC, Cooper DL, Lucente FE: Electromyography of masticatory muscles in craniomandibular disorders. *Laryngoscope*, 1991:101:150-157.
20. Fricton JR: Management of myofascial pain syndrome. In: Fricton JR, Awad E, eds. *Advances in Pain Research and Therapy Vol. 17.* New York: Raven Press Ltd., 1990.
21. Hench PK: Nonarticular Rheumatism, 22nd rheumatism review: Review of the American and English literature for the years 1973 and 1974. *Arthritis Rheum Suppl.* 1976;19:1081-1089.
22. Moldofsky H, Scarisbrick P, England R, Smythe H: Musculoskeletal symptoms and non-REM sleep disturbance in patients with "fibrositis" syndrome and healthy subjects. *Psychosom Med* 1975;37:341-351.
23. Yunus MB, et al.: Primary fibromyalgia (fibrositis): Clinical study of 50 patients with matched normal controls. *Semin Arthritis Rheum* 1981;11:151-171.
24. Wolfe F, et al.: The American College of Rheumatology 1990 criteria for classification of fibromyalgia: Report of the multicenter criteria committee. *Arthritis Rheum* 1990;33:160-172.
25. Yunus MB, Masi AT, Aldag JC: Preliminary criteria for primary fibromyalgia syndrome (PFS): Multivariate analysis of a consecutive series of PFS, other pain patients and normal subjects. *Clin. Exp. Rheumatol* 1989;7:63-69.

26. Scudds RA, et al.: Pain perception and personality measures as discriminators in the classification of fibrositis. *J Rheumatol* 1987;14:563-569.

27. Granges G, Littlejohn G: Postural and mechanical factors in localized and generalized fibromyalgia/ fibrositis syndrome. In: Vaeroy H, Merskey H, eds. *Progress in Fibromyalgia and Myofascial Pain.* Amsterdam: Elsevier Science, 1993.

28. Wolfe F, Cathey MA: The epidemiology of tender points: A prospective study of 1520 patients. *J Rheumatol* 1985;12:1164-1168.

29. Leavitt F, et al.: Comparison of pain properties in fibromyalgia patients and rheumatoid arthritis patients. *Arthritis Rheum* 1986;29:775-781.

30. Wolfe F: Fibromyalgia: The clinical syndrome. In: Bennett RM, Goldenberg DL, eds. *The Fibromyalgia Syndrome.* Philadelphia: W.B. Saunders Co., 1989.

31. Wolfe F: The clinical syndrome of fibrositis. *Am J Med* 1986;81:7-14.

32. Middleton GD, McFarlin JE, Lipsky PE: The prevalence and clinical impact of fibromyalgia in systemic lupus erythematosus. *Arthritis Rheum* 1994;37(8):1181-1188.

33. Caro XJ: Is there an immunologic component to the fibrositis syndrome? *Rheum Dis Clin North Am* 1989;15:169-186.

34. Clark S, Campbell SM, Forehand ME: Clinical characteristics of fibrositis Vol. II. A "blinded" controlled study using standard psychological tests. *Arthritis Rheum* 1985;28:132-137.

35. Hawley DJ, Wolfe F, Cathey MA: Pain, functional disability and psychological status: a 12-month study of severity in fibromyalgia. *J Rheumatol* 1988;15:1551-1556.

36. Hudson JI, Hudson MS, Plinter LF: Fibromyalgia and major affective disorders: a controlled phenomenology and family history study. *Am J Psychiatry* 1985;142:441-446.

37. Ahles TA, Yunus MB, Masi AT: Is chronic pain a variant of depressive disease? The case of primary fibromyalgia syndrome. *Pain* 1987;29:105-111.

38. Scudds RA, Tratschel LC, Luckhurst BJ, Percy JS: A comparative study of pain, sleep quality, and pain responsiveness in fibrositis and myofascial pain syndrome. *J Rheumatol (suppl)* 1989;19:120-126.

39. Singh BB, Berman BM, Hadhazy VA, Creamer P: A pilot study of cognitive behavioral therapy in fibromyalgia. *Altern Ther Health Med* 1998;4(2):67-70.

40. Sharpe M, Archard L, Banatvala J: Guidelines for research in chronic fatigue syndromes. *J R Soc Med* 1991;84:118-121.

41. Wessely S, Powell R: Fatigue syndromes: a comparison of chronic "postviral" fatigue with neuromuscular and affective disorders. *J Neurol Neurosurg Psychiatry* 1989;42:940-948.

42. Wessely S, Thomas PK: The chronic fatigue syndrome (Myalgic encephalomyelitis or Postviral fatigue). In: Kennard C, ed. *Recent Advances in Neurology Vol. 6.* Edinburgh: Churchill Livingstone, 1990.

43. Wessely S, Newham D: Virus syndromes and chronic fatigue. In: Vaeroy H, Merskey H, eds. *Progress in Fibromyalgia and Myofascial Pain.* Amsterdam: Elsevier Science, 1993.

44. Whelton CL, Salit I, Moldofsky H: Sleep, Epstein-Barr virus infection, musculoskeletal pain, and depressive symptoms. *J Rheumatol* 1992;19: 939-943.

45. Wessely S: The history of the postviral fatigue syndrome. *Br Med Bull* 1991;47:919-941.

46. Sigal LH: Summary of the first 100 patients seen at a Lyme disease referral center. *Am J Med* 1990; 88:577-581.

47. Hsu VM, Patella SJ, Sigal LH: Chronic Lyme disease as the incorrect diagnosis in patients with fibromyalgia. *Arthritis Rheum* 1993;36(11):1493-1500.

48. DeFreitas E, et al.: Retroviral sequences related to human T-lymphotropic virus type II in patients with chronic fatigue immune dysfunction syndrome. *Proc Natl Acad Sci* 1991;88:2922-2926.

49. Berg AM, Naides SJ, Simms RW: Established fibromyalgia syndrome and parvovirus B19 infection. *J Rheumatol* 1993;20:1941-1943.

50. Gow J, et al.: Enteroviral RNA sequences defected by polymerase chain reaction in muscles of patients with post-viral fatigue syndrome. *Br Med J* 1991;302:692-696.

51. Goldenberg DL: Fibromyalgia and other chronic fatigue syndromes: is there evidence for chronic viral disease? *Semin Arthritis Rheum* 1988;18:111-120.

52. Yunus MB, Dailey JW, Aldag JC: Plasma tryptophan and other amino acids in primary fibromyalgia: a controlled study. *J Rheumatol* 1992;19:90-94.

53. Pellegrino MJ, Waylonis GW, Sommer A: Familial occurrence of primary fibromyalgia. *Arch Phys Med Rehab* 1989;70:61-63.
54. Russell IJ, Michalek JE, Vipraio GA: Serum amino acids in fibrositis/fibromyalgia concentration. *J Rheumatol* (suppl.19) 1989;16:158-163.
55. Houvenagel E, Forzy G, Cortet B, Voncent G: 5-Hydroxy indole acetic acid in cerebrospinal fluid in fibromyalgia. *Arthritis Rheum* 1990;33(suppl):55.
56. Russell IJ, et al.: Platelet 3H-imipramine uptake receptor density and serum serotonin levels in patients with fibromyalgia/fibrositis syndrome. *J Rheumatol* 1992;19:104-109.
57. Crofford LJ, et al.: Hypothalamic-pituitary-adrenal axis perturbations in patients with fibromyalgia. *Arthritis Rheum* 1994;37(11):1583-1592.
58. Russell IJ, et al.: Elevated cerebrospinal fluid levels of substance P in patients with the fibromyalgia syndrome. *Arthritis Rheum* 1994;37(11):1593-1601.
59. Murphy RM, Zemlan FP: Differential effects of substance P on serotonin-modulated spinal nociceptive reflexes. *Psychopharmacology* (Berlin) 1987;93:118-121.
60. Bennett RM, Clark SR, Campbell SM, Burckhardt CS: Low levels of somatomedin C in patients with the fibromyalgia syndrome. *Arthritis Rheum* 1992;35(10):1113-1116.
61. Cuneo RC, Salomon F, Wiles CM, Hesp R, Sonksen PH: Growth Hormone treatment in growth hormone-deficient adults. Effects on exercise performance. *J Appl Physiol* 1991;70:695-700.
62. Crist DM, Peake GT, Loftfield RB, Kraner JC, Egan PA: Supplemental growth hormone alters body composition, muscle protein metabolism and serum lipids in fit adults: characterization of dose-dependent and response-recovery effects. *Mech Ageing Dev* 1991;58:191-205.
63. Bagge E, Bengtsson BA, Carlsson L, Carlsson J: Low growth hormone secretion in patients with fibromyalgia—a preliminary report on 10 patients and 10 controls. *J Rheumatol* 1998;25:145-148.
64. Moldofsky H, Scarisbrick P, England R, Smythe H: Musculoskeletal symptoms and non-REM sleep disturbance in patients with "fibrositis syndrome" and healthy subjects. *Psychosom Med* 1975;37:341-351.
65. Jacobsen S, et al.: Primary fibromyalgia: clinical parameters in relation to serum procollagen type III aminoterminal peptide. *Br J Rheumatol* 1990;29:174-177.
66. Granges G, Littlejohn G: Pressure pain threshold in pain-free subjects, in patients with chronic regional pain syndromes, and in patients with fibromyalgia syndrome. *Arthritis Rheum* 1993;36(5):642-646.
67. Russell IJ: Advances in fibromyalgia: possible role for central neurochemicals. *Am J Med Sci* 1998;315:377-384.
68. Goldenberg DL: Fibromyalgia syndrome: an emerging but controversial condition. *J Am Med Assoc* 1987;257:2782-2787.
69. Burda CD, Cox FR, Osborne P: Histocompatibility antigens in the fibrositis (fibromyalgia) syndrome. *Clin Exp Rheumatol* 1986;4:355-357.
70. Wallace DJ, et al.: Fibromyalgia, cytokines, fatigue syndromes and immune regulation. In: Fricton JR, Awad EA, eds. *Advances in Pain Research and Therapy Vol. 17.* New York: Raven Press, 1989.
71. Komaroff AL, Goldenberg D: The chronic fatigue syndrome: Definition, current studies and lessons for fibromyalgia research. *J Rheumatol* 1989;16(suppl.19):23-27.
72. Krueger JM, Karnovsky ML: Sleep and the immune response. *Ann NY Acad Sci* 1987;6:496-510.
73. Jacobsen S, et al.: Screening for autoantibodies in patients with primary fibromyalgia syndrome and a matched control group. *APMIS* 1990;98:655-658.
74. Tirelli U, Marotta G, Improta S, Pinto A. Immunological abnormalities in patients with chronic fatigue syndrome. *Scand J Immunol* 1994;40: 601-608.
75. Greene RL: *The MMPI-2/MMPI: An interpretive manual.* Boston: Allyn and Bacon, 1991.
76. Yunus MB, Ahles TA, Aldag JC, Masi AT: Relationship of clinical features with psychologic status in primary fibromyalgia. *Arthritis Rheum* 1991;34: 15-21.
77. Ellertsen B, et al.: MMPI in fibromyalgia and local nonspecific myalgia. *New Trends Exp Clin Psychiatry* 1991;7:53-62.
78. Ellertsen B, Troland K, Vaeroy H: Psychological assessment of patients with musculoskeletal pain. In: Vaeroy H, Merskey H, eds. *Progress in Fibromyalgia and Myofascial Pain.* Amsterdam: Elsevier Science, 1993
79. Taylor ML, Trotter DR, Csuka ME: The prevalence of sexual abuse in women with fibromyalgia. *Arthritis Rheum* 1995;38(2):229-234.

80. Simons DG: Referral phenomena of myofascial trigger points. In: Vecchiet L, et al., eds. *Pain Research and Clinical Management: New Trends in Referred Pain and Hyperalgesia Vol. 27.* Amsterdam: Elzevier Science, 1993;341-357.

81. Yunus MB: Towards a model of pathophysiology of fibromyalgia: aberrant central pain mechanisms with peripheral modulation. *J Reumatol* 1992;19:846-849

82. Bengtsson M, Bengtsson A, Jordfeldt L: Diagnostic epidural opioid blockade in primary fibromyalgia at rest and during exercise. *Pain* 1989;39:171-180.

83. Bengtsson A, Bengtsson M: Regional sympathetic blockade in primary fibromyalgia. *Pain* 1988;33:161-167.

84. Willis WD: The Pain System: The Neural Basis of Nociceptive Transmission. In: *Mammalian Nervous System.* Karger, 1985.

85. Guedj D, Weinberger A: Effect of weather conditions on rheumatic patients. *Annals of the Rheumatic Diseases* 1990;49:158-159.

86. Goldman BL, Rosenberg MD: Myofasial Pain Syndrome and Fibromyalgia. *Seminars in Neurology* Vol. II, 1991; 3:274-279.

87. Quimby LG, Block SR, Gratwick GM: Fibromyalgia: Generalized pain intolerance and manifold symptom reporting. *J Rheumatol* 1988;15:1264-1270.

88. Erickson PP, et al.: Symptoms and signs of mandibular dysfunction in primary fibromyalgia syndrome. *Swed Dent J* 1988;122:141-149.

89. Littlejohn GO: Fibrositis/fibromyalgia syndrome in the workplace. *Rheum. Dis. Clin. North Am.* 1989,15:45-60

90. Hedenberg L, Magnusson B, Ernberg M, Kopp S: Symptoms and signs of temporomandibular disorders in patients with fibromyalgia and local myalgia of the temporomandibular system. A comparative study. *Acta Odontol Scand* 1997; 55(6):344-349.

91. Goldenberg DL: Fibromyalgia, chronic fatigue syndrome, and myofascial pain syndrome. *Curr Opin Rheumatol* 1997;9(2):135-143.

92. Bennett R: Fibromyalgia, chronic fatigue syndrome and myofascial pain. *Curr Opin Rheumatol* 1998;10(2):95-103.

93. Thomas NR: The effect of fatigue and TENS on the EMG mean power frequency. In: Bergamini M, Prayer Galletti, eds. Pathophysiology of Head and Neck Musculoskeletal Disorders. *Front Oral Physiol Vol. VII.* Basel: Karger; 1990:162-170.

94. Arroyo JF, Cohen ML: Abnormal responses to electrocutaneous stimulation in Fibromyalgia. *J Rheumatol* 1993;20:1925-1933.

95. Bergamini M, Pantaleo T, Prayer Galletti S: Neurophysiological mechanisms involved in the mediation and control of musculoskeletal pain as a basis for the therapeutic approach. In: Coy R, ed. *Anthology of Craniomandibular Orthopedics Vol. III.* Illinois, Buchanan Pub., 1994.

96. Castelli S, et al.: Magnesium in the prophylaxis of primary headache and other periodic disorders in children. *Pediatr Med Chir* 1993;15(5):481-488.

97. Thomas J, et al.: Migraine treatment by oral magnesium intake and correction of the irritation of buccofacial and cervical muscles as a side effect of mandibular imbalance. *Magnes Rtes* 1994;7(2):123-127.

Evaluation of Patients with Facial Pain and/or Craniomandibular Disorders

D. Gary Wolford

Historically, temporomandibular joint disorders (TMD) involve specific clinical findings. In 1934 Costen[1] described what became temporomandibular joint (TMJ) syndrome to include (1) preauricular pain, (2) tenderness to palpation of the elevator muscles of the mandible, (3) decreased oral opening, and (4) TMJ noise. Joint noise during the period of 1970 through 1990 was specifically defined as a reciprocal clicking caused by displacement of the articulator disc anterior to the condylar head on closure and reducing to a normal position on opening. In 1969, Laskin[2] introduced the term myofascial pain disorders (MPD) to include patients who had preauricular pain, decreased opening, and pain to palpation of the elevator muscles of the mandible. Farrar and McCarty[3] defined internal derangements as a condition resulting from a tear of the discal ligament(s) that leads to reciprocal clicking in the temporomandibular (TM) joint. Reciprocal clicking refers to TM joint noise occurring during opening and closing. The opening click occurs at a greater incisal opening than the closing click. They also noted that with internal derangements radiographic imaging of the condyles showed posterior positioning in maximum occlusion.

Review of the literature revealed no generally accepted inclusive differential diagnostic paradigm. Bell[4] published "Categories of Temporomandibular Disorders" and placed hypomobility and growth disorders in the same category. He did not include subluxation of the condyle. The author will present clinical results which reveal that subluxation of the mandibular condyles occurs much more frequently than is reported in the literature. Over the last ten to fifteen years, temporomandibular joint disorders have become a "catch-all" term for dentists, physicians, and lay people. The best term to classify mandibular dysfunction is craniomandibular disorders. The following classification of craniomandibular disorders includes the majority of factors that can affect mandibular movement and function. The classification is the result of 30 years of clinical evaluation and treatment of patients with craniomandibular disorders. Additionally, this hierarchy should complement deficiencies in other classification schemes. More than 8000 patients have been evaluated.

The hierarchy to be presented is a functional classification system in which seven subdivisions represent pathology resulting from injury, dysfunction, or developmental abnormalities of specific craniomandibular anatomical sites.

Craniomandibular disorders include dysfunction, injury, inflammation, or developmental abnormalities of the muscles that move the mandible, discal ligament (which attaches the articular disc to the condyle) tears, intra-articular disorders, extra-articular disorders, capsular ligament (which hold the condyle in the glenoid fossa) tears, skeletal abnormalities, and traumatic injuries. Masticatory muscles move the mandible, and ligaments limit joint movement. The discal and capsular ligaments limit disc/condyle movement and condyle/fossa movement. If the medial and lateral discal ligaments are torn, there will be excessive movement of the articular disc with respect to condylar movement. If the capsular ligament is torn, the mandibular condyle will move anterior to the articular eminence on opening. A capsular ligament tear may involve fibers that limit anterior translation of the condyle. A tear of the capsular ligament does not imply a hole or defect of the ligament, but a distortion of the connective tissue matrix creating stretched, distorted capsular tissue. Skeletal malrelationships refer to abnormal maxillary and mandibular growth. Traumatic injuries refer to fractures of the jaws or teeth that are treated differently from all other subdivisions. Trauma that does not produce a fracture (whiplash, direct trauma) can produce dysfunction in all subdivisions.

An extensive review of the literature did not reveal any classification that included all of the following subdivisions.

Functional Classification of Craniomandibular Disorders

I. Masticatory Muscle Disorders (muscle pain)
   1. Protective Muscle Splinting
   2. Muscle Spasm Activity
   3. Muscle Inflammation
II. Disc Interference Disorders (internal derangements)
   1. Early Derangement
   2. Mid Derangement
   3. Late Derangement
   4. Dislocated Disc
III. Inflammatory Disorders of the Joint (joint pain)
   1. Synovitis and Capsulitis
   2. Retrodiscitis
   3. Inflammatory Arthritis
      A. Degenerative Arthritis
      B. Traumatic Arthritis
IV. Chronic Mandibular Hypomobilities (decreased movement of mandible)
   1. Contracture of Elevator Muscles
   2. Capsular Fibrosis
   3. Ankylosis
      A. Fibrous
      B. Osseous
   4. Coronoid Hyperplasia
V. Mandibular Hypermobilities (excessive movement of mandible)
   1. Subluxation
      A. Associated with Internal Derangement
      B. Disc Condyle Function Normal
   2. Spontaneous Dislocation of the Condyle
   3. Chronic (recurrent) Dislocation of the condyle
VI. Growth Disorders of the Jaws (skeletal malrelationships)
   1. Aberration of Development
      A. Vertical Maxillary Deficiency
      B. Vertical Maxillary Excess
      C. Apertognathia
      D. Asymmetry
   2. Acquired Change in Joint Structure
   3. Unilateral Condylar Hyperplasia
VII. Traumatic Injuries (fractures of the jaw and/or teeth)
   1. Fracture
      A. Open
      B. Closed
      C. Non-displaced
      D. Displaced
   2. Hemarthrosis

The Functional Classification of Craniomandibular Disorders is divided into seven categories, which are indicated by Roman numerals. Each of the subdivisions under the Roman numerals is listed in order of lesser to more severe conditions. Masticatory Muscle Disorders (I) are the dysfunctions of the elevator and lateral pterygoid muscles. Pure masticatory muscle disorders have no joint noise. Disc Interference Disorders (II)[3] typically have reciprocal clicks with the opening click occurring at a greater incisal opening than the closing click. Inflammatory Disorders (III)[4] are intracapsular disorders. Chronic Mandibular Hypomobilities (IV)[4] have decreased mandibular opening and are painless unless attempts are made to increase the range of movement. Mandibular Hypermobilities (V)[5] are excessive movement of the mandibular condyles. Growth Disorders (VI) refer to skeletal malrelationships between the maxilla and mandible, and in the author's opinion they should be evaluated in both maximum intercuspation and in myocentric position. Traumatic Injuries (VII) refer to fractures of the facial bones and hemarthrosis (intercapsular hemorrhage). Fractures are obviously treated differently than the conditions in categories I–VI. Hemarthrosis could be included in category III, but because it is an acute emergency, hemarthrosis is included in the trauma category. Trauma that does not produce a fracture, and that is not properly or successfully treated, can produce dysfunction in categories I–VI.

I. Masticatory Muscle Disorders (muscle pain)
1. Protective Muscle Splinting
2. Muscle Spasm Activity
3. Muscle Inflammation

Normal incisal opening is 50 mm (the distance between the incisal edge of the maxillary incisors to the incisal edge of the mandibular incisors on wide opening). Patients who open past 50 mm of incisal opening subluxate, as verified by fluoroscopy and axially corrected tomography in an unpublished study.[6] Patients with protective muscle splinting typically have an incisal opening which can be increased to 50 mm with gentle passive opening of the patient's lower jaw with finger pressure. Muscle spasm is defined when the incisal distance cannot be increased to 50 mm with finger pressure. Trigger points can be palpated in the masseter, medial pterygoid, and temporalis muscles. Muscle inflammation (myositis) most commonly occurs with pericoronitis of the mandibular third molars or as a result of multiple inferior alveolar nerve injections. The incisal opening is usually less than 30 mm and cannot be increased by finger manipulation. Lateral excursions are usually normal (10 mm) unless the lateral pterygoid muscle is involved in which case lateral excursions to the contralateral side will be decreased. Post injection myositis (PIM) usually starts 3–5 days after the injections and produces a marked reduction of incisal opening (less than 20 mm) and may take up to three months to resolve. PIM is seen in patients who have undergone multiple inferior alveolar nerve injections with the same needle.

II. Disc Interference Disorders (internal derangements)
1. Early Derangement
2. Mid Derangement
3. Late Derangement
4. Dislocated Disc

Patients with internal derangement have a reciprocal click on opening and closing. The opening click is always at a greater incisal opening than the closing click. The click is produced following a tear of the discal ligament(s) which attach the articular disc to the condylar head. The disc will move with respect to condylar movement, but it cannot be displaced if the discal ligaments are intact.[3] When discal ligaments are torn, the disc is normally displaced anteromedially to the condyle as a result of anteromedial tension or pull of the superior head of the lateral pterygoid muscle, and/or the posterior or posterosuperior position of the condyles within the glenoid fossa when in maximum intercuspation.

An anteriorly displaced disc with reduction (reciprocal click) will be positioned or displaced anterior to the condyle when the teeth are in maximum intercuspation. During opening the condyle translates anteriorly engaging the posterior aspect of the disc. As opening continues the condyle translates over the posterior portion of the articular disc producing a clicking noise (disc reduced) which may be felt and/or heard. On closure the disc will translate anterior to the condyle and produce a closing click (disc displaced anteriorly). In patients with a closed lock, the disc remains anterior to the condyle on opening, and there is no opening or closing click. Based on clinical evaluation of over 8000 patients, early derangement is defined as an opening click that occurs within 0–20 mm of opening, mid derangement between 20–35 mm of opening, and late derangement at an incisal opening greater than 35 mm. A dislocated disc (closed lock) is defined as a disc displacement that no longer reduces on opening. The patient will give a history of reciprocal joint clicking, but over time their TM joint noise disappeared. Opening is usually less than 35 mm in the chronic condition; however, this can be much less in an acute situation. A careful differential diagnosis must be formulated with a patient who has limited oral opening. Consideration between muscle inflammation, myositis, chronic hypomobilities, and a dislocated disc or a combination must be determined. Normal lateral excursions are 10 mm. Patients with myositis of the masseter and medial pterygoid will have a marked, limited opening, but their lateral excursions may be normal. In patients with a dislocated disc (closed lock), opening and lateral excursions will be restricted. This condition will permit the patient no more than 3–5 mm of lateral movement toward the contralateral (unaffected) side. They will have normal excursions in lateral movement toward the affected side.

III. Inflammatory Disorders of the Joint (joint pain)
1. Synovitis and Capsulitis
2. Retrodiscitis
3. Inflammatory Arthritis
A. Degenerative Arthritis
B. Traumatic Arthritis

Synovitis and capsulitis refer to inflammatory intracapsular pathology in which the patient has pain on wide opening and palpation of the temporomandibular joint with the teeth separated or with the mouth open wide. Retrodiscitis occurs when the patient has pain and discomfort on closing or when the condyle is manipulated posterosuperiorly. One must be very careful to rule out referred pain. Inflammatory changes in the joint include degenerative and traumatic arthritis. These will have radiographic evidence of loss of condylar contour, erosions, or sclerosis that may involve the anterior aspect of the glenoid fossa and condylar head when evaluated with axially corrected tomograms. Arthritic changes exhibit crepitus on opening and closing.

IV. Chronic Mandibular Hypomobilities (decreased movement of mandible)
1. Contracture of Elevator Muscles
2. Capsular Fibrosis
3. Ankylosis
A. Fibrous
B. Osseous
4. Coronoid Hyperplasia

These conditions limit mandibular opening and may reduce lateral excursions. The movements are painless unless an attempt is made to increase the opening. There are no joint noises in pure mandibular hypomobilities. Hypomobility may be the result of connective tissue disease (i.e., slceroderma or lupus erythematosis), following trauma (capsular fibrosis, fibrous and osseous ankylosis), and skeletal abnormalities (coronoid hyperplasia). It must be emphasized that these conditions are painless, but result in decreased opening and occasionally decreased lateral excursions. In unilateral cases, decreased condylar translation is limited, creating a decreased lateral excursion to the contralateral side. In the author's experience, coronoid hyperplasia is seen in patients with chronic internal derangements, chronic clenching, bruxism, and in patients with a posterior closure pattern.

V. Mandibular Hypermobilities (excessive movement of mandible)
1. Subluxation
A. Associated with Internal Derangement
B. Disc Condyle Function Normal
2. Spontaneous Dislocation of the Condyle
3. Chronic (recurrent) Dislocation of Condyle

Hypermobility is most commonly misdiagnosed as internal derangements. Subluxation results from a tear of the capsular ligament. Subluxation occurs when the mandibular condyle translates past the most dependent (most convex) portion of the articular eminence, with a resultant positioning (locking) beyond the articular eminence preventing the mandible from returning to maximum intercuspation. This may be diagnosed with fluoroscopy or tomograms of the temporomandibular joint. Subluxation is the most commonly misdiagnosed or undiagnosed craniomandibular disorder. This clinical presentation may require manipulation of the condyle. Subluxation of the condyle can occur with or without internal derangements. If subluxation occurs with an associated internal derangement, there will be two joint sounds on opening and two joint sounds on closing. This condition is very difficult to treat conservatively because both the discal and capsular ligaments have been torn. A subluxation of the condyle reduces when the condyle returns to the glenoid fossa on closure. With a dislocation, the condyle remains anterior to the articular eminence, and the patient is unable to close their teeth together. Manipulation of the mandible is necessary to reduce the dislocation. Some patients will show subluxation on opening, but not on lateral excursions. Others may show subluxation on lateral excursions, but not on opening.

VI. Growth Disorders of the Jaws (skeletal malrelationships)
1. Aberration of Development
A. Vertical Maxillary Deficiency
B. Vertical Maxillary Excess
C. Apertognathia
D. Asymmetry
2. Acquired Change in Joint Structure
3. Unilateral Condylar Hyperplasia

Vertical maxillary deficiency is defined clinically in a patient who does not show maxillary incisors with the teeth at rest or smiling. These individuals normally have a mandibular plane angle that is less than 25 degrees. Vertical maxillary excess is defined in patients who show maxillary mucosa above the maxillary anterior teeth when smiling. These patients generally have a mandibular plane angle greater than 30 degrees.

Apertognathia can be anterior, posterior, or a lateral open bite. Anterior apertognathia must be evaluated to rule out a skeletal or functional condition. Posterior apertognathia usually occurs after iatrogenic treatment for jaw dysfunction, excessive anterior mandibular growth, or with decreased posterior maxillary growth. Lateral apertognathia may be due to abnormal mandibular growth or tongue habit. Mandibular asymmetry will produce abnormal opening and closing. Acquired change in joint structure must be evaluated. The mandibular condyle adapts to pressure during mastication, and patients with posterior closure patterns may develop a bowing or anterior curvature of the condyle (hyperplastic changes). Unilateral condylar hyperplasia is one sided, post pubertal growth of the condyle, producing a mandibular asymmetry. Skeletal relationships should be evaluated in maximum intercuspation and on myotrajectory.

VII. Traumatic Injuries (fractures of the jaw and teeth)

1. Fracture

A. Open

B. Closed

C. Non-displaced

D. Displaced

2. Hemarthrosis

Traumatic injuries include fractures of the mandible, maxilla, zygoma, and teeth. These are usually treated with an attempt to return the patient to form and function. In the author's thirty years of experience, patients who sustain mandibular and/or midface fractures that are appropriately treated rarely develop craniomandibular disorders.

Hemarthrosis is the acute emergency that occurs when a patient sustains trauma to the mandible producing bleeding within the temporomandibular joint capsule. These injuries should be treated as an emergency with a soft mandibular bite guard. This will decrease continued trauma to the intracapsular structures that may occur during swallowing or other functional movements.

Benign and malignant neoplasms (primary or metastatic), infections, neuralgias, and odontogenic and non-odontogenic lesions are clinical entities seen in patients who present with facial pain. Thus, appropriate imaging is important to aid in the diagnosis, as well as eliminate other possible causes, of the pain and/or dysfunction. Panoramic radiography is recommended as a general screening radiograph.[7] A properly exposed panogram will reveal the relationship between the upper and lower teeth, and the maxillary sinuses, as well as image odontogenic and non-odontogenic lesions in the maxilla and/or the mandible. Styloid ligaments may be visualized (rule out Eagles syndrome), as well as coronoid hyperplasia, and maxillary and mandibular asymmetry. The panogram is not a satisfactory radiograph to evaluate condyle-fossa relationships. A modified panogram taken in a maximum opening position can reveal a subluxation of the mandibular condyles. The presence or absence of dental caries as an initiating factor in producing facial pain can be evaluated with the panogram. The panogram should be taken with the teeth in maximum intercuspation.

Since a large number of skeletal asymmetries and abnormal relationships are seen in patients with craniomandibular disorders, lateral cephalometric radiographs are taken on all patients who have craniomandibular disorders. This reveals the relationship of the maxilla to the mandible and to the cranial base, as well as the relationship of the maxillary and mandibular teeth. The cephalometric radiograph is taken with the teeth in maximum intercuspation and will show the relationship of the maxilla to the mandible (skeletal and dental), and it is used to identify skeletal asymmetry. With facial asymmetry, an A/P cephalometric radiograph can also be taken to document skeletal relationships.

In all patients with craniomandibular disorders, a submental vertex is recommended to allow for axially corrected tomograms. The initial tomograms are taken in 3 to 5 mm cuts depending on the width of the condylar head. This is determined by evaluating the submental vertex radiograph. There are three views taken in the sagittal plane with the teeth in maximum intercuspation and one in maximum opening. With axially corrected tomograms, the practitioner may easily determine condylar position in maximum intercuspation, and identify degenerative and/or proliferative changes of the condylar head, as well as sclerotic changes in the fossa and condyle.[7] Additionally, in the wide-open view, subluxation of the mandibular condyle can be confirmed.

Transcranial radiographs are used by many practitioners, but incorrectly interpreted. Since the angulation of the radiation source to the film passes downward through the temporomandibular joint, the radiograph shows the most lateral aspect of the glenoid fossa and the most lateral aspect of the condyle.[8] A transcranial film does not reveal an accurate relationship of the articulating surfaces and their relationship to one another.

Arthrograms are the most accurate radiographic evaluations of the disc-condyle relationship. The author has modified the technique by mixing 1:1 marcaine 0.5% and 1:100,000 epinephrine with contrast media. The discomfort is minimal with the addition of the marcaine. Additionally, the marcaine provides anesthesia to the retrodiscal tissue. Arthrography is the only radiographic modality that can identify a perforation of the disc and/or retrodiscal tissue. Utilizing arthrography, the practitioner can observe recapture of the disc and resurface the orthotic to maintain this position. Fluoroscopy is used with arthrography, allowing for evaluation of TM joint function and biomechanics.

Magnetic Resonance Imaging (MRI) has been proposed as an aid in diagnosing internal derangements of the TMJ. However, in the author's clinical experience, less than 30% of MRIs provide accurate information because the patients are lying flat on their back, as the study is performed. Many patients are aware that they do not have reciprocal clicking when lying down and that the clicking returns when they are in an upright position.

In a recent study of 125 consecutive facial pain patients diagnosed with internal derangements, 105 of the 125 patients had a subluxation, and none had been previously diagnosed with this condition. Additionally, 73% of the patients had a posterior or a posterosuperior positioning of the condyles in the glenoid fossa. No degenerative conditions were identified in this group.

Preliminary Clinical Results

125 Consecutive Facial Pain Patients

Evaluation of patients with facial pain and/or craniomandibular disorders may include the patient's chief complaint, detailed history, clinical examination, electromyography, computerized mandibular scanning, sonography, and appropriate radiographic evaluation. The information required may vary from patient to patient. There are more than 200 disease entities[9] that can produce facial pain and/or craniomandibular disorders. In the author's experience, approximately 20% of the disorders produce 99% of facial pain and/or craniomandibular disorders, and these are contained in the Functional Classification of Craniomandibular Disorders. A recent survey of 125 facial pain patients referred to my practice with a diagnosis of internal derangements were either misdiagnosed or incompletely diagnosed as to the condition producing their pain and/or dysfunction. There are many different published classifications of conditions that may produce orofacial pain. The most common disease entities that produce facial pain are craniomandibular disorders.

These patients were evaluated clinically and radiographically with axially corrected tomograms in maximum intercuspation. Surprisingly, none of the 125 patients had degenerative changes of their temporomandibular joints. Internal derangements were diagnosed clinically and with the use of computerized mandibular scanning. Subluxation was diagnosed with axially corrected tomograms and computerized mandibular scanning. Posteriorly positioned condyles were diagnosed utilizing axially corrected tomograms, as were hyperplastic condylar changes. The following diagnostic combinations were identified in the 125 patients *(Figure 1)*.

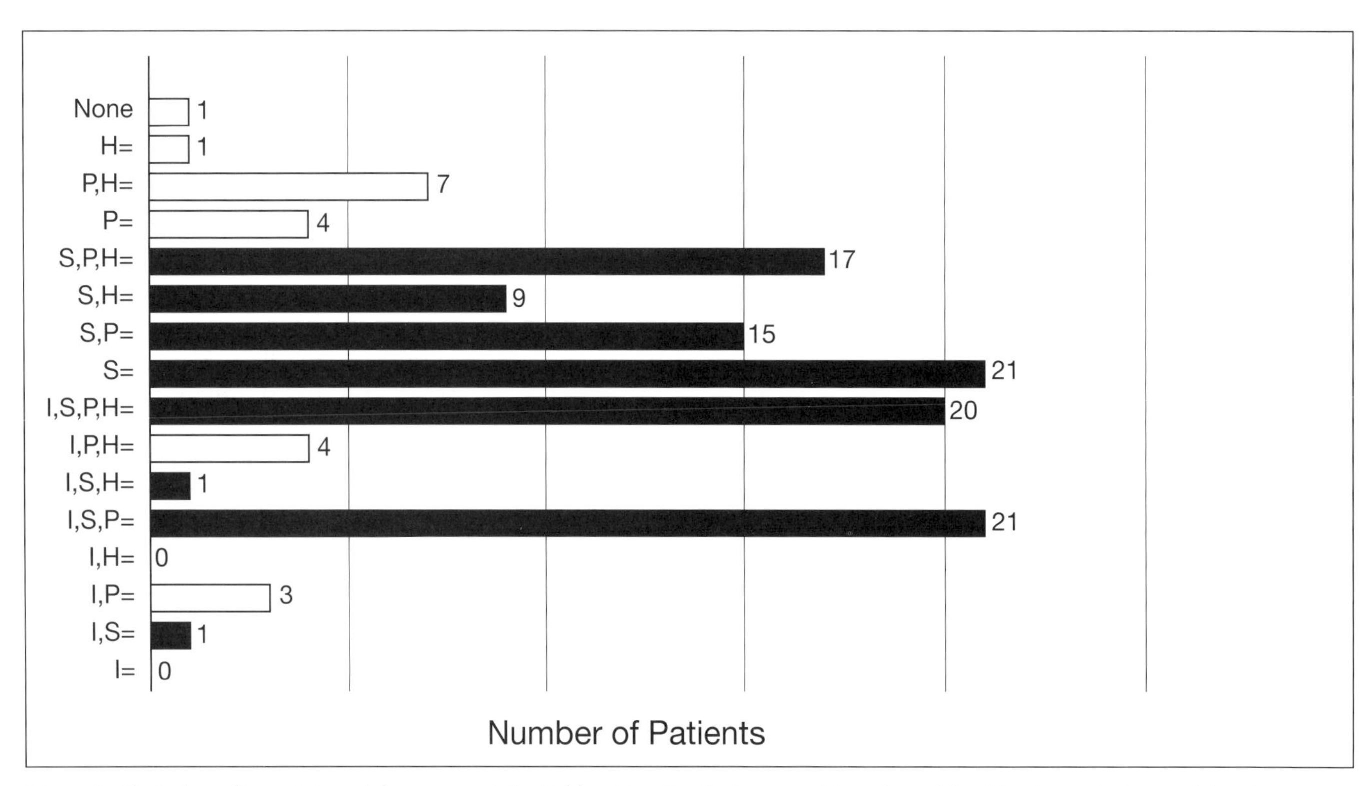

Figure 1. Clinical results. I = Internal derangement; S = Subluxation; P = Posterior positioned condyles; H = Hyperplastic condylar changes.

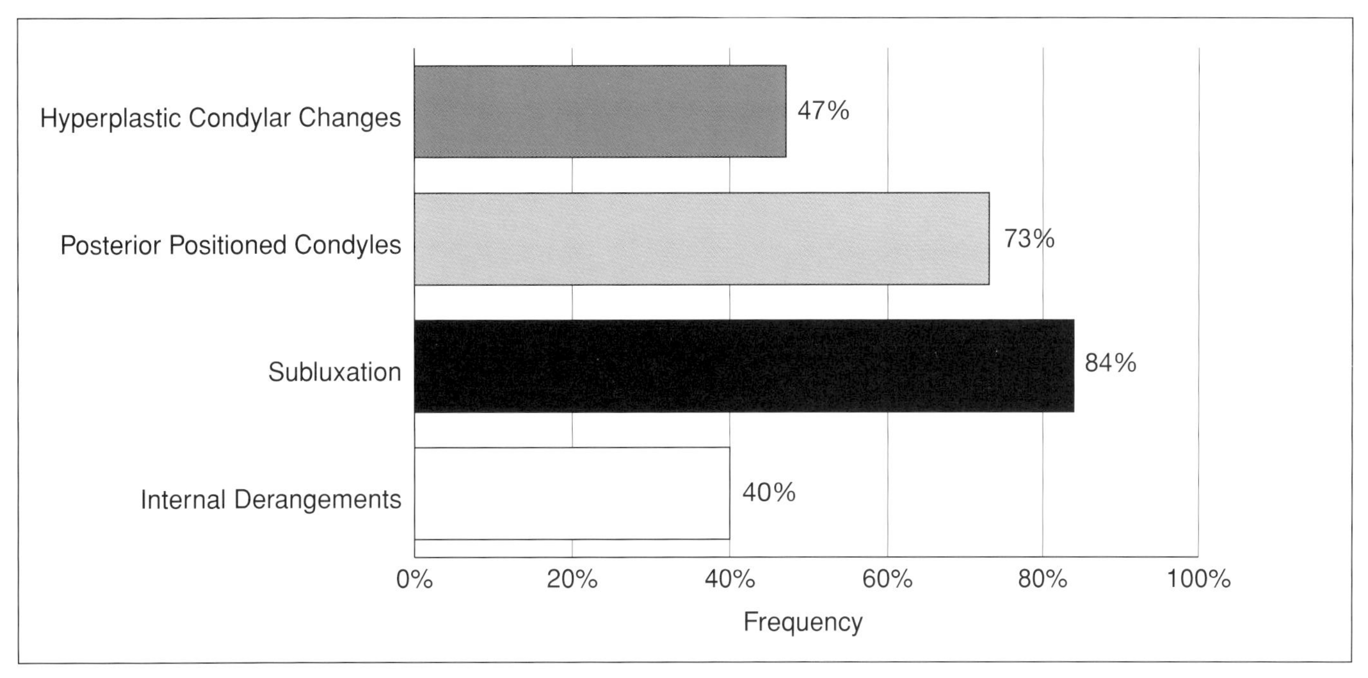

Figure 2.

As indicated in *Figure 1*, subluxation can occur as the sole disorder or in combination with various other dysfunctions/disorders. Subluxation is more common than reported in the literature and is often misdiagnosed as an internal derangement.

The frequencies of the diagnoses in the 125 patients are indicated in *Figure 2*.

None of the 125 patients in *Figure 2* with subluxation, posterior positioned condyles, or hyperplastic condylar changes were correctly diagnosed.

These patients were also evaluated with electromyography (EMG), computerized mandibular scanning (CMS), and sonography (ESG) [(K6-I, Myotronics-Noromed)]. The CMS scans obtained on each patient were scans 1–8 and 13. The EMG scans obtained were scans 9–12. The following muscles were evaluated:

1. Anterior temporalis—Ta
2. Posterior temporalis—Tp
3. Masseter—Mm
4. Digastric—Da

Correlation of scans 3, 4, 6, 8, and 12 are not included in this study.

Scan Definitions

Scan 1—Simultaneous sagittal and frontal registration of opening and closing movements of the mandible. This aids in diagnosing pathological closing patterns.

Scan 2—Simultaneous velocity and frontal-lateral movement in opening and closing to aid in the diagnosis of internal derangements, subluxation, deviation, bradykinesia, and dyskinesia of mandibular movement.

Scan 5—Measures sagittal and frontal mandibular closure patterns after masticatory muscle relaxation. Proper utilization will aid in the construction of a repositioning orthotic appliance to a physiologic position.

Scan 7—Simultaneous velocity and frontal-lateral movement in opening and closing following relaxation of the muscles of mastication.

Scan 9—Measures the resting activity of the muscles. This aids in determining hyper or hypotonicity prior to muscle relaxation.

Scan 10—Measures resting activity of the muscles following muscle relaxation. These values are compared with scan 9 and aid in treatment planning and in the decision to utilize muscle relaxants or not.

Scan 11—Measures clenching function of the masticatory muscles with natural teeth, control (cotton), and orthotic pre-relaxation.

Scan 13—Measures the opening, closing, lateral, and protrusive movements, and pre and post relaxation.

Scan 15—Records the sound vibrations emitted from the left and right joints and the corresponding mandibular movement (vertical and velocity) during opening and closing. The joint sounds can then be analyzed to assess the status of the temporomandibular joint.

I. Masticatory Muscle Disorders (muscle pain)
   1. Protective muscle splinting
      a. EMG
         1. Resting (scan 9)—variable
         2. Post pulse (scan 10)—normal
         3. Clench (scan 11)—centric occlusion (CO) less than control (cotton)

b. CMS
1. Decreased opening (scan 13) less than 50 mm.
2. Assisted opening (scan 13) to 45–50 mm.
3. Posterior closure (Scan 5)

c. ESG
1. No noise

2. Muscle Spasm Activity

a. EMG
1. Resting (scan 9)—variable
2. Post-pulse (scan 10)—normal
3. Clench (scan 11)—CO less than control

b. CMS
1. Decreased opening (scan 13) 25–35 mm, cannot assist to 50 mm
2. May or may not have a deviation on opening
3. Posterior closure (scan 5)

c. ESG
1. No noise

3. Muscle Inflammation (myositis)

a. EMG
1. Resting (scan 9)—variable
2. Post pulse (scan 10)—variable, usually elevated
3. Clench (scan 11)—may not increase with control

b. CMS
1. Marked decreased opening (scan 13) 0–20 mm
2. Cannot increase opening with assistance (scan 13)
3. May not have posterior closure pattern (scan 5)
4. Normal lateral excursion (scan 13) 10 mm, if the lateral pterygoid muscles are not involved

c. ESG
1. No noise

II. Disc Interference Disorders (internal derangements)

1. Early derangement (opening click 0–20 mm)

a. EMG
1. Resting (scan 9)—variable
2. Clench (scan 11)—decreased Mm function, increased Mm function with control

b. CMS
1. Opening click (scan 2) 0–20 mm
2. Closing click (scan 2)—closer to occlusion than opening click
3. Abnormal opening and closure (scan 1)
4. Posterior closure to myotrajectory (scan 5)

c. ESG
1. Opening noise at a greater incisal opening than closing noise

2. Mid derangement (Opening click 20–35 mm)

a. EMG
1. Resting (scan 9)—Ta elevated, Mm variable
2. Clench (scan 11)—decreased Mm function, increased Mm function with control

b. CMS
1. Opening click (scan 2) 20–35 mm
2. Closing click (scan 2)—closer to occlusion than opening click
3. Abnormal opening and closing (scan 1)
4. Posterior closure to myotrajectory (scan 5)

c. ESG
1. Opening noise at a greater incisal opening than closing noise.

3. Late derangement (opening click 35–50 mm)

a. EMG
1. Resting (scan 9)—Ta elevated, Mm variable
2. Clench (scan 11)—Ta, Mm decreased; Tm, Mm increased with control

b. CMS
1. Opening click (scan 2) 20–35 mm
2. Closing click (scan 2)—closer to occlusion than opening click
3. Abnormal opening and closing (scan 1)
4. Posterior closure to myotrajectory (scan 5)

c. ESG
1. Opening noise at a greater incisal opening than closing noise

4. Dislocated disc (closed lock)

a. EMG
1. Resting (scan 9) increased Ta, Tp, Mm
2. Clench (scan 11) minimal values Ta, Mm

b. CMS
1. Decreased opening click (scan 13) 20–35 mm
2. Decreased lateral excursions (scan 13)—0–7 mm
3. May not have posterior closure (scan 5)

c. ESG
1. No noise

III. Inflammatory Disorders of the Joint (joint pain)

a. EMG
1. Variable

b. CMS
1. Variable

c. ESG
1. Variable

IV. Chronic Mandibular Hypomobilities (decreased movement)

a. EMG
1. Resting and clenching values (scans 9 and 11)—normal

b. CMS
1. Decreased opening (scan 13)

2. Closes on trajectory (scan 5)
3. Decreased lateral excursions (scan 13)

c. ESG

1. No noise

V. Mandibular hypermobilities (excessive movement)

1. Subluxation

a. EMG

1. Resting (scan 9)—variable Ta, Tp, usually elevated
2. Clenching (scan 11)—Usually normal

b. CMS

1. Subluxation (scans 1, 2, 7, and 13)
2. Opening greater than 50 mm (scan 13)
3. Lateral excursions greater than 10 mm (scan 13)
4. May have opening less than 50 mm if associated with muscle spasm of Ta and Mm

c. ESG

1. Variable

VI. Growth Disorders of the Jaws (skeletal malrelationships)

Not measured

VII. Traumatic Injuries

Not measured

Summary

Presented is a Functional Classification of Craniomandibular Disorders with diagnostic guidelines, which is a compilation of clinical and objective data gathered from the evaluation and treatment of patients suffering from facial pain of various origins. The clinical study presented demonstrated that of 125 patients the most common craniomandibular disorder was subluxation. This is rarely diagnosed by dental or medical practitioners. These results indicate that the clinician must be cautious to carefully consider subluxation as the primary disorder or in combination with other conditions which commonly affect the craniomandibular apparatus, particularly internal derangement. Furthermore, the allied application of computerized instrumentation (EMG, CMS, and ESG) with radiographic imaging greatly strengthens the assessment and diagnostic differentiation of patients with craniomandibular disorders.

As diagnostic guidelines develop, we expect to have the capability to more accurately diagnose clinical conditions, enabling the clinician to develop more effective and efficient treatment. Having this ability will enable the dentist to increase the quality of care and treatment provided, as well as provide treatment outcome assessments.

Bibliography

1. Costen JB: Syndrome of sinus and ear symptoms dependent upon disturbed function of the temporomandibular joint. *Ann Otol Rhinol Laryngol* 1934;43:1-5.
2. Laskin DM: Etiology of the pain-dysfunction syndrome. *J Am Dent Assoc* 1969;79:149-153.
3. Farrar WB, McCarty WL: *A Clinical Outline of Temporomandibular Joint Diagnosis and Treatment, 7th Ed.* Montgomery, Ala.: Normandie Publications, 1982.
4. Bell WE: *Temporomandibular Disorders—Classification, Diagnosis, Management, 3rd Ed.* In: Bell WE, ed. Chicago: Medical Publishers, Inc.; 1990;273-280.
5. Sarnat BG, Laskin DM: *The Temporomandibular Joint: A Biological Basis for Clinical Practice.* Philadelphia: W.B. Saunders Company; 1992;374-375.
6. Wolford DG: Unpublished study.
7. Okeson JP, ed.: *Orofacial Pain; Guidelines for Assessments, Diagnosis and Management.* Quintessence Publishing Company; 1996;32.
8. Miles DA, VanDis ML, Jensen CW, Ferretti AB: *Radiographic Imaging for Dental Auxiliaries, 2nd Ed.* Philadelphia: W.B. Saunders Company; 1993;186-188.
9. Moses AJ: The Gold Standard, personal communication.

Chewing Cycle Analysis

Andrea Deregibus and Pietro Bracco

I. Overview of Craniomandibular Dysfunction (CMD)

Craniocervical-mandibular disorders, also known as craniomandibular disorders (CMD) or temporomandibular disorders (TMD), are odontologic pathologies that have recently gained much attention. These disorders are considered by some researchers to be "new" pathologies as a result of modern lifestyles. In fact, stress is considered by some to be one of the major factors causing these disorders. However, more appropriately, we can reasonably believe that the increase, both relative and absolute, of people suffering from these disorders is not only due to a more thorough diagnosis from the dentist, but also because patients and health care professionals have become more aware of these conditions.

Many of these disorders are not intracapsular temporomandibular joint disease as many health professionals have traditionally believed, but extra-capsular pathology. Also, from a biomechanical and/or functional perspective, mandibular posture plays a major role in the onset and progression of CMD since the temporomandibular joints and mandibular movements are biomechanically and neurologically integrated with head and neck biomechanics and neurophysiology. Furthermore, the definition of CMD is questionable because it is not possible to limit it as an exclusive oral pathologic process. It is necessary to consider CMD as a disorder involving the head, neck, and shoulders, as well as the cervical spine.[1]

The definition of CMD is so nonspecific that the American Academy of Orofacial Pain in its guidebook[2] defines it as "a generic term that applies to a number of clinical problems involving the temporomandibular joint with its associated structures or both." In the text *Cranio-Mandibular Dysfunction*,[3] Hansonn and co-authors define CMD as "... an action combining pain in the joints, head, neck, and shoulders, muscular fatigue, articular noises, and limitation of the jaw movement with or without limitation of the movement of the cervical back-bone. ..." Gola and co-authors[4] assert that "... Algo (dysfunctional) Syndrome of the Stomatognathic Apparatus (Syndrome Algo-Dysfonctionnel de l'Appareil Manducateur SADAM) indicates problems with masticatory function adapting to a dysfunctional or a parafunctional accentuated by a psychic or a systematic disorder. ..." The National Institute of Health/National Institute of Dental Research stated in a 1996 report that there is no etiologic or biologic explanation for temporomandibular disorders. There is much confusion that continues to cloud the issue of head, neck, and face pain.

Currently, the potential to diagnose cranio-mandibular disorders has improved since we are now able to take advantage of the traditional basic clinical examination, radiologic imaging (X-ray, CAT scan, MRI) and/or electronic and non-electronic instrumentation to analyze the stomatognathic system. Biomedical instrumentation has given the profession the ability to objectively measure physiologic processes of the stomatognathic system. Certain aspects of this data have only recently begun to be studied, and its complete meaning is somewhat vague. Clinical application of this data used to define healthy from unhealthy is difficult. In many cases, normal may actually be regarded as unhealthy, hence, the high presence of false positives so often used to detract from the value of biomedical instrumentation. This could be linked to the inability of instrumentation to identify the progression of CMD, or with the identification of stages between health and disease.[1,5,6]

This science remains in a state of change. For example, just when we feel that normal anatomy and physiology of the temporomandibular joint apparatus is understood, it is determined that muscle fibers from the masseter and the anterior temporalis muscles insert into the temporomandibular joint disc. The isolation of these fibers complicates understanding the physiologic movement of the disc and generates further questions in a field of macroscopic anatomy which seemed to offer no additional surprises.[7,8,9]

In a field where it is difficult to define normal or physiologic, it becomes even more complicated to define the meaning of pathologic. To consider pain as the "gold standard" or the determining factor to dictate treatment is dangerous and limiting. Many pathologic processes may progress for years without producing any pain; however, destruction of structures may be an ongoing process, as well as limitation of its function.

To confuse this issue further, it must be considered that over the last fifteen years at least five different systems to classify these pathologies have been proposed,[1] yet an unequivocal definition of CMD has not been achieved. Furthermore, etiologic factors are being discussed along with the possibility that non-symptomatic active forms could exist, as well as other precipitating factors which could transform a silent form of the disease into a clinically active form.

Therefore, this field continues to evolve, remaining in a constant state of change. What we "believe" we understand is continuously put to the test. The certainty of multiple etiologic factors of CMD in combination with its extreme symptom variability makes it very difficult to combine data obtained by various authors to develop any clear meaning of CMD. In fact many signs and symptoms when considered singularly are not clearly pathologic, however, combined may yield a number of diseases. Consequently, it is possible to build an endless number of theoretical sample groups. From this perspective, even the concept of "normal" is related to the composition of the reference sample being studied, which is dependent upon the type of subjects comprising the study. Many errors exist in the literature since it has been based on an undefined standard. So the expression "gold standard," which seems to be very clear, is relative to the subjects studied. Many authors maintain that when instrumentation is used as an aid in diagnosis an unusually high percentage of positive results occur, resulting in a high percentage of false positive diagnoses.[10-12] This has resulted with those who are critical of practitioners who utilize biomedical instrumentation since no standard boundary defining healthy and unhealthy has been defined. This problem creates the question: which factors, signs, and symptoms do we consider when developing a diagnosis? It is impossible to know if individuals are diagnosed as false positive or false negative relative to a healthy versus a sick population.

Since the linearity of these instruments and the repeatability of the tests have been validated, we should attribute the high presence of potentially false positives to both the difficulty to read and interpret the graphs and the inadequacy of clinical procedures to identify the initial pathology.

We know how gnathographic instruments display mandibular movement, but a detailed analysis of the functional capacity of the stomatognathic organ cannot be ignored which would include the analysis of mandibular range of motion and the capacity of musculature to contract and relax. The analysis to be introduced will assess the actual chewing capacity and also extrapolate the functional capacity of the intrinsic muscles and mandibular motion. The analysis of the chewing capacity or, more importantly, the functional capacity of the stomatognathic organ during mastication, comes from testing the so-called masticatory cycles. Masticatory tests in which standardized foods are chewed are to be performed to understand the functional capacity of muscles, articulation, and the compensatory possibilities that exist.

In recent years, clinicians have a renewed interest in the study of mastication. However, the use of masticatory cycles to diagnose gnathologic conditions is criticized because this examination requires the use of a screen, a magnet, surface electrodes, or instrumentation even more invasive to the mouth. Another criticism concerns the lack of spontaneity of movement. For example, some researchers believe that the recording of the masticatory cycles is very much influenced by the recording instruments since it is an automatic spontaneous movement. One must recall that the analysis of chewing cycles is not the study of a natural movement, but it is the study of the trajectory or the pattern that the mandible follows during mastication of a standardized bolus, creating repeatable conditions.

Spontaneous mandibular movements are not replicatable. These movements should be carefully avoided when conducting chewing cycle analysis because they are not repeatable and cannot be standardized. Testing should be standardized in order for a test to have diagnostic meaning. The masticatory cycles that are recorded, particularly those with a hard bolus, can be compared with a stress test electrocardiogram or with an Oral Glucose Tolerance Test (OGTT). These types of tests allow us to very clearly identify tissue capacity for response, as well as the compensatory mechanisms of the organism.

The dynamic and electromyographic variables associated with mastication are many and only the newest electronic systems allow computation of a large volume of data, yielding the possibility of acquisition and analysis of all data simultaneously. The authors have developed and tested a software program (Chewing Cycles Analysis or CCA) that analyzes data obtained by the K6I kinesiograph (Myo-Tronics Research Inc.). Data is acquired via Scan 8 using the Jankelson's protocol.[13] Scan 8 of Janckelson's protocol is the simultaneous registration of mandibular motion in the sagittal and frontal planes with simultaneous EMG for vertical positioning. Tracing sweeps are recorded concurrently with real time mandibular movement. Hence, it is possible to add a new dimension to the neuromuscular diagnosis, analysis, and evaluation of the stomatognathic system and, particurlarly, masticatory function.

In this paper, our goal is to provide basic information on the physiology of mastication, and the possibility of using chewing cycles analysis to aid in making a diagnosis. Furthermore, we present software developed for the K6I kinesiograph (Myo-Tronics Research Inc.) which will allow for the use of this instrument in the analysis of masticatory cycles.

II. Outline of The Masticatory Physiology

A) Neurologic Control

Mastication is a series of highly coordinated mandibular motions involving various elements of the stomatognathic system whose aim is to break-up and crush food and prepare it for digestion. In order for this function to occur in the most harmonious way, a coordinated movement is necessary between the right and the left temporomandibular joints and masticatory muscles; between the postural and power muscles, and joints. Mastication is one of the most important functions of the mandibular motion.

Mastication is a reflex and semiautomatic activity, with rhythmical cycles. It is possible to distinguish three phases of the masticatory cycle; 1) the opening, 2) the closing, and 3) the power phase. During the last phase, the power developed by the muscle increases to perform a particular task. During mastication the neurologic control of mandibular motion is fundamental. In fact, the planning of mandibular movements reflects coordination with movements of both tongue and other orofacial muscles. During movement, improper or uncoordinated movements between these structures might cause extensive damage.[14] It is possible to divide the neurologic control of mandibular motion into three levels:

1) simple reflex arc-like system
2) cortical and cerebellar control
3) limbic control

The innervation of the mandibular muscles has some particular features that distinguish these muscles from the limb musculature. The proprioceptive afferents from the mandibular elevator muscles have their cell bodies in the mesencephalic nucleus located in the brain stem. These cells receive a great variety of nerve afferents, either centrally or peripherally. These afferents not only arrive from the oral field, but also from extraoral fields. Afferent pathways may arise from dental pulp receptors, periodontal ligaments, skin, and mucous membranes. All take part in programming mandibular motility *(Figure 1)*. Furthermore, afferent information is received from receptors placed within the temporomandibular joint. These receptors have particular importance in providing fundamental information about the position and the movement of the joint itself, as well as nociception. These receptors and their afferent pathways, including the mesencephalic centers, the muscles, and their motoneurons, are a part of common neurologic circuitry. This is the basis for the automatic reflex and rhythmic activity of mandibular movement.[15,16,17] Scientific studies report that laboratory animals are able to redevelop efficient masticatory activity following decortation.[18]

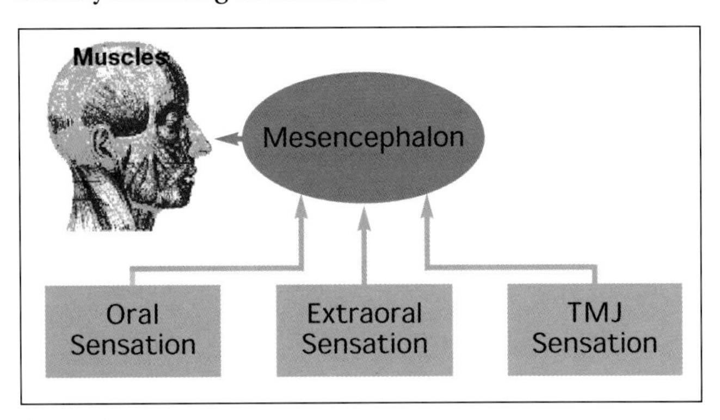

Figure 1.

The rhythmic activity of the circuitry that has been described is integrated and modulated by superior centers, which is the second level of activity *(Figure 2)*. This second level is composed of two structures:

1) A creator center of masticatory motor patterns which resides in the brain stem. This center is the pattern generator.
2) Structures at superior levels direct the general mechanism of motility. These structures are in the motion areas of the brain cortex, the ganglion of the brain stem, and the cerebellum.

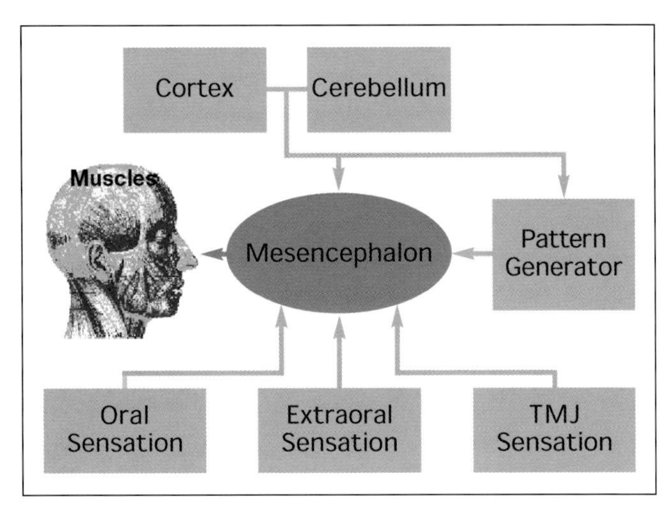

Figure 2.

The capacity of programming refined movements is due to the integration of these two latter structures, as well as the capacity to learn and to apply new motion strategies. This is extremely important from our point of view. These new motion strategies can be inserted on, or can totally substitute that made by the pattern generator and by those at the first level. The first level is the automatic reflex.

It is known that movements routinely performed are the result of a learning process that began at birth and continues throughout life.[19,20] Learned movements result from "motor memory" or engrams. Changing motor strategy may occur for two reasons: 1) to increase the motor ability as a normal occurrence, and 2) to compensate for injury or disease which creates deficits within the organism requiring a behaviorial modification to adapt to new unexpected situations. For instance, if a person leaves a stone in his shoe for days or weeks, he is obliged to develop new walking patterns and strategies of coordination for the muscular activity. This is an avoidance mechanism. These new model strategies or engrams are applied to avoid trauma to the foot.[16,17]

When dealing with orofacial pain, one must remember that the teeth, periodontal fibers, temporomandibular joint, and the muscles are supplied by nociceptors. Pain creates the development and the application of new strategies controlling rhythmic masticatory activity. The two described structures on this level are delegated to learn and perform this new motor strategy. This is under superior cortico-cerebellar control. Another consideration of primary interest when considering motion pathology relates to emotions, which structurally reside within the limbic system *(Figure 3)*. Every sensation that arrives from the periphery has a result that can be pleasant or unpleasant. This affective response is influenced by our experience and can be modulated in very different manners in different individuals. One's psychological status helps explain the different motor responses which may develop in different individuals. In this way, a pleasant sensation can harmonize a movement and an unpleasant sensation may depress movement. Limbic system efferents, modulated by emotional afferents, make the third level of control and the variation seen with masticatory rhythmicity. In our particular case, there is a difference when eating a refined dish in a nice restaurant compared to eating a sandwich standing in a street. In these two cases, the masticatory rhythmicity and cyclic activity will have different effects for different sensations arriving in the limbic system.

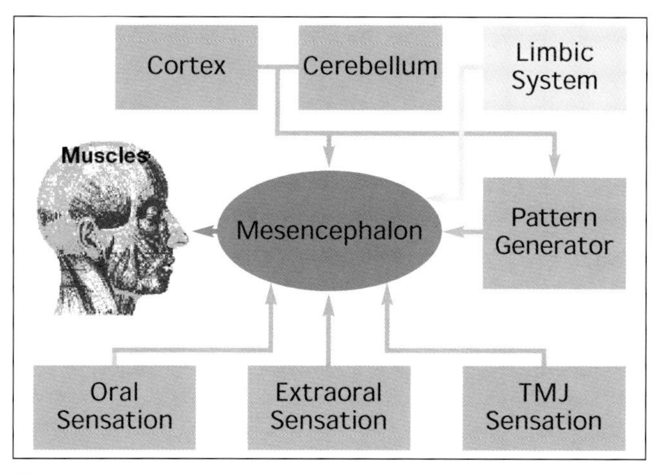

Figure 3.

Summarizing, we can say that a structure governing reflex masticatory control exists. The ability to change movement is under superior corticocerebellar control and limbic control which can modulate movement.

It is important to remember that mastication may occur as a reflex or a voluntary act, similar to respiration. It may be influenced by the will. Another important characteristic is the type of movement voluntarily performed during every masticatory cycle. A ballistic movement occurring on closing from maximum opening towards maximum closing cannot be influenced. The only possible participation is the interruption of the movement.[14]

B) The Physiological Aspect of the Chewing Cycles

A physiologic masticatory cycle is a movement with an elliptical shape, like a teardrop, and it includes three phases; an opening phase, a closing phase, and a power phase.[21]

1. The first phase is the opening phase.
2. The second phase is the closing phase, with the capture of the bolus.
3. The third phase is the power phase, with crushing and tearing of the food.

Figure 4 shows an illustration of the masticatory cycle. In a normal masticatory cycle, the patient opens and closes, opens and closes, and so on, in a teardrop fashion. In *Figure 5,* the tear drop shaped movement is reduced, occurring near occlusion. In this situation, the mandible makes a slipping movement with the bolus between the teeth as the food is crushed. As will be seen later, as chewing continues, every cycle becomes shorter and more narrow than the previous. In this way a masticatory cone is formed. Moreover, the shape of this cone varies in relation to the type of bolus chewed. The temporomandibular joints, discs, and masticatory muscles have to perform a well coordinated movement to perform this tear-like movement. If one of the components does not act properly, the form of the movement will be changed in its opening and/or closing shape.

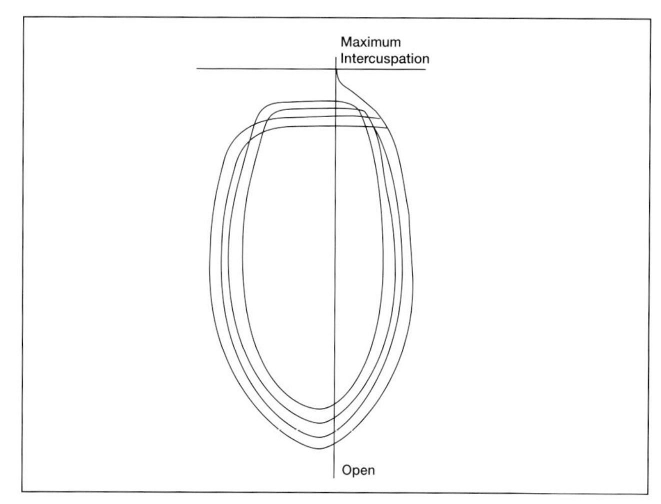

Figure 4. Scheme of a masticatory cycle.

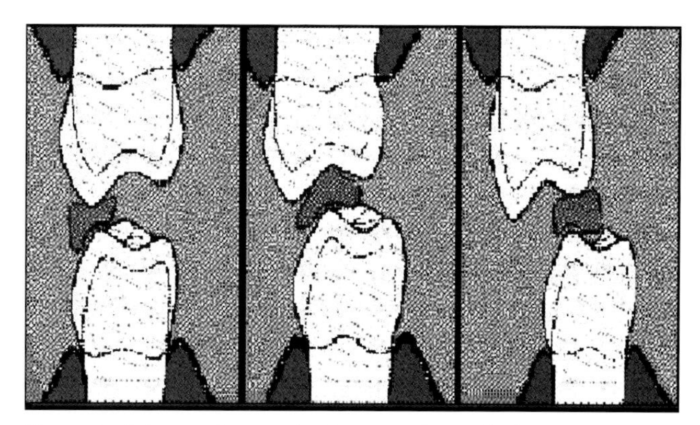

Figure 5. Scheme of a mastication near the occlusion.

1) Definitions

First, we should consider the masticatory cycle from the frontal plane. In this plane, we are visualizing the subject from their left side, the face is positioned toward the left, and their back toward the right. Furthermore, we visualize the working side as the side on which the food will be chewed and the non-working side as contralateral to the working side. Therefore, if a patient is chewing on his right, the working side is the patient's right side, and the non-working is the patient's left side. When observed from the front and as the patient chews on the right side, a clockwise cycle is created. A counter-clockwise cycle is created when the patient chews on his left side. In a masticatory cycle, we are able to distinguish the apex of the masticatory cycle as the most occlusal part, and the body as the drop of the cycle *(Figure 6)*.

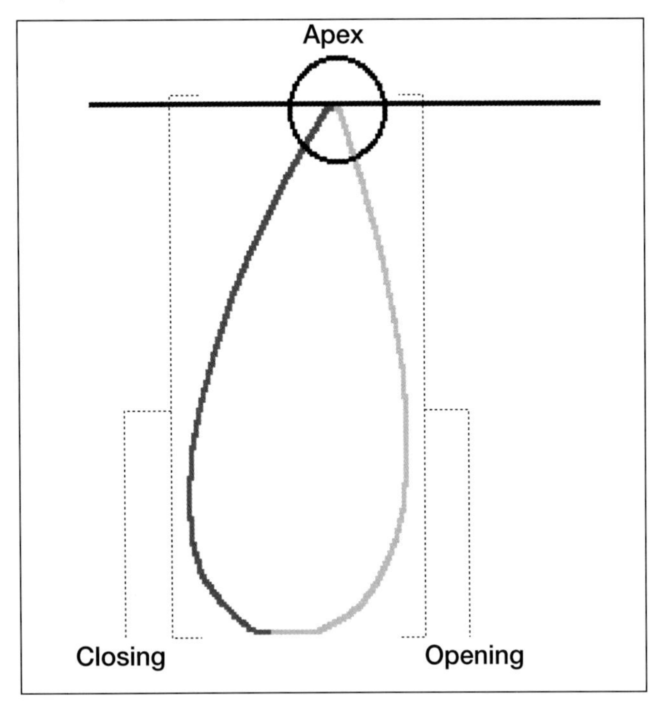

Figure 6. Apex of the cycles.

The two or three most occlusal millimeters of the cycles represent the apex of a masticatory cycle. At the apex, we can distinguish the shape and position regarding the point of maximal intercuspation. In the body, we can distinguish width, height, and an axis. The width of the cycles *(Figure 7)* is the maximum distance between the opening and the closing traces, and the height of the cycle *(Figure 8)* is the distance between the occlusal pause and the turning point, or where opening coincides with closing. It is possible to trace a line, the axis of the cycle, that joins the occlusal pause with the point where opening becomes coincidental with closing *(Figure 9)*. The horizontal portion nearest to occlusion is called occlusal pause. In this part of the chewing cycle, crushing of food occurs. The apex of the cycles is influenced in its characteristics by the occlusal components and by the interrelationship between neuromuscular and articular components. The body of the cycle is influenced by its height, width, general shape, and axis of both the neuromuscular and articular characteristics.

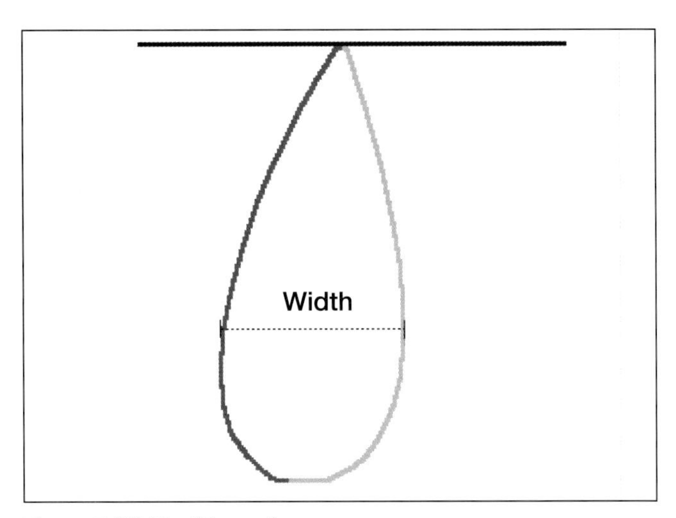

Figure 7. Width of the cycles.

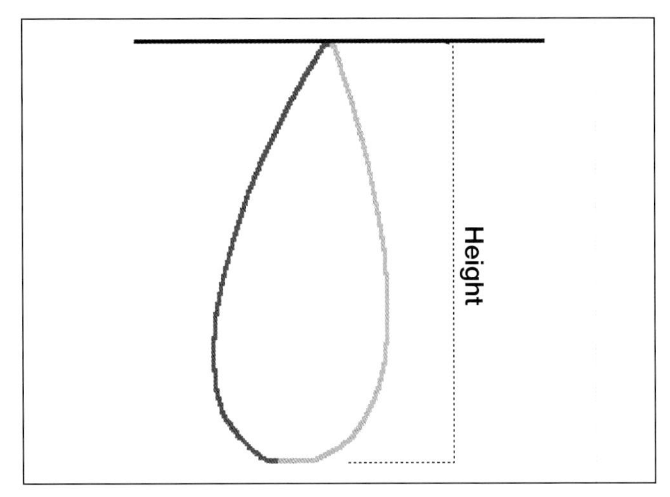

Figure 8. Height of the cycles.

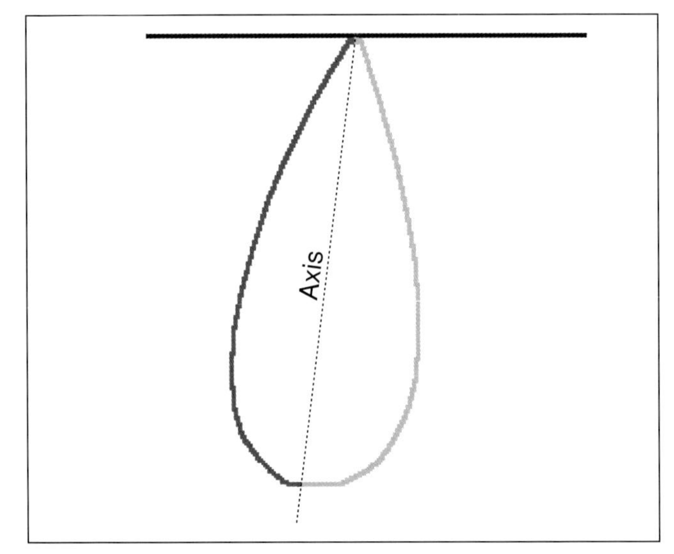

Figure 9. Axis of the cycles.

2) Aspects on the Frontal Plane

Now let us inspect the physiologic masticatory cycle that initially develops in the frontal plane. In the schematic picture of *Figure 10,* the illustration depicts a patient chewing on the right side. During opening, the mandible translates toward the non-working side with a curvilinear movement. The concavity faces the working side. As the opening phase is completed, the jaw moves to the working side with an almost horizontal movement The length of movement is influenced by the food type. As food hardness increases, mandibular movement toward the working side increases. Therefore, as the closing phase begins, the jaw is brought to occlusion with a curvilinear movement and its concavity turned to the non-working side *(Figure 11).*

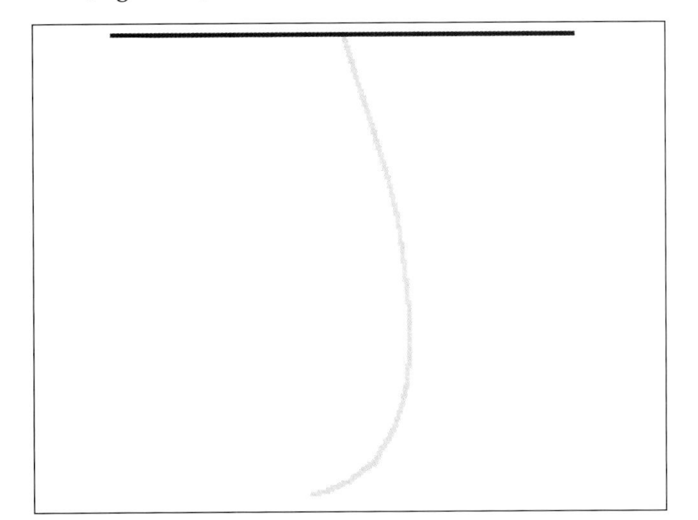

Figure 10. Opening phase of the cycles.

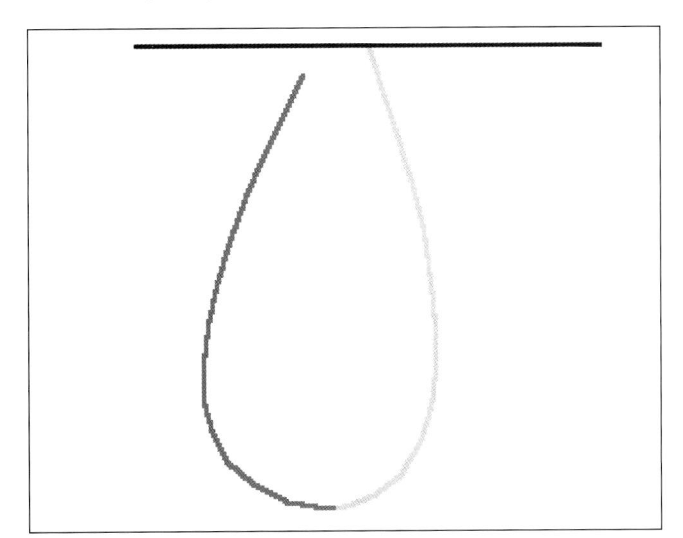

Figure 11. Closing phase of the cycles.

When the mandible is near centric occlusion, making an almost horizontal movement, the mandible moves to the non-working side and begins a new cycle *(Figure 12).* During this part of the movement, the food is crushed and, the softer the bolus, the closer the mandible will move toward centric occlusion. It is not important if the bolus was soft or hard in the beginning. Furthermore, the softer the bolus, the shorter is the occlusal pause. This same characteristic (bolus softness) also influences the width and the height of the cycles. The soft bolus creates a narrow and short cycle *(Figure 13),* and the hard bolus creates a large and high cycle *(Figure 14).*

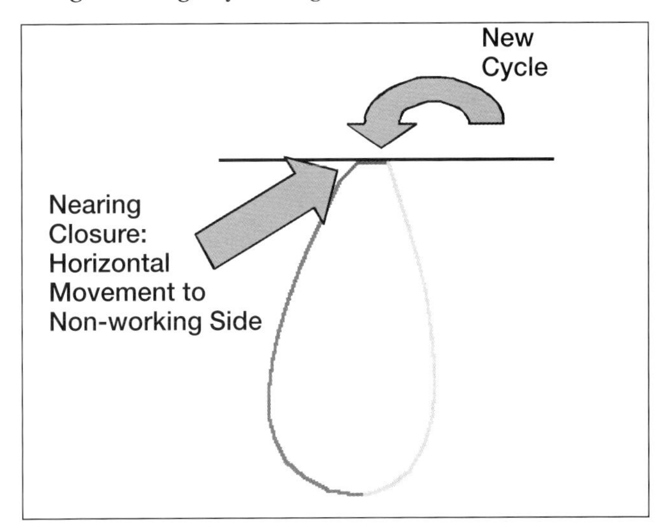

Figure 12. Occlusal pause of the cycles.

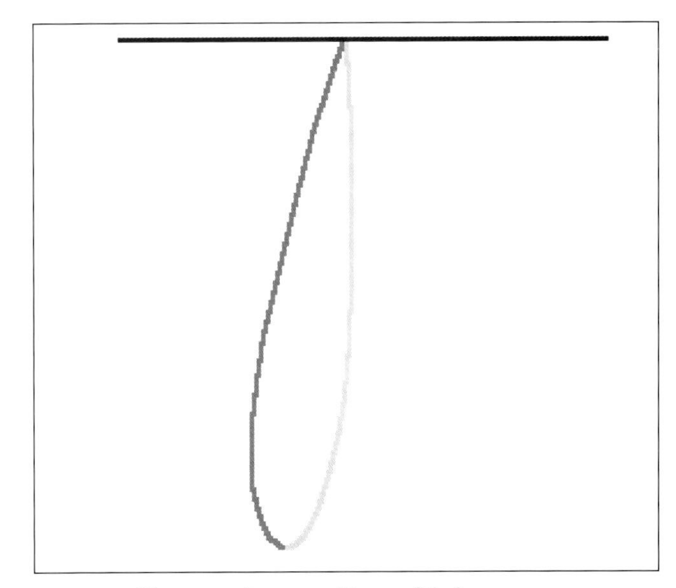

Figure 13. Narrow cycles created by a soft bolus.

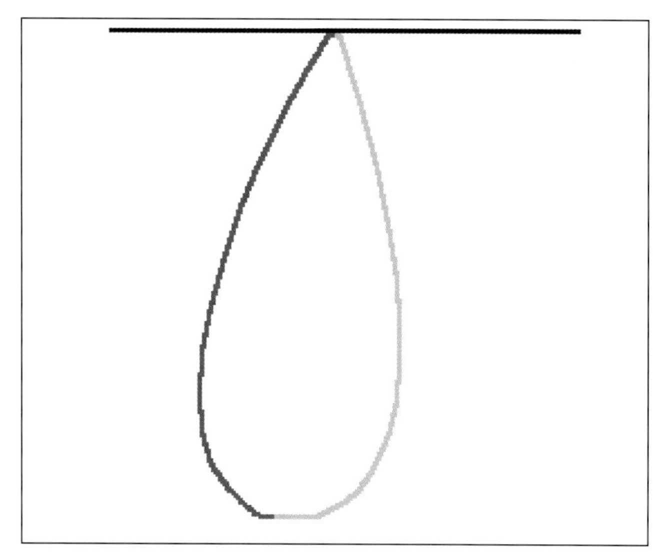

Figure 14. Large cycles created by a hard bolus.

In a physiologic cycle, the cycle axis is inclined towards the working side. In case of right side mastication, the axis has a right axial inclination, and, with left mastication, the axis is inclined toward the left. Axis inclination increases with bolus hardness. *(Figures 15 and 16). Table I* summarizes the characteristic of the cycles from frontal plane influenced by the hardness of the bolus.

Table I
Characteristics of the cycles influenced by the type of bolus

	Hard bolus	Soft bolus
Movement at the end of the opening	Long	Short
Dimension of the cycle	High and large	Short and narrow
Occlusal phase	Long	Short
Axis	Much inclination	Little inclination

It is important to understand joint mechanics in order to assess the transformation of the cycles analyzed on the frontal plane from a physiologic and pathologic perspective. As previously stated, during the opening phase, the jaw tends to move towards the non-working side *(Figure 17A, B)*. During this mandibular shift, the condyle of the working side tends to move, eccentrically from the glenoid fossa. At the end of the opening phase, the working side condyle tends to seat in the glenoid fossa and the jaw moves towards the working side *(Figure 17C)*. During this phase of the movement, the condyle of the non-working side tends to move eccentrically from the glenoid fossa *(Figure 17D)*. In the closing phase, the condyle of the non-working side re-seats in the glenoid fossa at the occlusal pause, and a new cycle begins *(Figure 17E)*.

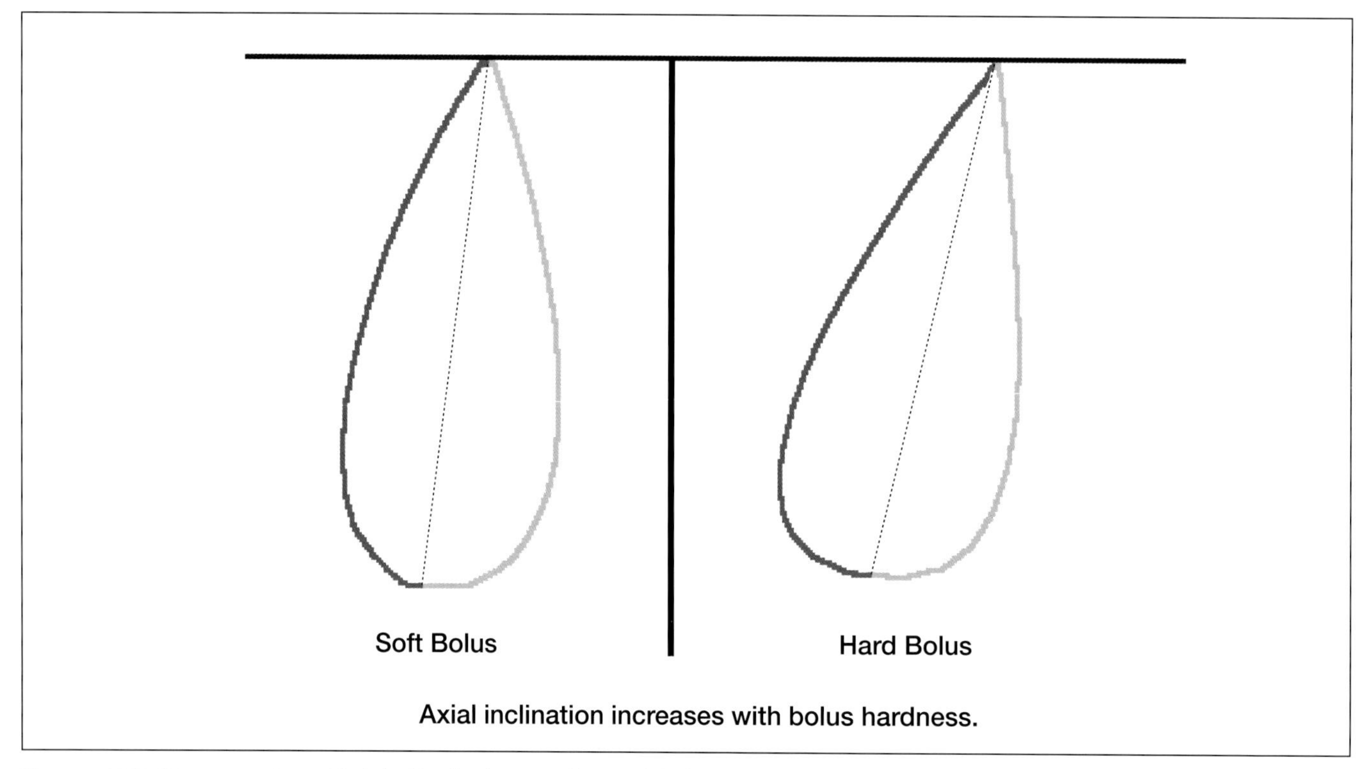

Figures 15 (left) and 16 (right). Little inclined axis created by a soft bolus (left) and much inclined axis created by a hard bolus.

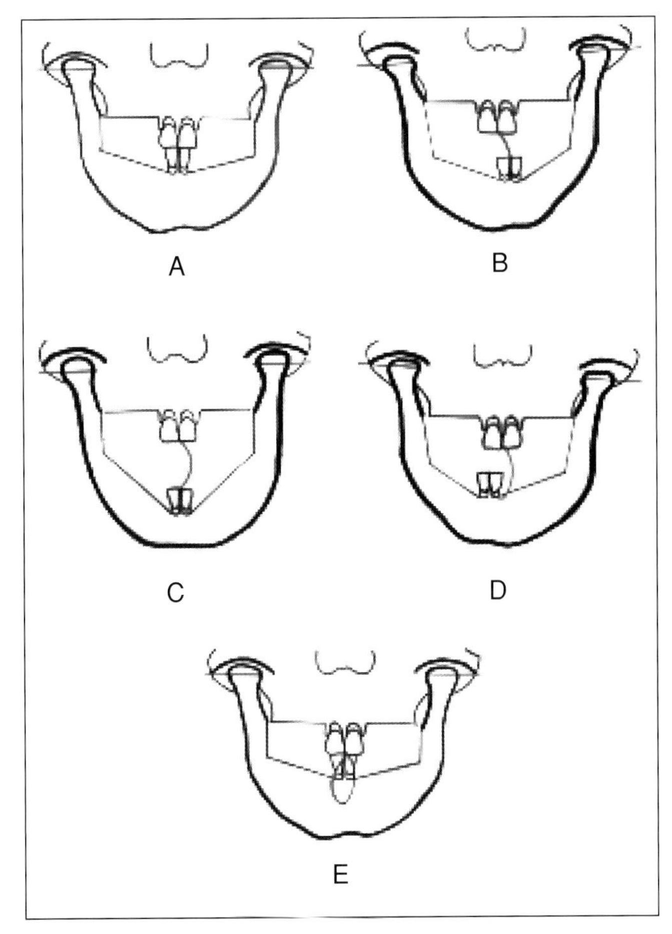

Figure 17.

It is obvious that any anomaly of function of either joint will influence the opening and closing phase of the cycle. Any disorder of the right joint will primarily influence the opening phase of right chewing and the closing phase of left chewing.

3) Aspects on the Sagittal Plane

In the sagittal plane, the influences linked with the bolus are much smaller, and obviously the cycle resembles Scan 1 or Scan 13 of K6I kinesiograph (MyoTronics-Noromed Inc.). We remember that Scan 1 is the simultaneous sagittal and frontal tracing of a single open/close cycle. Furthermore, Scan 13 is the simultaneous sagittal and frontal trace of a single movement of protrusion, opening and closing, and lateral movements as demonstrated by Posselt's envelope of motion. The greatest difference in this phase occurs during opening, where it is clearly visible that a protrusive component is linked to the overjet. In fact, the mandible moves forward to find the incisal contact. The closing trace follows a parallel path and generally returns to centric occlusion.

C) Principles of Interpretation of the Mastication Through the Examination of the Masticatory Cycles

In the previous section, we have described the physiology of masticatory cycles. In this section, we will try to supply information on interpretation of the pathologic aspects of masticatory cycles. Qualitative analysis is commonly performed. One tries to estimate how pathologic masticatory cycles are different from the physiologic. The width, height, axis inclination, and position of the apex are evaluated. The symmetry of movement is evaluated, that is: how much difference exists between right and left cycles (shape, dimension etc.) of the masticatory cycles executed with the same kind of bolus, and how much difference exists between soft bolus and hard bolus. This is evaluated for several masticatory cycles. Presently, numerical norms for the diagnostic parameters for using means of the masticatory cycles do not exist. In fact, the dimensions of the cycles are not only influenced by anomalies of masticatory muscles and joints, but also by the size of the patient. This means that as a patient's height and weight increases, you will find masticatory cycles that are greater in height and width.

The degree of repeatability or, if you prefer, the degree of variability, is also evaluated. We have found that masticatory movement has a ballistic type of behavior. At the end of the opening movement, muscular contraction restrains the opening movement causing the jaw "to shoot" towards the occlusion. The closing tracing is variable and depends on anatomical and bolus characteristics. Therefore, with this phenomenon, we can see the variability of the movement. The more we move away from centric occlusion, the more the tracing becomes variable *(Figure 18)*. On the contrary, if the jaw tracings are repetitive *(Figure 19)*, this means that the anatomy would influence the jaw to follow the same trajectory. For example, the inflammation due to an osteoarthritis can create pain during the jaw movement. In this case, the jaw will always move in the same trajectory to avoid pain. These anatomical variations of movement will indicate changes of a pathological nature. From these considerations, the diagnosis of muscular and/or articular involvement may be formulated, including which joint is primarily involved.

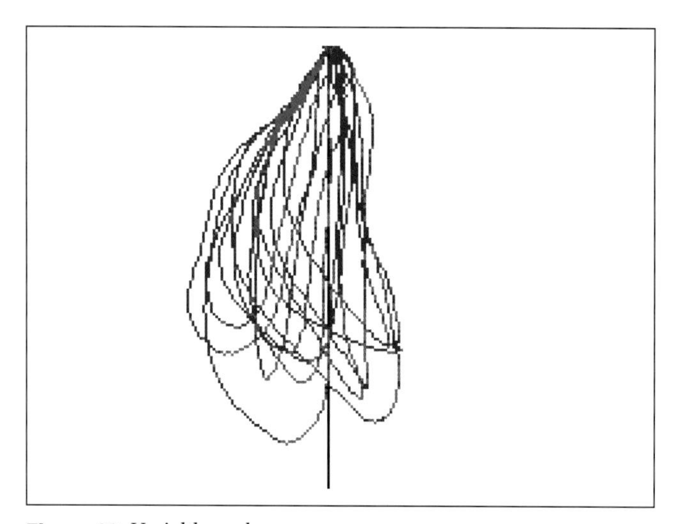

Figure 18. Variable cycles.

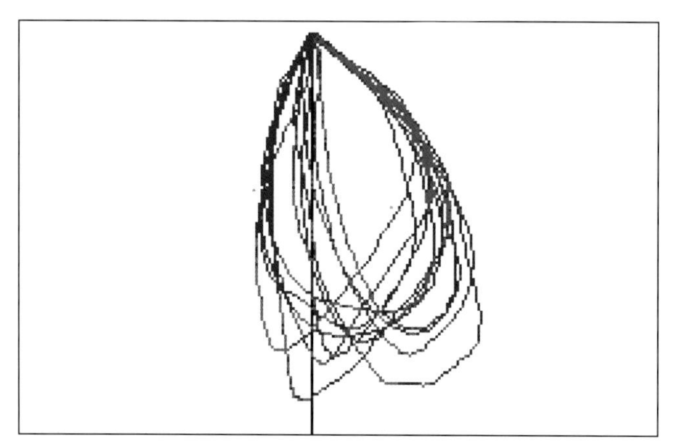

Figure 19. Repetitive cycles.

To better understand the next section, we need to provide additional definitions. Chewing cycles can be examined as specific cycles or as average cycles. Specific cycles are a graphic representation of the cycles as they have been performed by the patient *(Figure 20)*. This is a group of opening and closing movements that begin at the zero point, or with teeth in occlusion, and end after ten continuous seconds of data acquisition. They can be examined one at a time or superimposed to study the masticatory pattern. Moreover, specific cycles may be analyzed in terms of shape and form as previously described, or they may be analyzed in time and form similar to a Scan 3 from the K6I kinesiograph (Myotronics-Noromed Inc.). Scan 3 is a real time recording of the spatial position of the mandible, measured in vertical, lateral, and anteroposterior planes. Using this scan gives one the ability to analyze the patient's accommodative rest position, as well as the movement that the mandible makes when traveling from accommodative rest position to the habitual centric occlusion.

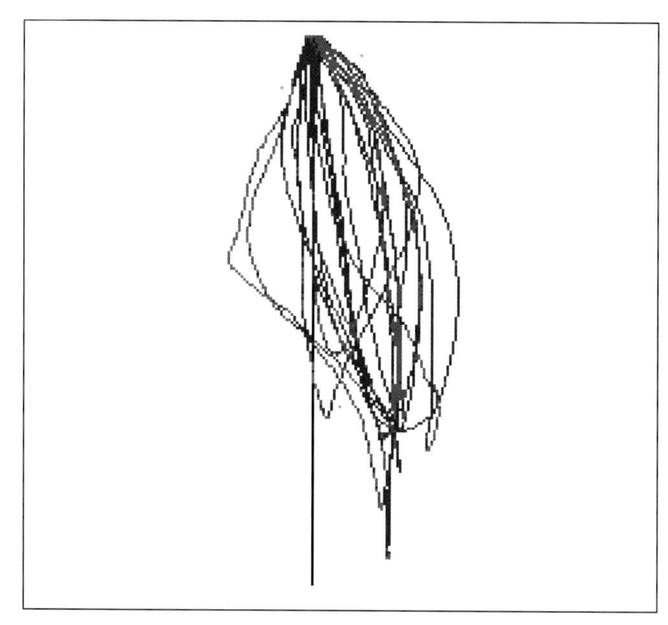

Figure 20. Example of specific cycles.

A suitable algorithm is used to calculate the probable cycle from the specific cycles. This is the average or mean cycle *(Figure 21)*. Clustering all the homogeneous masticatory acts (i.e., all the right cycles with soft bolus) makes the calculation of the average cycle with a total of six different possibilities. From this calculation, the first two cycles performed by the patient during each masticatory act are erased. These two cycles are known as testing cycles. In these two cycles, the patient carefully tests the consistency of the bolus.

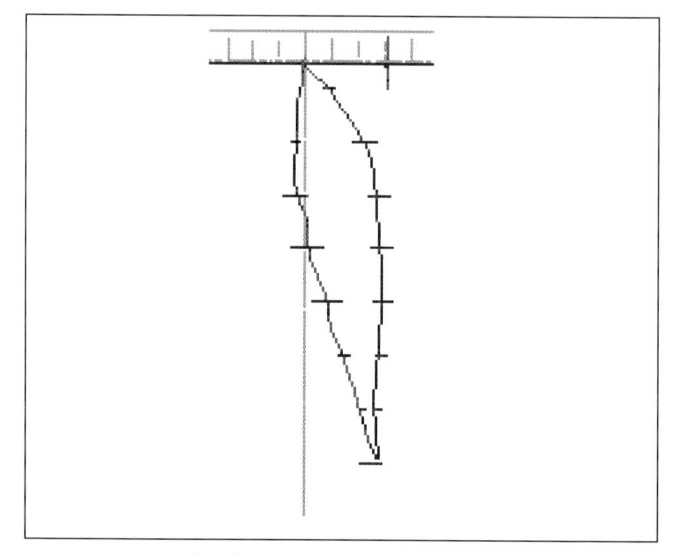

Figure 21. Example of average cycles.

Furthermore, the anomalous (or erratic) cycles are not used. An anomalous movement *(Figure 22)* is a short and quick inversion of the trace which could be described as a long and complete opening movement interrupted by brief closure. Usually the erratic cycles are due to bolus recovery or unexpected pain. The anomalous cycles are not used to calculate the average cycles because they may impact the shape of the averaged cycle, but they are analyzed as specific cycles. Most information is gained by studying the frontal plane, since the working asymmetries between the right and left components (muscles and TM articulations) mainly influence the frontal aspect of the cycles.

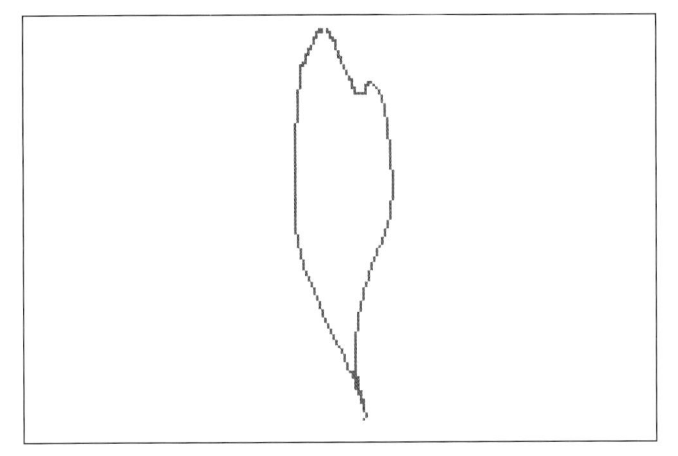

Figure 22. Example of anomalous cycle.

The aspects that are examined can be outlined and summarized as follows:

1. general shape of specific cycles
2. overlap of specific cycles
3. aspect of the averaged cycles
4. standard deviation
5. width of cycles
6. height of cycles
7. inclination of the axis of the cycles
8. position of apex
9. the closing direction

It is necessary to examine the previous points and the possible relationships involving multiple combinations. It is important to remember that this is just a scheme, and the diagnosis must be made considering the meaning that can be drawn from the several aspects of different masticatory cycles. The *general shape* of the specific cycles supplies indications as to whether there is good muscular equilibrium and normal joint movement. Every cycle may have its particular characteristics, but when comparing cycles it is possible to recognize the same pattern of movement. The less recognizable the pattern, the more variable the cycles, indicating that the patient is unsure. This insecurity can be due to muscular or articular pain, pain from the teeth, or from stress. In this last case, the pattern becomes regular as masticatory cycles are recorded.

Aspects of the *specific cycles* which overlap give indications of muscular and articular equilibrium. The more that single cycles overlap, the more repetitive the movements, indicating a high level of articular problems demonstrated by the movements. In these cases, the jaw will follow the same trajectory to avoid or to reduce pain. If the tracing is repetitive during opening and closing, both the articulations are involved. On the contrary, if there is involvement of only one joint, this can provoke repetitive movements in the opening phase with ipsilateral chewing and during the closing phase of contralateral chewing. In the absence of dental problems, if the cycles are greatly variable with extremely different shapes, it is possible to conclude that the difficulty lies in the equilibrium and coordination of the muscles. The degree of specific cycles which overlap influences the standard deviation of the cycles' mean. As the cycles become more repetitive, the standard deviation becomes less. As the cycles vary and become more dispersed, the standard deviation will become greater.

Averaged cycles supply a great deal of information regarding the clinical condition. Usually the tracing is examined with regards to estimated height and width of the cycles, position of the axes, and the differences in mastication when comparing soft and hard boluses. *Standard deviation* supplies indications on the repetition of the masticatory cycles. Highly repetitive cycles yield lower standard deviations while highly variable and dispersed cycles yield higher standard deviations. The *width of the cycles* supplies indications concerning both the level of muscular contraction and/or joint(s) involvement. In both cases, alteration of the inclination of the axis will be present due to muscular and/or articular involvement. As the muscles become more contracted, the cycles will become narrower; as the muscles become more relaxed, the cycles will become wider. In the later situation, the axis of the cycles will be much more vertical both in right and in left chewing. Decreased ability of articulations to execute mediotrusion to avoid pain results in narrower cycles. Previously, it was stated that a problem in the right joint mainly influences the opening phase of right chewing and the closing phase in left chewing. This means that the opening tracing of right mastication and the closing tracing of left mastication will be less concave, therefore, closer to the axis of the cycles. The *height of the cycles* supplies indications of the muscular contracture. As muscle contraction increases, the height of the cycles is reduced. Increased muscle relaxation results in cycles tending to have a greater height.

The *axis inclination* of the cycles supplies interesting findings from patients with joint disorders. The first apparent problem in executing mediotrusion is a straightening of the axis of mastication made contralaterally to the involved joint. Increasing joint pathology may cause a more vertical axis. In the case of large lesions, the axis is tilted towards the involved joint, rather than towards the contralateral side.

Therefore, a lesion in the right joint causes a straightening of the axis in left mastication, but if the lesion is extensive, the axis of left mastication will be tilted toward the right rather than the left. It is obvious that these last three parameters (height, width, inclination of the axis) are closely linked together. There is a relationship between all three parameters, and all are affected when masticatory cycles are altered.

The *cycle apex* supplies indications of both dental and articular changes. The cycle apex lies within two or three occlusal millimeters of the masticatory cycle. The apex is composed by a closing and opening portion. Physiologically, the closing motion is toward the working side and the opening motion is toward the non-working side. The shape of the apex is influenced by the type of bolus chewed, the steepness of the canine guidance, and the degree of the dental abrasion. Its position is influenced by many factors, for example, the presence of laterally deflecting premature contacts or an articular disc displacement with reduction (ADDwR). The analysis of the position of the apex is made by looking at the averaged tracing. In normal conditions, when chewing a soft bolus, the apex of the masticatory cycles coincides with the point of intercuspal position (zero point); chewing a hard bolus causes the apex of the masticatory cycle to be moved below intercuspation because of the interposition of the bolus. The apex position of the cycles is more influenced in its position by a hard bolus rather than from a soft bolus. For example, the mastication of a hard bolus on the side with a TM joint disc displacement may cause the reduction of the disc. In this case the apex of those cycles will be positioned toward the involved side. Moreover, mastication of a hard bolus in presence of a deflecting premature contact causes the movement of the apex in the opposite direction in comparison to that due to a premature contact. Any masticatory effort executed with a hard bolus by a patient with a premature contact that moves the jaw towards the left will always move the apex to the right.

We have said that the clockwise or counter-clockwise direction of cycles is dependent upon the side of mastication. In fact, physiologically, right side chewing creates masticatory cycles with clockwise direction, and a bolus chewed on the left creates masticatory cycles with counter-clockwise direction. The *closing direction* of the cycles can become reversed; during right side chewing the direction creates counter-clockwise cycles, and during left chewing, clockwise cycles can occur such as in a cross-bite situation. When occlusion is considered, the direction of the cycles may become reversed as a result of generator pattern control to allow for the opposition of a greater amount of dental surfaces. These types of cycles are called reversed cycles. This type of cycle can be totally reversed during both opening and closing, partially reversed or with crossover. Sometimes the shape of the cycle is regular and compatible with the type of mastication that the patient is executing, but as occlusion is approached a crossover and reversal of direction occurs. These occurrences may be due to teeth slipping through the bolus or to articular vibrations where there is minimal movement of the TM disc. If this type of cycle reversal occurs very rarely during the examination, it must be concluded that it is due to the bolus; however, if this reversal occurs frequently during the examination, it must be concluded that it is due to articular conditions. Therefore, articular problems also must be considered if this type of cycle reversal occurs with the presence of decreasing cycle width and concurrent anomalies on the axis position. The opening portion of the cycles has not been discussed, since the literature and clinical observations seem to indicate that opening does not give information additional to that previously discussed. All the information that can be gained by studying opening is included in the other portions of the cycles.

III) Study of Chewing Cycle

A) Brief History of Old and New Methodologies

Because of the complexity of chewing cycles, the study of mastication is a relatively recent occurrence. The first studies began in the 1950s utilizing cinematography. In 1956, Silverman[22] used this method to describe the cyclic tear-like shape of masticatory cycles formed as opening approached maximum vertical opening followed by the mandible moving toward the working side during closing. The author also described the "slipping" of cuspal inclines to reach maximum intercuspation. In 1958, Mongol,[23] using the same technique, reached similar conclusions. Subsequently, in 1964 Cannon built a system which later became known as the Replicator or Jaw Replicator.[24] This system was composed of an apparatus that was attached to the facial surfaces of the mandibular teeth, leaving the occlusal surface completely uncovered. Through transducers, this apparatus was able to determine and display mandibular movement with six degrees of freedom: three translatory and three rotational movements. Data was stored in a computer enabling it to be utilized at a later time. The mock patient was attached to this apparatus allowing the chewing cycle to be observed. In 1966, Gibbs[25] used the Replicator on a sample of 185 subjects, including subjects of both sexes and all ages. Both physiologic and pathologic masticatory parameters were defined. The pathological aspects studied included the presence of dental abrasion or premature contacts.

Today the methodologies used to estimate the masticatory capabilities could be outlined in three categories:
1) electromechanical methodology
2) optometrical methodology
3) magnetometric methodology

The instrument utilizing the electromechanical methodology is the axiograph.[26] This has been modified with the insertion of transducers. This modification allows monitoring mandibular movement three-dimensionally, enabling one to reconstruct mandibular trajectory during mastication. This is the technique used by Slavicek.[27,28] It requires an apparatus to be fixed to the gingival part of the vestibular surface of the mandibular teeth, which alters the harmonic movement during chewing since several grams of weight must be added to the mandible. This creates a disadvantage by potentially overloading the muscles. The great advantage with this methodology is the possibility of reconstructing jaw movement at any point in space.

In the optometric methodology, a television camera follows the movements of lighted points placed on the mandible. These points of light may be bright or small reflecting ambient points of light. Movement of the lights yields a three-dimensional picture of mandibular movement. Signals are sent from the cameras to a computer that reconstructs the path that the lights create in space. Reflecting points may be fixed to the mandible or to a fixed structure on the vestibular surface of lower incisors. These methods were used by Palla[29,30] and Ostry.[31-33] As in the electromechanical methodology, the great advantage is ability to reconstruct, three-dimensionally, the movement of the mandible at any point.

In the magnetometric methodology, a small magnet is fixed to the mandibular incisors, and an antenna is fixed to the head of the patient. This antenna receives movement of magnet, three-dimensionally. Examples of this methodological system are the K6I kinesograph (MyoTronics-Noromed), Sirognatograph (Siemens), and Bio-Pack (BioResearch). The great advantage of magnetometric methodology is the absolute freedom of this system. With the exception of the facial surfaces of the mandibular anterior teeth, nothing is attached to the teeth. Therefore, chewing may be considered normal.

The only disadvantage is the system's inability to record rotational movements. From a mechanical point of view, it is possible to deduce and reconstruct the movement of any point of a body if the movement of one point of that body is known. However, it is essential to know the characteristic of the movement of this point in six degrees of freedom; that is, three translatory and three rotational movements. In our specific case, we know very well the movement of the incisal point in only three degrees of freedom (translation). From this incisal point, it is impossible to reproduce the movements of other points of the mandible, for example, the condyles.

B) Proof of Validity of Masticatory Cycles in the Evaluation of Dysfunction

One of the major criticisms in this area of research is the inability to consistently register chewing cycles. Furthermore, does this kind of analysis provide any further information to the diagnosis of the craniomandibular disorders? Some believe that the chewing cycles are greatly influenced by multiple variables, including the kind of food, the occlusal status, etc.

Research reported in this area analyzes differences between healthy and dysfunctional subjects or on groups treated with various techniques using chewing cycle analysis as the discriminant. In these works, the most widely used parameters are velocity and other dynamic parameters such as height and width of the cycles. On the contrary, it was not possible to find works in which authors were able to distinguish between a healthy and dysfunctional population using the chewing analysis.

Using the Replicator, Gibbs[34-36] found a bias in the averaged values, but not in the variability of the measurements. Moreover, a group of researchers led by Howell and Klineberg[37,38] has conducted a study that demonstrated a lack of variability in chewing cycles or a great repeatability when chewing the same kind of food in 15 out of 20 patients for 40 parameters being analyzed. The remaining 5 patients had a great repeatability in 36 parameters. The possibility of utilizing the chewing cycles in diagnosis was proposed by Proschel,[39] who developed a classification system using the frontal plane of the cycle. This system enabled him to correlate dysfunctional states with certain kinds of movement.

Kuwahara[40-51] demonstrated the different pathways between working and non-working condyles in dysfunctional patients. He observed how each distinct chewing pattern appeared to be associated with a specific TM disorder. Differentiation of patients with internal derangement from patients without internal derangement could be accomplished using the position of the turning point (point where the opening became the closing) and velocity. He could differentiate patients with unilateral TM joint derangements from patients with bilateral internal derangements. Wilding and Lewin[52] analyzed patients with poor and good masticatory activity. They were able to observe that good masticatory activity is linked to a wide bilateral chewing cycle with a predominantly lateral path of closure and minimal changes in velocity.

To summarize, one can find how different aspects of the chewing cycle may be used to define health and dysfunction. In dysfunctional subjects, you may have a deviation to one side, a large variability or absolute repeatability in movement, minimal distance between the opening and the closing traces, decrease in vertical opening, and variation in the opening and/or closing velocity. This is found both with soft and hard boluses.

C) Use of Jaw Tracking K6-I in the Registration of Masticatory Cycles

For nearly 15 years, the authors have been in the process of developing and making application of a very detailed protocol for gnathologic analysis. This protocol is currently being utilized on all of the authors' patients at the end of orthodontic therapy. This protocol allows the author to evaluate the degree of dysfunction on pathologic patients and to determine the effectiveness of treatment. Our protocol also consists of a neuromuscular examination according to Jankelson's diagnostic protocol[13] and a masticatory analysis according to Lewin's original standard protocol,[21,53,54] modified by the authors.

Until recently, the K-5 and K6-I manufactured by Myo-Tronics Research Inc. was used in neuromuscular evaluation and the original Sirognatograph by Siemens was used for the analysis of chewing cycles. The software for the Chewing Cycle Analysis was written by an Italian software engineer under the authors' supervision and was released in 1985. This software enabled the authors to analyze mandibular dynamic movements and electromyography (EMG) simultaneously, evaluate the specific and mean cycles, evaluate the standard deviation, and divide clockwise from counterclockwise cycles.

In 1987, the authors made their first trial utilizing only one instrument for both the neuromuscular analysis and chewing cycle analysis. A K-5 system (Myo-Tronics Research Inc.) was adapted to our software. Later, specifications for the K6-I (Myo-Tronics Research Inc.) appeared to be more linear, having less distortion than the Sirognatograph. A test was developed to evaluate the linearity between these two instruments. To assure precise, repeatable measurements with comparable test conditions, both instruments were evaluated at the Department of Experimental Physics at the University of Torino in collaboration with the Dental School. To summarize our results, we concluded that K6-I has good reproducibility of all points, especially within the most significant volume of data. The K6-I had good precision, and the most linear distortions occurred only at the outer borders, generally not reached by large excursions of the mandible.[55]

Initially, Myo-Tronics Research Inc. developed a software utility package linked to its program. This made it possible to analyze chewing cycles using the K6-I. In 1993, we demonstrated the utility of this software. In *Figure 23 (below)* you can see an example of the chewing cycle analysis. At the top of the window there is a smaller box containing the specific cycles and at the bottom of the box are mean cycles.

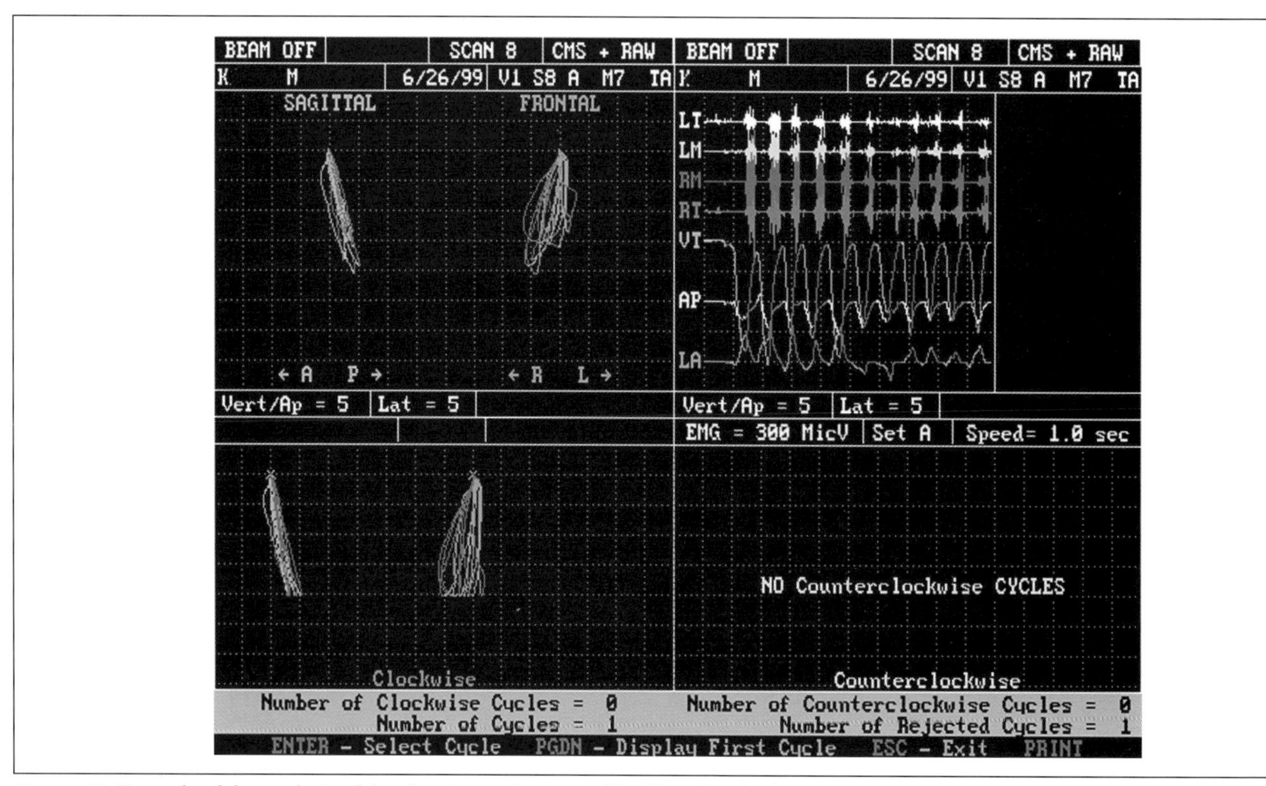

Figure 23. Example of the analysis of the chewing cycles created by Myo-Tronics in 1993.

Subsequently, the authors developed additional software to use in conjunction with the K6-I program. This gave the ability to evaluate acquired and stored data, as well as perform an in-depth analysis of the dynamics of EMG activity during mastication. In *Figures 24, 25, and 26,* you can see screens representative of the program. In *Figure 24,* there are the specific cycles for spacial analysis. In *Figure 25,* there are specific cycles for the analysis of real-time EMG, and *Figure 26,* shows averaged cycles with standard deviations. A new algorithm for both mean and standard deviation is used. The dynamic and electromyographic data acquisition lasts 10 seconds, and the results are saved on hard disk under chewing cycle (Scan 8). This scan is thc simultaneous registration of the mandibular trace (CMS) and electromyographic activities (EMG) in sweep mode. We have chosen a period of 10 seconds because it proved to be ideal for recording a sufficient number of chewing strokes without interference of the swallowing act.

Patients are asked to deliberately chew on the right side, then on the left side, and last the patient is directed to chew freely. Each is done three times, alternating the different kinds of masticatory acts in order to influence the patient as little as possible. Electromyographic activity of eight groups of muscles is collected simultaneously, typically from the anterior temporalis, masseter, anterior digastric, and posterior temporalis.

IV. Exam Execution

A) Choice of the Bolus

In performing chewing cycle analysis, the choice of the bolus is very important. A standard bolus is necessary to insure repeatability in the examination. It has already been said that chewing cycles allow one to evaluate, although in limited conditions, the functional capabilities of the musculature and joints. The characteristics of the bolus (hard or soft) cause different effects on muscles and joints. For example, a soft bolus, chewed for a long time, can arouse pain in joints with inflammation, and it can also produce spasm in tired overloaded muscles. In the same way, a hard bolus cannot be effectively chewed by muscles in spasm. A hard bolus may also allow for reduction of the disc if the displacement happens very close to the occlusion.[21] This principle for reducing a displaced disc is based on simple lever mechanics. In order to properly examine muscles and joints, we must evaluate them in different situations, using different types of boluses, one soft and one hard.

Literature on chewing cycles[21,30,56] includes the use of several types of boluses, e.g., peanuts, cheese, carrots, sweets, bread, biscuits, etc. Certain boluses may create deflections that can invalidate the examination: a bolus that breaks suddenly or one that forms irregular points can produce a nociceptive response in the patient. A bolus with a strong taste, such as cheese, can stimulate thirst; a very acidic bolus can

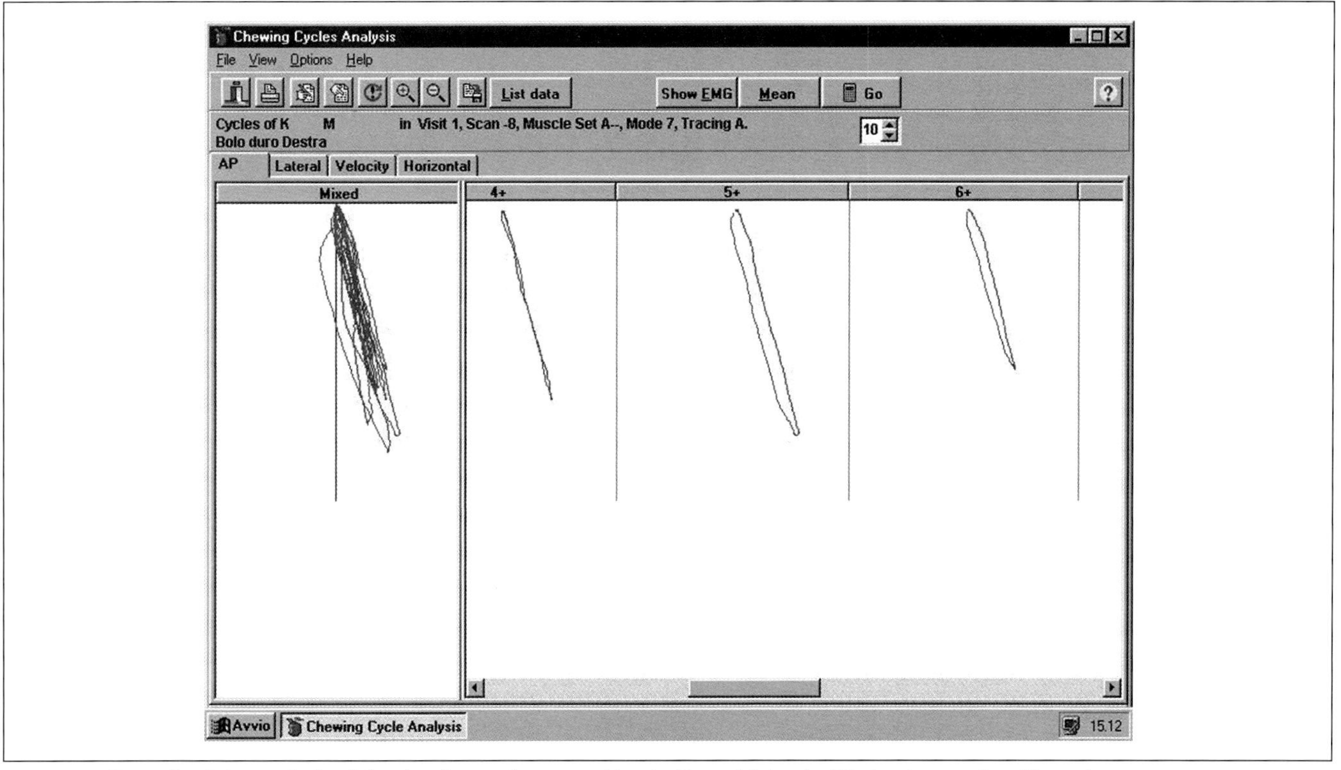

Figure 24. Example of the analysis of the chewing cycles created by the Dental School of Torino in 1997. Specific cycles.

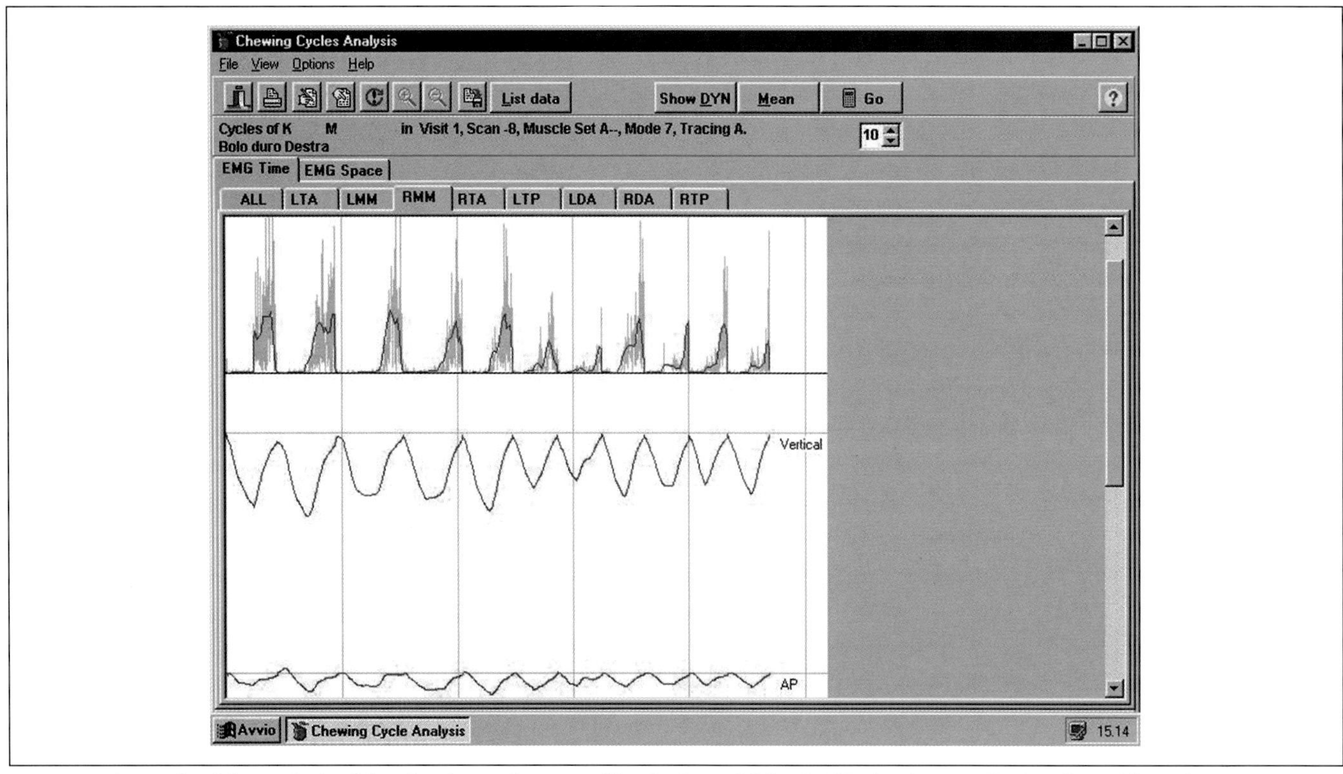

Figure 25. Example of the analysis of the chewing cycles created by the Dental School of Torino in 1997. EMG and specific cycles.

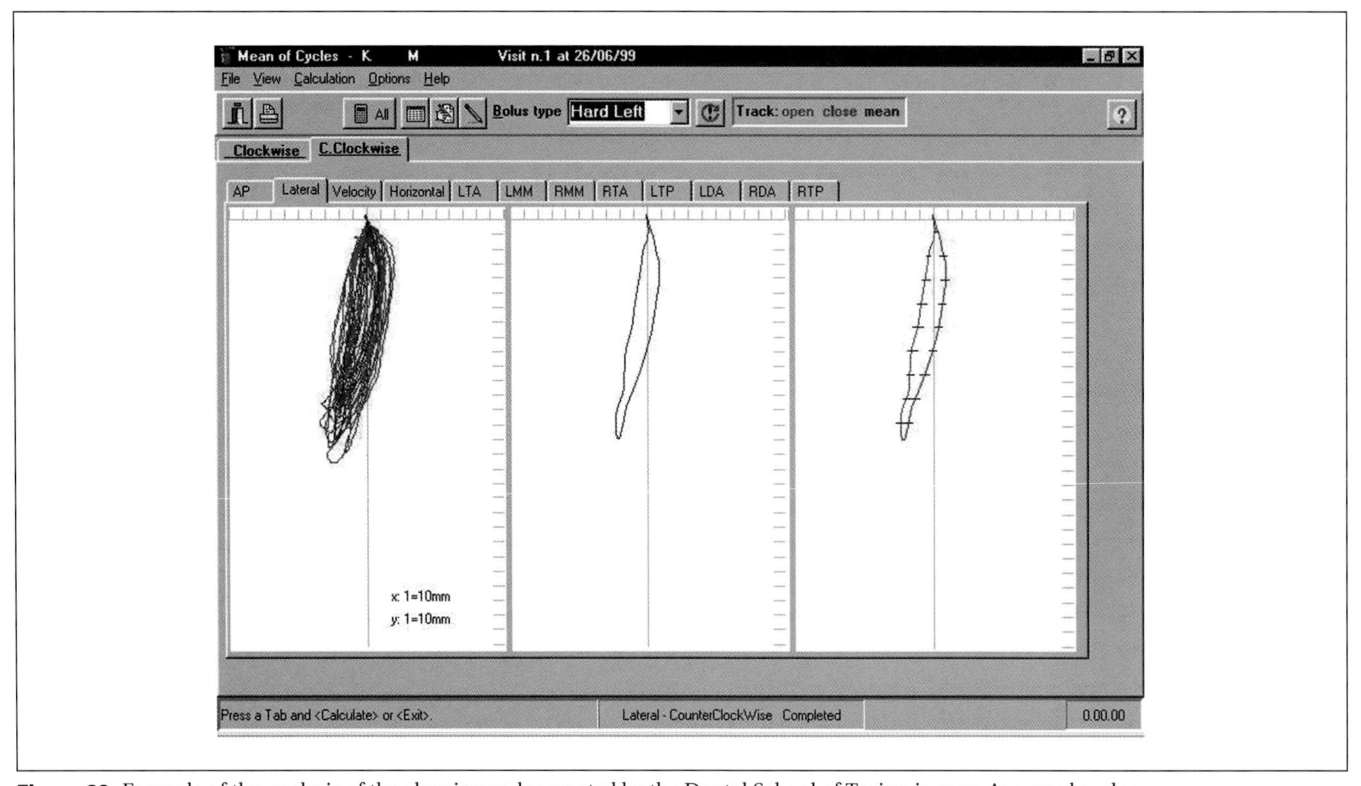

Figure 26. Example of the analysis of the chewing cycles created by the Dental School of Torino in 1997. Averaged cycles.

increase salivation. In addition, boluses that suddenly change their consistency (some biscuits or sweets) do not supply the correct information we need from that type of bolus.[21,56]

1) Boluses of Choice

It is suggested to use boluses with similar shapes, dimension, and hardness. The latter is categorized in two manners.

a) Soft bolus. It is suggested to use chewing gum that does not stick to the teeth and does not have a strong taste.
b) Hard bolus. It is suggested to use hard toffee with a standard shape, dimension, and taste. The ideal dimension might be one to two centimeters, depending on whether an adult or a child is being examined.

These dimensions hopefully allow ten seconds of chewing without provoking the stimulus of swallowing.

2) Boluses to Avoid

Boluses that are:

1) too hard which cannot be easily bitten or may create pain in the patient's teeth.
2) too large and cannot be easily placed between dental arches.
3) "explosive" (as peanuts and biscuits) or break suddenly are not well controlled by the patient.
4) of a strong taste may influence chewing.

B) Choice of the Sequence

The choice of the sequence of chewing acquisition is as important as the choice of the bolus.

It has been noted that a soft bolus may overload muscles while a hard bolus may overload the TM joints, causing pain.[21] It is best to first record cycles with a soft bolus and then record cycles with a hard bolus. It must be remembered that, during a healthy masticatory act, the contralateral TM joint to the working side translates most. When chewing a soft bolus, such as chewing gum, muscles are more loaded on the same side of chewing. When chewing a hard bolus, muscles of both sides are loaded; but the more widespread the pathology of the chewing side, the more the muscles of the opposite side are loaded. As a consequence, when considering the bolus choice, it is important to alternate the chewing side. In case of pain, provoked either by a single tooth or by a particular movement, the patient acquires protective mechanisms for avoiding that particular movement or that particular trajectory. Therefore, it is important to analyze all movement possibilities to determine an alternate sequence, if needed.

The patient is invited to chew, first on his right, then on his left, and last to chew freely. This sequence is then repeated. The free chewing is as important as right and left forced chewing. This allows identification of the preferred/less painful side. The right-left-free sequence must be repeated three times for a total of eighteen trials to have a sufficient number of chewing cycles (30 to 40) to calculate an average cycle.

C) Contraindications

The chewing cycle analysis is a non-invasive examination; therefore, some contraindications exist.

They fall within one of the following groups:

1. tooth decay and/or periodontal disease
2. fixed orthodontic appliances
3. missing posterior teeth involving one or both arches
4. dentures in one or both arches
5. acute locking and non-healed fractures.

Tooth decay or periodontal disease may create a pulpal reaction or pain affecting the results. If there is a large number of decayed teeth, even though there is no pain, portions of the bolus may be retained within the lesions, forcing the patient to make anomalous movements for recovery. The presence of a fixed orthodontic appliance is a contraindication since the bolus could lodge within the brackets and wires, forcing the patient to make anomalous movements to recover it. Missing a large number of teeth (four or five teeth in one jaw) is a contraindication since the patient cannot chew efficiently. Complete dentures are also contraindicated because of instability which could invalidate the examination. An acute closed lock and unconsolidated mandibular fractures are absolute contraindications. In fact, chewing with these conditions creates intense pain, invalidating the examination.

V. Conclusion

In this paper, the authors wished to show neurological and mechanical problems linked to chewing cycles.

Diagnostic opportunities of chewing cycle analysis have also been presented. Attention was focused on the possibility of discriminating which joint is primarily involved in the pathology. Interpretation of data considered in this paper came either from a review of the scientific literature or from many years of experience in this field.

The authors suggest that daily use of this new diagnostic facility could be useful in both diagnosis and monitoring of therapy. In fact, it must be remembered that the aim of therapy for the dysfunctional patients is not only the resolution of pain, but also the improvement of the functional capabilities.

Bibliography

1. Kaplan AS, Assael LA: *Temporomandibular disorders: diagnosis and treatment.* Philadelphia: W.B. Sauders Co., 1991.
2. The American Academy of Orofacial Pain: *Temporomandibular Disorders: Guidelines for Classification, Assessment and Management.* Chicago: Quintessence Publishing, 1993.
3. Hansson T, Honee W, Hesse J: *Craniomandibulaire Dysfunktie.* Brussel: Samson Stafleu Publishing, 1986.
4. Gola R, Chossegros C, Orthlieb JD: *Syndrome Algo-Dysfonctionnel de l'Appareil Manducateur (SADAM).* Paris: Masson, 1992.
5. Katzberg RW, Westesson PL: *Diagnosis of the Temporomandibular Joint.* Philadelphia: W.B. Saunders Co., 1993.
6. Lund JP, Widmer CG, Feine JS: Validity of diagnostic and monitoring tests used for temporomandibular disorders. *J Dent Res* 1995;74(4):1133-1143.
7. Piette E: Anatomy of the human temporomandibular joint. An updated comprehensive review. *Acta Stomat Belgica* 1993;90:103-127.
8. Gola R, Chossegros C, Orthlieb JD: Appareil discal de l'articulation temporo-mandibulaire. *Rev Stomatol Chir maxillofac* 1992;93:236-245.
9. Scheffer P, Roucayrol AM, Boudon Brière De L'isle R: Les insertions musulaires sur le disque temporo-mandibulaire. Implications physiologiques. *Rev Stomatol Chir maxillofac* 1992;93:246-251.
10. Mohl ND, McCall WD, Lund JP, Plesh O: Devices for the diagnosis and treatment of temporomandibular disorders. Part I: Introduction, scientific evidence and jaw tracking. *J Prosthet Dent* 1990;63:198-201.
11. Mohl ND, Lund JP, Widmer CG, McCall WD: Devices for the diagnosis and treatment of temporomandibular disorders. Part II: Electromyography and sonography. *J Prosthet Dent* 1990;63: 332-336.
12. Mohl ND, Ohrbach RK, Crow HC, Gross AJ: Devices for the diagnosis and treatment of temporomandibular disorders. Part III: Thermography, ultrasound, electrical stimulation and EMG biofeedback. *J Prosthet Dent* 1990;63(4):472-477.
13. Jankelson R: *Neuromuscular Dental Diagnosis and Treatment.* St. Louis: Ishiyaku EuroAmerican Publisher, 1990.
14. Anderson DJ, Matthew SB: *Mastication.* Bristol: Wright, 1976.
15. Kandel ER, Schwartz JH, Jessel TM: *Principles of Neural Science.* Amsterdam: Elsevier, 1991.
16. Luschei ES: Neural mechanisms of mandibular control: mastication and voluntary biting. In: Brooks VB. *Handbook of Phisiology, Section I: The Nervous System, Vol. 2, Motor Control.* Bethesda: American Physiological Society; 1981;1237-1274.
17. Kaas JH: Plasticity of sensory and motor maps in adult mammals. *Annu Rev Neurosci* 1992;14: 137-167.
18. Kawamura Y: *Frontiers of Oral Physiology Vol. 1: Physiology of Mastication.* Basel: S. Karger, 1974.
19. Tanji J: The supplementary motor area. *Neurosci Res* 1994;19:251-268.
20. Thach WT, Goodkin HP, Keating JG: The cerebellum and the adaptive coordination of movement. *Annu Rev Neurosci* 1992;15:403-442.
21. Lewin A: *Electrognathographics: Atlas of Diagnostic Procedures and Interpretation.* Chicago: Quintessence Publishing Co., 1985.
22. Silverman SI: Denture prosthesis and the functional anatomy of the maxillofacial structures. *J Prosthet Dent* 1956;6:305-331.
23. Nagle RJ, Sears VH: *Dental Prosthetics.* St. Louis: The C. V. Mosby Co., 1958.
24. Cannon DC, Reswick JB, Messerman T: Instrumentation for the investigation of mandibular movements. *Engineering Design Center Report EDC* 1964;4-64-8.
25. Gibbs CH, Messerman T, Reswick JB: The case gnathic Replicator for the investigation of mandibular movements. *Engineering Design Center Report EDC* 1966;4-66-14.
26. Theusner J, Plesh O, Curtis D, Hutton JE: Axiographic tracings of temporomandibular joint movements. *J Prosthet Dent* 1993;69:209-215.
27. Piehslinger E, Celar AG, Celar RM, Slavicek R: Computerized Axiography: principles and methods. *J Craniomandib Pract* 1991;9:354-355.
28. Slavicek R: Clinical and instrumental function analysis for diagnosis and treatment planning. Part VIII: Case studies in Cardiax. *J Clin Orthod* 1989;23(1):42-47.

29. Krebs M, Gallo LM, Airoldi RL, Palla S: A new method for three-dimensional reconstruction and animation of the temporomandibular joint. *Annals of the Academy of Medicine*, Singapore. 1995;24:11-16.

30. Gallo LM, Airoldi GB, Airoldi RL, Palla S: Description of mandibular finite helical axis pathways in asymptomatic subjects. *J Dent Res* 1997;76:704-713.

31. Ostry DJ, Vatikiotis-Bateson E, Gribble PL: An examination of the degrees of freedom of human jaw motion in speech and mastication. *J Speech Language Hearing Res* 1997;40:1341-1351.

32. Ostry DJ, Munhall KG: Control of jaw orientation and position in mastication and speech *J Neurophysiol* 1994;71:1528-1545.

33. Guiard-Marigny T, Ostry DY: A system for three-dimensional visualization of human jaw motion in speech. J *Speech Language Hearing Res* 1997;40:1118-1121.

34. Gibbs CH, Lunden HC, Mahan PE: Movements of the mandibular condyles during chewing. *J Dent Res* 1980 (Special Issue B);59:915.

35. Gibbs CH, Lundeen HC: *Advances in Occlusion.* Boston: John Wright-Publishing, 1982.

36. Gibbs CH, Lupkiewicz SM, King GJ, Keeling SD, Jacobson AP: Analysis of repeated-measure multicycle unilateral mastication in children. *Am J Orthod Dentofac Orthop* 1991;99:402-408.

37. Howell GT, Johnson CWL, Ellis S, Watson IB, Klineber GI: The recording and analysis of EMG and jaw tracking. I. the recording procedure *J Oral Rehab* 1992;19:595-605.

38. Howell PGT, Ellis S, Johnson CWL, Watson IB, Klineberg I: The recording and analysis of EMG and jaw tracking. II. reproducibility of jaw tracking. *J Oral Rehab* 1993;20:33-43.

39. Proschel P: An extensive classification of chewing patterns in the frontal plane. *J Craniomandib Pract* 1987;5:56-63.

40. Kuwahara T: Clinical study on the relationship between chewing movements and temporomandibular joint abnormalities (Summary). *Jour Osaka Univ Dent Soc* 1989;34(1):64-105.

41. Kuwahara T, Miyauchi S, Maruyama T: Condylar movements during mastication (Summary). *Jour Osaka Univ Dent Sch* 1989;29:87-102.

42. Kuwahara T, Miyauchi S, Maruyama T: Characteristics of condylar movements during mastication in stomatognathic dysfunction. *Int J Prosthodont* 1990;3(6):555-566.

43. Kuwahara T, Miyauchi S, Maruyama T: Clinical classification of the patterns of mandibular movements during mastication in subjects with TMJ disorders. *Int J Prosthodont* 1992;5(2):122-129.

44. Yoshioka C, Ogawa H, Kuwahara T, Takashima F, Maruyama T: The relationship between the mandibular movements during speech and specific types of malocclusions. *Jour Osaka Univ Dent Sch* 1993;33:39-44.

45. Kuwahara T, Yoshioka C, Ogawa H, Maruyama T: Effect of malocclusion on mandibular movement during speech. *Int J Prosthodont* 1994;7(3):264-270.

46. Kuwahara T, Bessette RW, Maruyama T: A retrospective study on the clinical results of temporomandibular joint surgery. *J Craniomandib Pract* 1994;12(3):179-183.

47. Kuwahara T, Bessette RW, Maruyama T: The influence of postoperative treatment on the results of temporomandibular joint meniscectomy. Part I: Comparison of mandibular opening and closing movements. *J Craniomandib Pract* 1994;12(4): 252-258.

48. Kuwahara T, Bessette RW, Maruyama T: Chewing pattern analysis in TMD patients with and without internal derangement: Part I. *J Craniomandib Pract* 1995;13(1):8-14.

49. Kuwahara T, Bessette RW, Maruyama T: Chewing pattern analysis in TMD patients with and without internal derangement: Part II. *J Craniomandib Pract* 1995;13(2):93-98.

50. Kuwahara T, Bessette RW, Maruyama T: Chewing pattern analysis in TMD patients with unilateral and bilateral internal derangement. *J Craniomandib Pract* 1995;13(3):167-172.

51. Kuwahara T, Bessette RW, Maruyama T: The influence of postoperative treatment on the results of TMJ meniscectomy. Part II: comparison of chewing movement. *J Craniomandib Pract* 1996;14(2):121-131.

52. Wilding RJ, Lewin A: The determination of optimal human jaw movements based on their association with chewing performance. *Arch Oral Biol* 1994;39:333-343.

53. Bracco P, Viora E, Deregibus A, Piancino MG: Presentazione dell' hardware e del software dell' ultima generazione per l'elaborazione dei dati sirognatografici ed elettromiografici. *RIS* 1990;58:27-34.

54. Bracco P, Deregibus A: A new program and clinical protocol for recording and analysis of chewing stroke patterns with precision and accuracy. ICCMO VIII International Congress Banff (Canada), October 1993.

55. Pane R: (Graduation Thesis). *Progettazione e sviluppo di un sistema di taratura per un kinesiografo mandibolare.* University of Torino (Italy), 1991.

56. Moller E: The Chewing Apparatus. *Acta Physiologica Scandinavica* 1966;69:280.

CLINICAL

The Fallibility of MRI Assessment as a Gold Standard in the Diagnosis of Craniomandibular Dysfunction Arising From Macrotrauma

Norman R. Thomas, Martyn R. Thomas, and N. Richard Thomas

Introduction

Considerable controversy exists in the literature over the accuracy of diagnostic tests in the determination of the status of the temporomandibular joint. Accuracy rates for subjective clinical diagnosis of internal derangement have ranged between 59% and 90% utilizing arthrography of the jaw joint as gold standard.[1-8]

Watt-Smith et al.[9] and Isberg et al.[10] contradicted these figures, but their studies were undertaken on highly selected patients. Their studies lead to the conclusion that arthrography and magnetic resonance imaging of the jaw joints did not provide any additional information useful to the diagnosis or treatment.

In our experience, with over 2,000 motor vehicle jaw joint trauma cases, it is usual for independent medical examiners to reject other clinical diagnoses based upon their own subjective clinical findings. They will often reject objective findings of others based on published works,[11-14] who have also utilized subjective assessment in addition to unsatisfactory statistical analysis.[15-16]

Magnetic resonance imaging has been shown to be superior to arthrography in the diagnosis of disc position, although less satisfactory in assessing adhesions and perforations.[17-19] Katzberg et al.[20-21] described the remarkable temporomandibular joint (TMJ) meniscus imaging by non-invasive and speedy magnetic resonance imaging. Recently, arthrography or MRI of the TMJ have been used as a gold standard to assess the accuracy of the clinical diagnosis of internal derangement and arthrosis.[22] It was concluded that the diagnostic accuracy of clinical assessment of the TMJ was 43% and hence unreliable. Langberg[23] has suggested that computerized mandibular scanning (CMS) is a valid adjunct to magnetic resonance imaging for the diagnosis of internal derangement of the temporomandibular joint. But the reliability of MRI/CMS was not assessed against the surgical findings in this study.

In a study involving 69 patients, Westesson and Paesani[24] determined that 28 asymptomatic volunteers had MRI evidence of disc displacement in one or both joints with no prior or existent TMJ symptoms, including jaw or ear pain, jaw dysfunction, jaw joint locking, maximal mouth opening of 40 mm or more, lateral excursions of more than 5 mm, and absence of joint sounds as evaluated by palpation and auscultation through the full range of mandibular motion. The asymptomatic patients showed no MRI evidence of decreased signal in the retrodiscal tissues.

In a later study by Sano and Westesson,[25] T2 signal intensity from the retrodiscal tissue was found to be increased in painful joints.

From these studies, it was indicated that painful joints have a higher degree of vascularity in the retrodiscal tissues compared with non-painful joints, and that disc position was not significantly related to signal intensity of the retrodiscal tissues.

Citing the studies of Kurita et al.,[26] Holmlund et al.,[27] Scapino,[28] Isaacson et al.,[29] Isberg et al.,[30] and Hall et al.[31] it was concluded by Sano and Westesson[25] that alteration occurs in the posterior disc attachment as a result of altered jaw function. Since altered jaw function is readily assessed by computerized, mandibular scan, it was decided to compare CMS and MRI observations in patients exhibiting unresolving retrodiscal pain and scheduled for jaw joint surgery.

Methodology

Twenty-one patients (42 joints) with an average age of 31.3 years who had suffered mandibular whiplash in a motor vehicle accident were submitted to careful physical examination, including TMJ and masticatory muscle palpation, occlusal analysis, maximal incisal opening, and review of history.

Surgery

The patients were subjected to computer mandibular scanning and MRI imaging of the jaw joints prior to surgical intervention. The surgical findings provided the gold standard for comparison with other findings.

Computerized mandibular scanning is a state-of-the-art electronic jaw tracking procedure that can indirectly depict disc displacement. In this modality, the mandible deviates sequentially in the direction of the disc dislocation and is accompanied by abnormal jaw joint sounds, reduced velocity parameters, and restricted range of jaw movements. Joint hypermobility was diagnosed by increased joint translation (A/V ratio) and by the presence of joint sounds as the condyle translated across the articular eminence. Masticatory myoelectrical potentials recorded were amplified 1000 times. A Fast Fourier Transformation (FFT) was applied and the resulting spectrum analyzed for mean power frequency (MPF) to determine the physiological rest position. EMGs were taken during 10 second intervals of maximal clench pre- and post-TENS.[34]

Disc displacements with reduction (RDD) were most often recaptured by an orthopedic repositioner formed to occlusal registrations produced by masticatory muscle relaxation through bilateral transcutaneous electrical neural stimulation (TENS) of the pre-auricular motor points.[32-33] In these cases, it was retrospectively found at joint surgery that joint adhesions were correlated with failure to resolve pain and dysfunction by orthotic therapy. In those cases where joint dysfunction and pain persisted, range of jaw joint movement, jaw tracking, and sonography[35-36] were correlated and compared with surgical findings in trial studies.

Jaw joint sounds were recorded utilizing electrosonography[35-36] of the varying joint conditions and compared with surgical findings in trial studies of surgerized temporomandibular joints. Peak frequencies at 50–100 Hz were taken as a positive indication of joint adhesions. Joint arthrosis[36] based on CMS and joint surgery findings were obtained by double blind assessment. The MRI findings were known to the surgeon prior to surgery.

Tomography

Temporomandibular joint tomography was found to be unreliable not only for providing only minimal thin sectional views through the joint, but also because it was found that joint space was inconsistently related to actual disc position as determined by surgical findings. Hence tomography of the jaw joint as a diagnostic tool was discounted in this study.

Magnetic Resonance Imaging

Magnetic resonance imaging of the temporomandibular joints incorporated bilateral surface coils (6x8 cm) at 1.5 Tesla on corrected sagittal and coronal planes through the jaw joints at closed mouth and open mouth conditions using 3 mm thickness consecutive slices T_1 weighted.

Results

Surgery revealed that 42 (100%) of the jaw joints demonstrated varying joint pathology including non-reducing disc displacement NDD (15), reducing disc displacement RDD (21), hypermobile discs HD (2), distorted discs DD (2), and joint adhesions JAds (42). *See Table I.*

Table I

	Surgical Findings	MRI Assessment
Normal	0	13
NDD	15	6
RDD	21	21
HD	2	2
DD	2	—
JAds	42	—
Total Joints	**42**	**42**

Magnetic resonance imaging failed to observe adhesions in any of the 42 joints which were shown to be present surgically. Locked discs (NDD) were missed in nine joints. In one case, a reducing displaced disc (RDD) was not diagnosed by two radiologists, but on further reading was found by a third radiologist to be displaced.

Non-reducing discs were frequently incorrectly diagnosed on MRI as normal or as reducing discs. Thus overall sensitivity and specificity in identifying disc displacement were grossly inadequate when compared against surgical findings. *See Table II.*

Table II

	Surgical Findings n=42	MRI Findings n=42
Sensitivity (disc displacement)	100%	75%
Specificity (disc displacement)	100%	60%
Overall sensitivity (joint pathology)	100%	69%
Overall specificity (joint pathology)	100%	44%

Computer Mandibular Scan Findings

By contrast, abnormal jaw tracking, altered jaw posture following TENS, abnormal velocity scan, decrease in terminal velocity (less than 150 mm/sec), abnormal joint sonography (200–600 Hz), and altered MPF of masticatory EMG pre- and post-TENS were completely correlated with the surgical findings *(Table I).*

Discussion

The findings from our study indicate that MRI is not an adequate gold standard for assessing jaw joint pathology. Computerized mandibular scan in contrast was highly correlated with the surgical findings and is therefore considered a superior non-invasive diagnostic procedure for differentiating jaw joint pathology from healthy jaw joint physiology.

The major defect of MRI studies appears to be due to the present inability to diagnose joint adhesions. Surprisingly, there was also considerable error in differentiating non-reducible disc displacement from reducible disc displacement by MRI. This may be due to the morphological changes that occur in the retrodiscal tissues with the passage of time, hence providing difficulty for the radiologists in the differentiation of the retrodiscal tissue bulge from the posterior band in the 12 o'clock position which is in agreement with the MRI studies by Westesson and Paesani.[24] They demonstrated altered signal in the retrodiscal tissues in 12% of symptomatic patients as opposed to none in the asymptomatic patients.

On the other hand, Sano and Westesson observed higher T2 signals in the retrodiscal tissues of painful jaw joints from which it was concluded that retrodiscal tissue inflammation is present in temporomandibular joint pain. Since the lateral pterygoid muscle and retrodiscal tissue function reciprocally, it is readily understood why physiopathological changes in the retrodiscal tissue may be a feature of altered jaw joint and masticatory function. Certainly the lateral pterygoid muscle activity interrelates with the anterior temporalis and posterior superficial masseter activity through feedback from muscle spindle function.[37-40] Consideration of the pre- and post-TENS mean power frequencies of the electromyogram of masseter and temporalis muscles enables diagnostic differentiation of disc lock from other types of disc condyle dissociations and muscle fatigue.

The failure of MRI to differentiate certain types of temporomandibular disorders in the in vivo condition vis a vis cadaveric material is undoubtedly related to gravitational effects on active craniomandibular and craniocervical tissues. Feedback from head, neck, and jaw muscles via muscle spindles and other proprioceptors will be affected by the supine status of the patient in the MRI chamber. Thus, directional and compressive forces in the active jaw joint differ from those in the prone position with consequent alteration in disc position and tissue fluid pressure. In contrast to this, in the cadaver the jaw is not fluid-filled and supple, thus the muscular forces ostensibly do not change with position of the specimen. The extent of joint compression will also be affected by the status of muscle fatigue, which does not of course occur in cadaveric material.

Joint adhesions as demonstrated by the sonographic signal limited at 50–100 Hz and jaw muscle mean power frequency as indicative of muscle fatigue were the most constant correlative findings of jaw and jaw joint pain. Joint pain as well as mean power frequency of the myoelectric signal in masseter and temporalis muscles were returned to healthy levels by six months following jaw joint surgery.

Bibliography

1. Roberts CA, Tallents RH, Espeland MA, Handelman SL, Katzberg RW: Mandibular range of motion versus arthrographic diagnosis of the temporomandibular joint. *Oral Surg Oral Med Oral Path* 1985;62:244-251.
2. Roberts CA, Tallents RH, Katzberg RW, Sanchez-Woodworth RE, Espeland MA, Handelman SL. Comparison of arthrographic findings of the temporomandibular joints with palpation of the muscles of mastication. *Oral Surg Oral Med Oral Path* 1987; 64:275-277.
3. Ibid. Comparison of internal derangement of the TMJ with occlusal findings. *Oral Surg Oral Med Oral Path* 1987; 63:645-650.
4. Ibid. Clinical and arthrographic evaluation of the location of temporomandibular joint pain. *Oral Surg Oral Med Oral Path* 1987;64:6-8.
5. Ibid. The clinical predictability of internal derangements of the temporomandibular joint. *Oral Surg Oral Med Oral Path* 1991;71:412-414.
6. Anderson GC, Schuffman EL, Schellhas KP, Fricton JR: Clinical vs. arthrographic diagnosis of TMJ derangements. *J Dent Res* 1989;68:826-29.
7. Kozeniauskas J: TMJ the diagnostic dilemma. *Aust Orthod J* 1988;10;213-216.
8. Kozeniauskas J, Ralph W: Bilateral arthrographic evaluation of unilateral TMJ pain and dysfunction. *J Pros Dent* 1988;60:98-105.
9. Watt-Smith S, Sadler A, Baddeley H, Renton P: Comparison of arthrogram and MRI of TMJ's with operative findings. *Brit J Oral Max Fac Surg* 1993;31:139-143.
10. Isberg A, Stenstrom B, Isaacson G: Frequency of bilateral temporomandibular joint disc displacement in patients with unilateral symptoms: A five year follow-up of the asymptomatic joints. *Dent Maxiofac Radiol* 1991;20:73-76.
11. Mohl ND, McCall WS, Lund JP, Pleash O: Devices for the diagnosis and treatment of temporomandibular disorders. Part I. Introduction, scientific evidence and jaw tracking. *J Prosthet Dent* 1990;63:198-201.
12. Mohl ND, Lund JP, Windmer CG, McCall WD: Devices for the diagnosis and treatment of temporomandibular disorders. Part II. Electromyography and Sonography. *J Prosthet Dent* 1990; 63:332-336.
13. Mohl ND, Ohabach RK, Crow HC, Gross AJ: Devices for the diagnosis and treatment of temporomandibular disorders. Part III. Tomography, ultrasound, electroneural stimulation and EMG biofeedback. *J Prosthet Dent* 1990;63:472-477.
14. Mohl ND: Current status of diagnostic modalities. Scientific Frontiers in Clinical Dentistry—An update at the National Institute of Dental Research. Bethesda, MD. April 15-16, 1993.
15. Levitt SR, McKinney MW: Appropriate use of predictive values in clinical decision making and evaluating diagnostic tests for TMD. *J Orofacial Pain* 1994;8:298-308.
16. Christensen LV, Ash MM: Remarks on probability theory and TMJ diagnosis. *J Oral Rehab* 1992;19:561-567.
17. Westesson P-L, Bronstein SL, Liedberg J: Temporomandibular joint: Correlation between Smyle-Contrast, video arthrography and postmortem morphology. *Radiology* 1986;160:767-771.
18. Tasaki MM, Westesson P-L: Temporomandibular joint diagnostic accuracy with sagittal and coronal MR imaging. *Radiology* 1993;186:723-729.
19. Rao VM, Farole A, Karasick D: Temporomandibular joint dysfunction correlation of MR imaging, arthrography and arthroscopy. *Radiology* 1990;174:663-667.
20. Katzberg RW, Bissete RW, Tallents RH et al: Normal and abnormal temporomandibular joint: MR imaging with surface coil. *Radiology* 1986;158:183-189.
21. Katzberg RW, Schneck J, Robarts D, Tallents RH et al: Magnetic resonance imaging of the temporomandibular joint meniscus. *Oral Surg Oral Med Oral Path* 1985; 59:332-335.

22. Paesani D, Westesson P-L, Halata MP, Tallents RH, Brooks SL: Accuracy of clinical diagnosis for TMJ internal derangement and arthrosis. *Oral Surg Oral Med Oral Path* 1992;73:360-363.

23. Langberg GJ: Computerized mandibular scanners, A valid adjunct to magnetic resonance imaging for the diagnosis of internal derangement of the temporomandibular joint in pathophysiology of head and neck musculo-skeletal disorders. In: Bergamini M, Prayer Galletti S, eds. *Pathophysiology of Head and Neck Musculoskeletal Disorders.* New York: Karger; 1990;52-66.

24. Westesson P-L, Paesani D: MR imaging of the TMJ. Decreased signal from the retrodiscal tissue. *Oral Surg Oral Med Oral Path* 1993;76:631-635.

25. Sano T, Westesson PL: Magnetic resonance imaging of the temporomandibular joint. Increased T2 signal in the retrodiscal tissue of painful joints. *Oral Surg Oral Med Oral Path* 1995;79:511-516.

26. Kurita K, Westesson PL, Stenby NA et al: Histologic features of the temporomandibular joint disc and posterior disc attachment comparison of symptoms free patients with internal derangement. *Oral Pathology* 1989; 67:635-43.

27. Holmlund AB, Gynther GW, Reinholt FP: Disc derangement and inflammatory changes in the posterior disk attachment of the temporomandibular joint. *Oral Surg Oral Med Oral Pathol* 1992;73:9-12.

28. Scapino RP: Histopathology associated with malposition of the human temporomandibular joint disc. *Oral Surg Oral Med Oral Pathol* 1983;55:382-397.

29. Isaacson G, Isberg A, Johansson AS, Larson O: Internal derangement of the temporomandibular joint: radiographic and histological changes associated with severe pain. *J Oral Maxillofacial Surg* 1986;44:771-778.

30. Isberg A, Isaacson G, Johansson AS, Larson O: Hyperplastic soft tissue formation in the temporomandibular joint associated with internal derangement. *Oral Surg Oral Med Oral Pathol* 1986;61:32-38.

31. Hall MB, Brown RW, Baughman RA: Histological appearance of the bilaminar zone in internal derangement of the temporomandibular joint. *Oral Surg Oral Med Oral Pathol* 1984;58:378-381.

32. Jankelson B, Savian CW, Crane PF, Radke JC: Kinesiometric Instrumentation: A new technology. *J Am Dent Assoc* 1975;90:834-840.

33. Jankelson RR: *Neuromuscular dental diagnosis and treatment.* St. Louis: Ishiyaka EuroAmerica Inc.; 1989.

34. Thomas NR: The effect of fatigue and TENS on masticatory EMG mean power frequency. In: Bergami M, Prayer Galletti S, eds. *Pathophysiology of Head and Neck Musculoskeletal Disorders.* New York: Karger; 1990;7:162-170.

35. Electrosonography. *Clinical Manual.* Seattle: Myotronics Inc., 1990.

36. Combadazou JC, Combelles PR: The efficiency of sonography in the diagnosis of joint disorders. In: Coy R, ed. *The Anthology of Craniomandibular Orthopedics.* 1992 2:207-214.

37. Griffen CI, Munro RR: Electromyography of the jaw closing muscles in the open-close clench cycle in man. *Arch Oral Biol* 1969;14:141-149.

38. Honee GLJM: An investigation on the presence of muscle spindles in the human lateral pterygoid muscle. *Ned Tijdschr Tandheel Kunde* 1966;73(3):43-48.

39. Portela-Gomes F: L'innervation proprioceptive due muscle pterygoidien externe chez l'homme et chez lapin. *Cr Ass Anat* 1963;119:1093-1097.

40. Gill HI: Neuromuscular spindles in human lateral pterygoid muscles. *J Anat* 1971;109:157-167.

Clinical Technique for Determining Appropriate Orthopedic-orthodontic Mechanics as Verified by the Quint-sectograph, K6-I Mandibular Kinesiograph, and Advanced Sassouni Analysis: A Case Report

Gregory Bixby

Overview

Cephalometric analysis has long been utilized to assess skeletal relationships that may be affected by orthodontic therapy. This paper describes a technique in which the clinician may incorporate the influences of the neuromuscular system on skeletal relationships. This analysis protocol may be used to facilitate biomechanics employed during orthodontic therapy.

Normally one should be able to open their mouth 45 mm to 60 mm without lateral deviation, measured from maxillary to mandible anterior incisal edges. Lateral mandibular movements should be 12 mm.[1] In addition to the above criteria, when the condyle is imaged with corrected tomography (Quint-sectograph), it should reside within the Gelb 4–7 position[2] and it should never violate the critical 3 mm of posterior joint space when the teeth are in centric occlusion.[3] If the first few millimeters of jaw opening are strictly a rotational phenomenon,[4] then

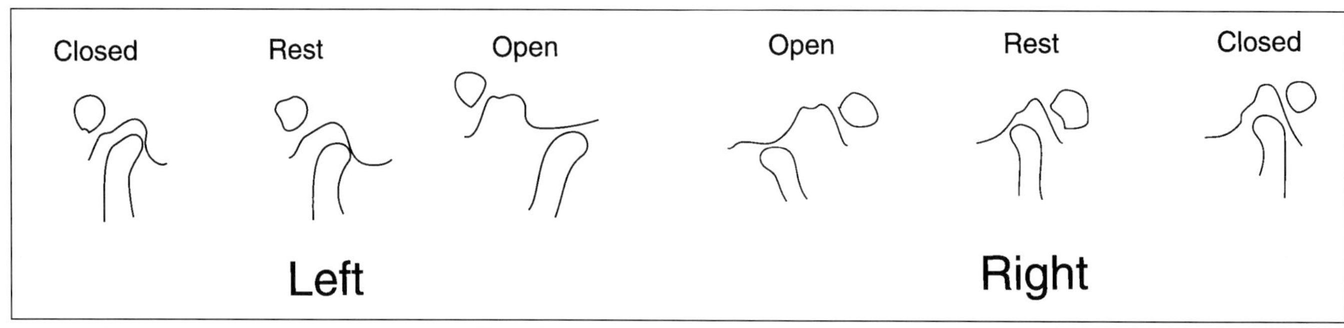

Figure 1. Pre-treatment tracings of temporomandibular joint tomograms taken in center occlusion, rest, and open positions.

there should be no discrepancy in condylar position on tomograms between centric occlusion and rest position when there is an acceptable freeway space of 1.5 mm to 2.0 mm.[5] When collecting initial orthodontic records, one must be alert to the patient who displays a discrepancy between centric occlusion and the rest position. This may indicate that the lateral pterygoid is in a state of hyperactivity.[3] Traditional cephalometric analysis,[6,7] which requires that the teeth be in centric occlusion when records are taken, is obviously of little diagnostic value in a patient who demonstrates muscular dysfunctions. Current orthodontic cephalometric analysis recognizes problems associated with this hard tissue concept.[8-10] It is at this point that the author utilizes biomedical instrumentation to evaluate craniomandibular relationships as verified by electromyographic (EMG) evaluation following application of low-frequency transcutaneous electrical neural stimulation (TENS) (Myotronics-Noromed, Tukwila, WA). Low-frequency TENS is used to establish a neuromuscular position. A biphasic pulse wave with a duration of 0.5 milliseconds, a variable amplitude from 0 to 25 milliamps, and a frequency of 1 pulse every 1.5 seconds is applied to the branches of the facial and trigeminal nerves for 45 minutes. Resting muscle EMG activity is recorded before and after TENS. When proper EMG levels are established, a K6-I kinesiograph (Myotronics-Noromed) is used to track and verify a stable mandibular position. Once a stable mandibular position is gained with appropriate EMG values, a bite position is recorded along the myotrajectory with 1.5–2.0 mm of freeway space.[11] At this neuromuscular position, tomographic images are again taken to verify that the mandibular condyles are in their appropriate relationships within the glenoid fossae and that no discrepancy exists between centric occlusion and the neuromuscular condylar positions.[12] It is at this craniomandibular relationship that an additional lateral skull radiograph is taken (Quint-sectograph). This radiograph is then traced according to the advanced Sassouni cephalometric analysis.[13-17]

Case Report

The following case will present the utilization of this technique on an adult Caucasian female, 34 years and 8 months of age. This patient presented with vertigo, tinnitis, ear fullness, stuffiness, and loss of hearing in the right ear. Her symptoms began approximately two years earlier and had intensified, causing her to seek a medical opinion and possible treatment. Her primary care physician conducted a routine medical screening exam and developed a working diagnosis of sinusitis. She was medicated with a decongestant. Following a one-month period of treatment, she returned to her physician with no improvement of her symptoms. She consequently was referred to an otolaryngologist. MRI was ordered to rule out intracranial or sinus neoplasms. MRI findings were negative, and she was subsequently diagnosed with Meniere's Disease.[18] She was informed that there is not a current cure for this ailment and 40,000 to 50,000 people suffer from this condition annually.[19]

This patient was subsequently referred to the author for evaluation. A craniomandibular disorder was diagnosed, as well as additional symptoms disclosed which included stiff neck, shoulder pain, and occasional numbness of both hands and the fingertips. These symptoms may be commonly associated with craniomandibular disorders.[20,21]

Lateral skull radiographs were taken and traced according to the principles of the Sassouni Plus technique in centric occlusion. Tomograms were taken in the centric occlusion, rest, and maximum open positions *(Figure 1)* followed by cephalometric analysis. Low-frequency TENS was applied to the patient for 45 minutes, and a bite relationship was taken at a myocentric position *(Figure 2)* utilizing a K6-I mandibular kinesiograph as previously described. Additional tomograms were taken at myocentric, rest, and maximum open positions and traced *(Figure 3)*. An orthotic was constructed for the patient at the myocentric position. She was instructed to wear this 24 hours per day. This patient returned for a three-week follow-up appointment, at which time all symptoms had subsided.

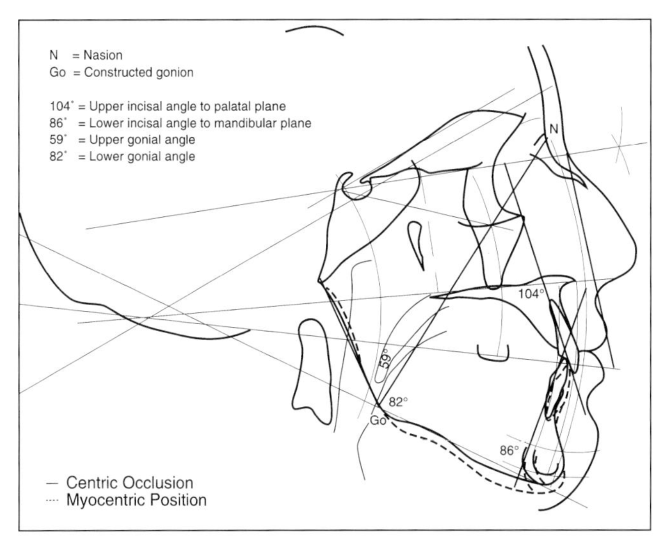

Figure 2. Sassouni cephalometric analysis at myocentric position.

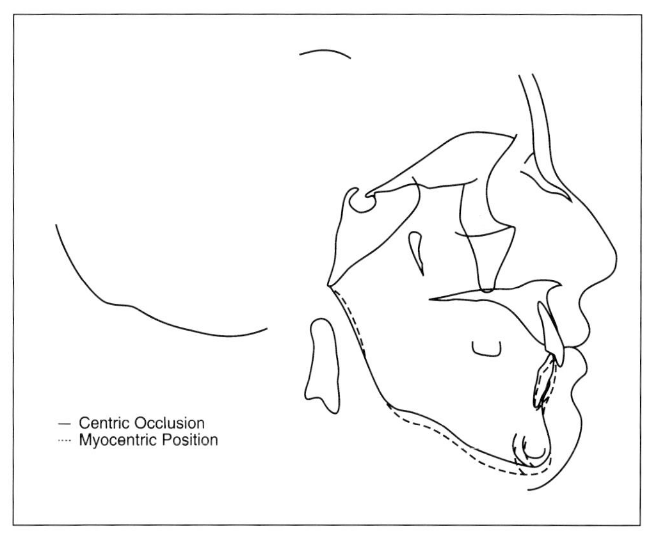

Figure 4. Lateral skull tracings in centric occlusion and myocentric position.

Since this patient's overlay Sassouni Plus analysis indicated that the ramal position remained the same following TENS application, there was an apparent change in the posterior borders. Pogonion actually became more normally positioned since the patient had a pronounced mental protuberance.

The lower lip posture remained exactly the same on both lateral skull radiographs, indicating that lower lip posture is more dependent on the upper incisal angle as opposed to the lower incisal angle. Note how the lower lip is nearly perfect following TENS *(Figure 4)*, resulting in no discrepancy between myocentric and rest position on the tomograms *(Figure 3)*. Consequently, orthopedic appliances were constructed in this position to correct transverse discrepancies while maintaining this vertical dimension. This case was then verticalized, utilizing a verticalizing orthodontic appliance, and is now being finished with Roth straightwire orthodontics.

Discussion

The preceding clinical case demonstrated that when treating the orthodontic patient the establishment of optimal muscle tone and function with proper placement of the condyles within the glenoid fossae is critical to provide an environment that will minimize orthodontic relapse, pain, and dysfunction. This is accomplished through the development of a comprehensive treatment plan utilizing a comprehensive clinical exam, radiologic imaging, and biomedical instrumentation.

When tracing lateral skull radiographs for orthopedic/orthodontic therapy, it becomes very obvious to the neuromuscular clinician that this technique will dramatically change the appliance selection and the mechanics used to treat the case, as opposed to a case treated in habitual occlusion.

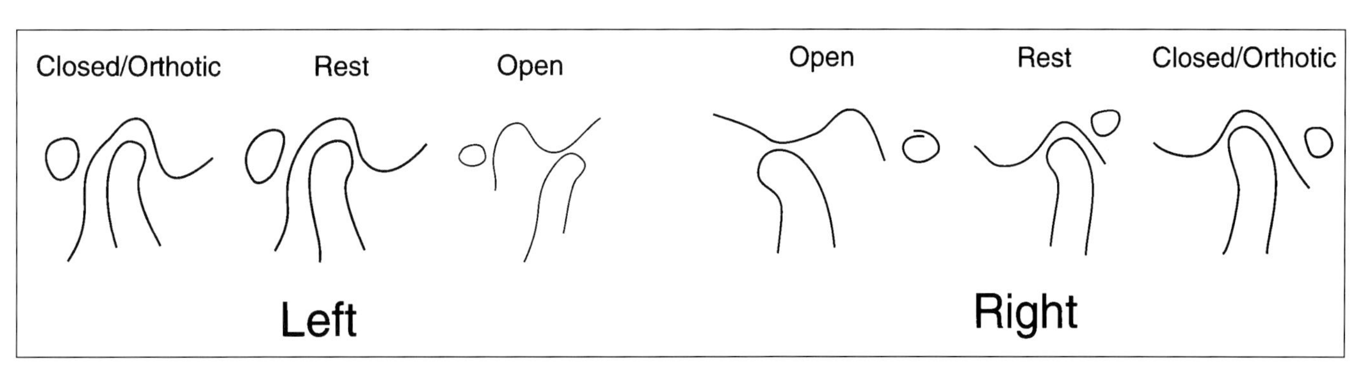

Figure 3. Tomographic tracings of the temporomandibular joints in myocentric position, rest, and maximum opening.

References

1. Stack BC: *Advanced TMJ Diagnosis to Splint Construction.* 1990, 93-115.
2. Gelb H: Effective management and treatment of the craniomandibular syndrome. In: Gelb H, ed. *Clinical Managment of Head, Neck and TMJ Pain and Dysfunction.* Philadelphia: W. B. Saunders Co.; 1977;314-320.
3. Witzig IW, Spahl TJ: Eliminating the NRDM/SPDC phenomenon: physiology put right again. In: Witzig WW, Spahl TJ, eds. *The Clinical Management of Basic Maxillofacial Orthopedic Appliances.* St. Louis: Mosby Yearbook, Inc.; 1991;287-411.
4. Spahl TI: The Fact Appliance. *Funct Orthod* 1998;15(2):4-23.
5. Melkonian RW: Relationship of Condylar Position and Vertical Freeway Space as Measured on the Quint Sectograph and the K6I Mandibular Kinesiograph. In: Coy R, ed. *Anthology of Craniomandibular Orthopedics Vol 2.* Collinsville, Illinois: ICCMO; 1992;239-246.
6. Perry HT: Principles of occlusion applied to modern orthodontics. *Dent Clin N Am* 1969;13:581-590.
7. Keller D: Orthotics; An Essential Orthodontic Diagnostic Tool. *J Gen Orthod* 1996;7(3):1-30.
8. Grummons D: *Orthodontics For the 7W/7MD Patient.* Scottsdale: Wright and Co., 1994.
9. Jankleson RR: *Neuromuscular Dental Diagnosis and Treatment.* St. Louis: Ishiyaku EuroAmerica, Inc., 1990.
10. Callader J: Orthodontic application of the mandibular kinesiograph. *J Clin Orthod* 1984;18(10):710-718.
11. Mazzoco MW: Physiology of Occlusion Seminar. Seattle, Washington: Myotronics Research Inc., 1996.
12. Cooper BC: Craniomandibular disorders. In: Cooper BC, Lucent EK; eds. *Management of Facial, Head and Neck Pain.* Philadelphia: Saunders; 1989;153-254.
13. Beistle R: Advanced Sassouni. Midwest Facial Symposium. Columbus, Ohio: S.W.O.S., 1996.
14. Magill T: *Sassouni Plus Cepholometric Analysis, Next Step Orthodontics.* Denver, Colorado: S.W.O.S., April, 1998.
15. Beistle RT: Sassouni Plus. *Funct Orthod* 1984;1(1): 39-48.
16. Gerber JW: *Orthodontic Course Manual.* 1987.
17. Personal Communication with Richard Beistle.
18. Bjorne A: Cervical signs and symptoms in patients with Meniere's Disease: A controlled study. *J Craniomandib Pract* 1998;16(3):194-202.
19. Stahle J, Stahle C, Arenberg IK: The incidence of Meniere's Diease. *Arch Otolaryngol* 1978;104: 99-102.
20. Steigerwald D, Verne S , Young D: A retrospective evaluation of the impact of joint arthroplasty on the symptoms of headache, neck pain, shoulder pain, dizziness and tinnitis. *J Craniomandib Pract* 1996;4:46-54.
21. Travell JS, Simons DG: *Myofacial Pain and Dysfunction—The Trigger-point Manual.* Baltimore: The Williams and Wilkins Co., 1983.

Clinical Application of TMJ Viscoelasticity Analyzer

Mitsuhiro Tatsuta, Masahiro Tanaka, and Takayoshi Kawazoe

Introduction

It has been reported that soft tissues of the temporomandibular joint (TMJ) region influence the position and movement of the condyles. Development of magnetic resonance imaging (MRI) has recently made possible the visualization of these tissues, especially the articular disc. This has permitted accurate diagnosis of TMJ disorders. While MRI primarily provides positional information, analysis of biomechanical (viscoelastic) properties of the region gives additional valuable diagnostic information on the function and pathological changes in soft tissues.

It has been reported that the human body possesses the properties of viscosity and elasticity. The analysis of viscoelastic properties has been carried out in periodontium for the index of tooth mobility.[1,2] There have been few studies on the biomechanical properties of the soft tissues of the TMJ region. Some authors have examined the relationship between peripheral joint mobility and the range of mandibular movements,[3,4] and there have been some attempts to measure the viscoelasticity of the TMJ. However, no quantitative method has been established for assessing the biomechanical properties of this region.

The diagnosis in patients with temporomandibular disorders has been primarily estimated through inquiry about the clinical course, palpation of masticatory muscles, and imaging. However, these methods depend upon a patient's or operator's subjectivity, which is affected by one's experience and sensibilities. In order to assess patients objectively, recording and analyzing of jaw movements and electromyographic signals of masticatory muscles were performed.

We have already developed a TMJ viscoelasticity analyzer[5] for non-invasive estimation of the biomechanical properties of the TMJ region. This system measures the mobility of the mandible and presumes the viscoelasticity of the TMJ region. In the initial type of system, we applied random vibration on the mandibular incisors and detected acceleration and resistance force when applied to the mandibular central incisors. However, we could not measure the TMJ viscoelasticity in case of loss of mandibular central incisor. Therefore, we applied random vibration on the chin and detected acceleration and force from the chin. We feel that information on biomechanical properties of the TMJ region should be useful not only for examining patients with temporomandibular disorders (TMD), but also for judging treatment outcomes.

In this paper, we introduce the TMJ viscoelasticity analyzer and describe viscoelastic parameters of the TMJ region in normal volunteers and patients with temporomandibular disorders (TMD) calculated from the TMJ Viscoelasticity Analyzer.

Materials and Methods

TMJ Viscoelasticity Analyzer

Figure 1 is a schematic diagram of the TMJ Viscoelasticity Analyzer, which estimates the viscoelastic properties of the TMJ region. It is composed of a device for measuring mechanical mobility and a data analysis unit that includes a personal computer. Random vibrations of 30–1000 Hz were applied through the chin by a portable vibrator with a small built-in impedance head.

Input acceleration and force response at the driving point were monitored by an impedance head fitted with two piezoelectric elements. Sampled signals were fed into an analog-to-digital (A/D) converter and processed by the Fast Fourier Transform (FFT) algorithm. The sampling interval is set at 333 μsec to obtain a frequency spectra below 1 kHz. Fast Fourier Transform processing was performed for 256 data points that are averaged 16 times at a frequency resolution of about 11.8 Hz. A digital data processing board was used for rapid FFT processing. During measurements, the preload fluctuation was also sampled by an A/D converter coupled to a personal computer.

With this apparatus it is possible for the examiner to measure mechanical mobility at a higher preload accuracy by checking the time course of preload fluctuations on the monitor, and this must be kept at 200±20 gf (gram force). All operations can be done by one examiner since the analyzer is equipped with a foot-switch to trigger operation of the personal computer.

Each volunteer was comfortably seated in a dental chair in an upright position. Measurement conditions were as follows: the Camper's plane was kept parallel to the floor, the vibrating direction was parallel to the Camper's plane in a midsagittal plane, and

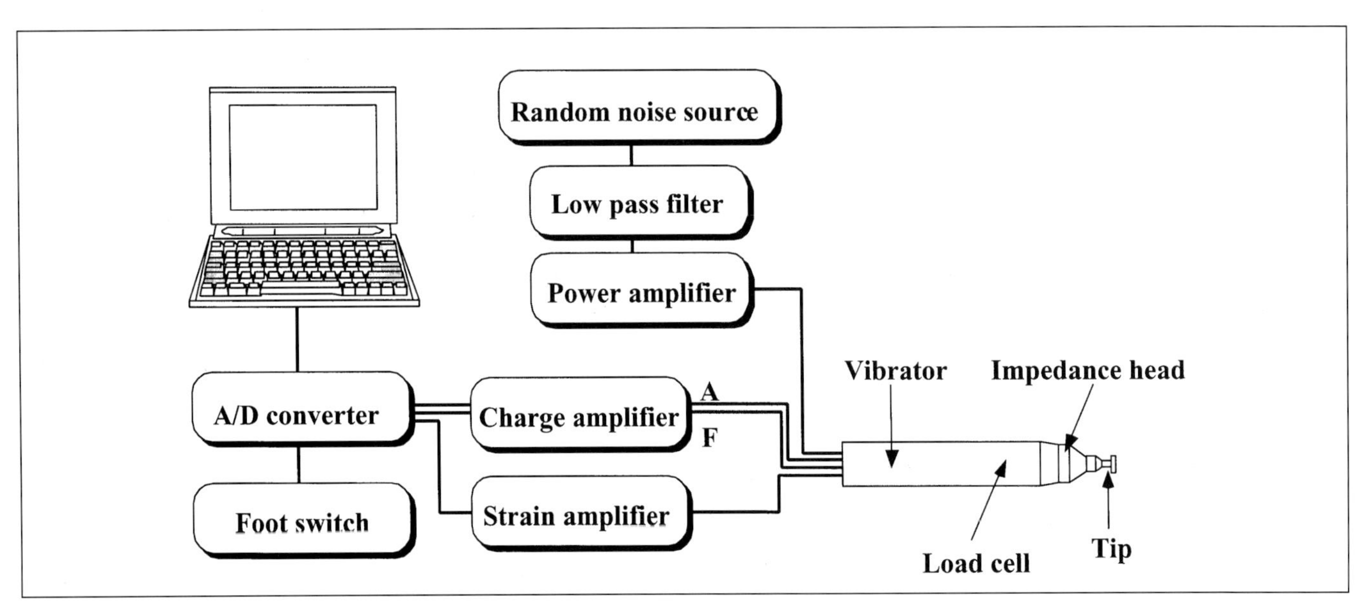

Figure 1. Schematic diagram and measuring conditions of the TMJ viscoelasticity analyzer.

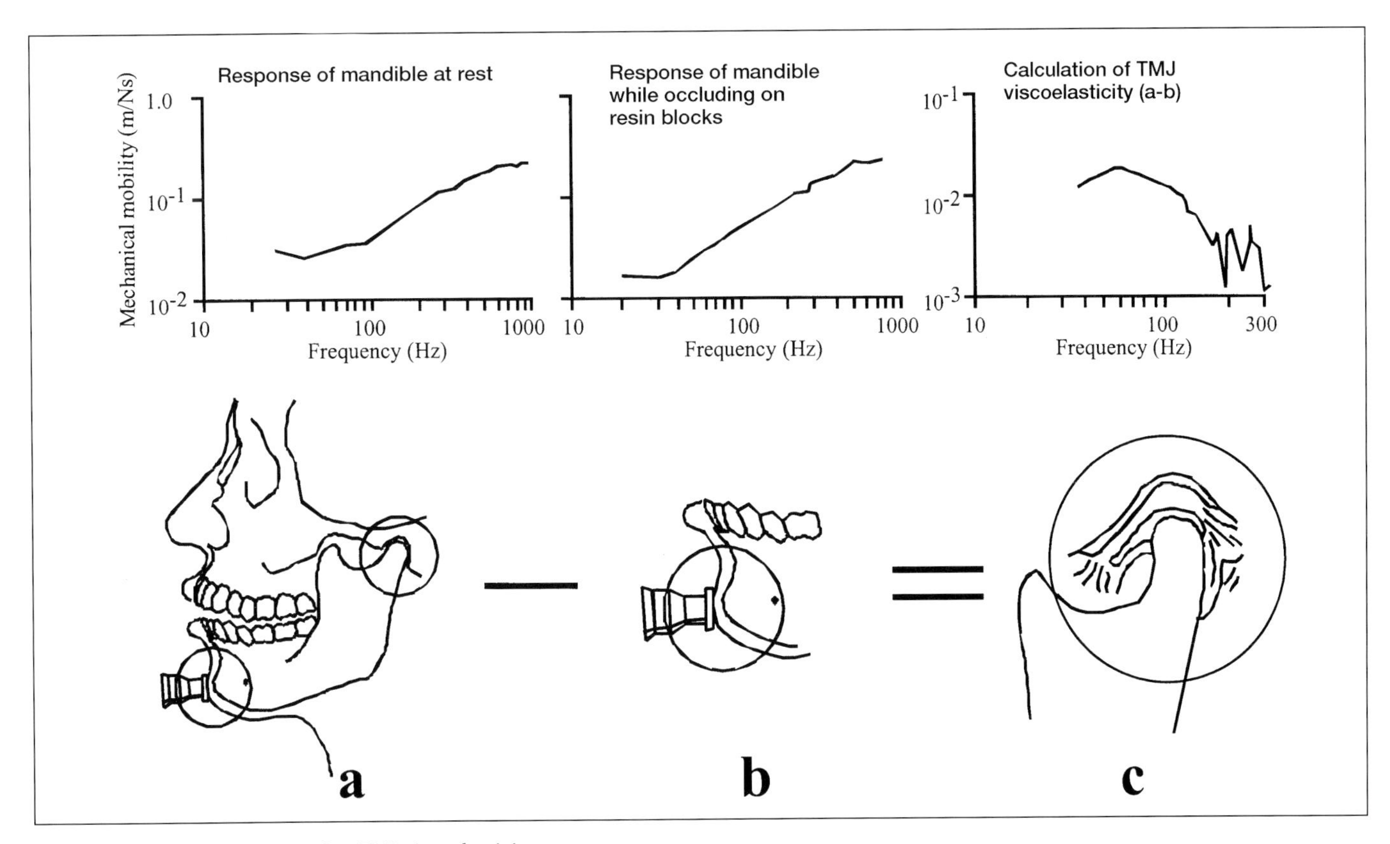

Figure 2. Procedure in measuring TMJ viscoelasticity.

measurements were recorded five times at each position (rest and bite positions).

Figure 2 illustrates the procedure when measuring TMJ viscoelasticity. First, the soft tissues of the TMJ region were randomly vibrated through the chin. The mechanical mobility spectrum which provided information about viscoelasticity of the chin and the TMJ region was obtained *(Figure 2a)*. Secondly, the volunteers were instructed to occlude on resin blocks (1.0 mm in height at the first molar) to prevent condylar movement and measurements were carried out again. This provided the mobility spectrum which provided the viscoelasticity of the chin *(Figure 2b)*. Mechanical mobility of the TMJ region was determined by subtracting the second data from the first *(Figure 2c)*.

First, a dynamic mechanical model of the TMJ region was developed, which is shown in *Figure 3*. Accordingly, it is possible to determine the modeling parameters c (viscosity), k (elasticity), and m (mass) using graphical techniques. The mechanical parameters for this model were determined with a personal computer based on findings generated by automatically fitting a curve to mobility spectra (curve-fitting method using least squares method). We assessed the viscoelasticity of the TMJ region with three biomechanical parameters: viscosity, c; elasticity, k; and mass, m.

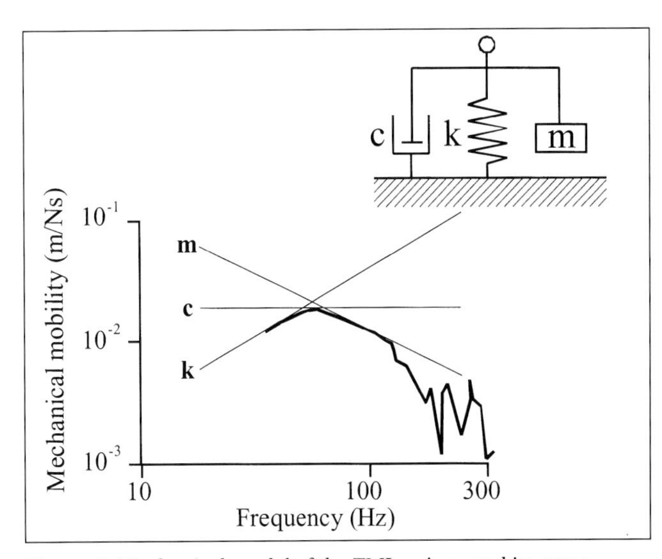

Figure 3. Mechanical model of the TMJ regions and its curve fitting on the mobility spectrum.

In this study, measurements were carried out using the TMJ viscoelasticity analyzer.

Measurement in Normal Subjects

Twenty-four healthy volunteers (12 males and 12 females), mean age 25.8 years, participated in this study. None had a history of functional disturbances in the masticatory system or any signs or symptoms,

Table I
List of patients with temporomandibular disorders

Patient		Chief Complaint	TMJ Symptom	Muscle Symptom	Behavior
Male:	#1	Trismus	Tenderness, clicking (L)	Pain	None
	#2	Occlusal instability	Clicking (L)	Pain	Bruxism
	#3	Muscle pain	None	Pain	None
	#4	TMJ sound	Clicking (R)	None	None
	#5	Muscle pain	None	Pain	Bruxism
Female:	#6	Trismus	None	None	None
	#7	Trismus	Tenderness, clicking (RL)	None	None
	#8	Trismus	Tenderness, clicking (RL)	Pain	None
	#9	TMJ sound	Clicking (R)	None	None
	#10	TMJ sound	Clicking (RL)	Pain	None

such as limited opening or tenderness to palpation of temporomandibular joint or masticatory muscles. Measurements were carried out between 2 PM and 6 PM, more than two hours after eating.

Sex differences were statistically examined using Mann-Whitney U test and normal ranges (mean ±2SD) were prepared for the following study.

Measurement in Patients with Temporomandibular Disorders

Using data obtained from the normal subjects as a standard, we analyzed 10 patients (five male and five female, mean age 26.4 years) with temporomandibular disorders. *Table 1* summarizes signs and symptoms of the patients at their first visit. Almost all patients had a sense of discomfort of masticatory muscle and TMJ noise. Occlusal analysis showed no missing teeth in all patients.

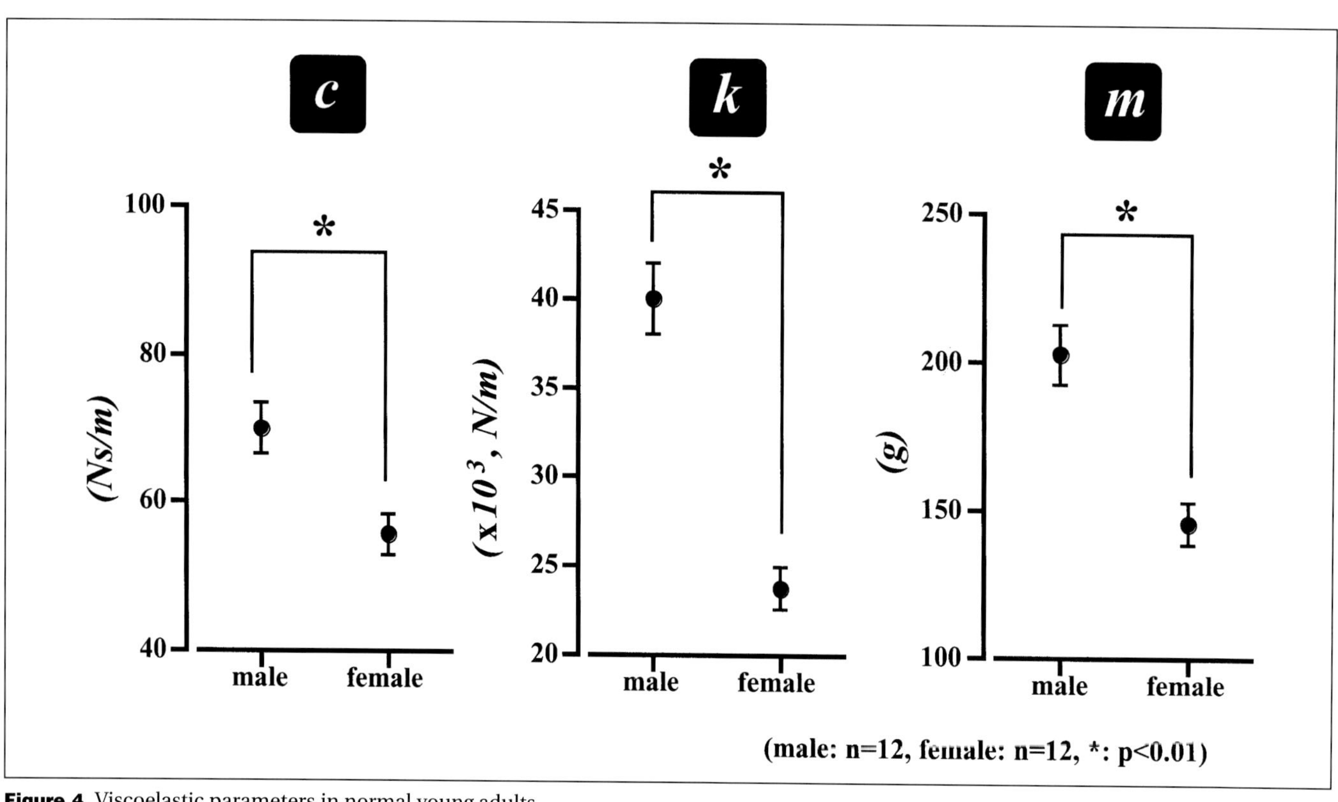

Figure 4. Viscoelastic parameters in normal young adults.

Change with Treatment in Patients with Temporomandibular Disorders

We selected two typical patients with good treatment prognosis from the list shown in *Table 1 (Patient #1 and #6)*. Temporomandibular joint viscoelasticity and clinical symptoms were evaluated during treatment with stabilization occlusal splint therapy and occlusal adjustment.

Results

Measurement in Normal Subjects

Figure 4 illustrated the viscoelastic properties in normal young adults. Normal volunteers indicated specific ranges in all viscoelastic parameters. Each viscoelastic parameter of the TMJ region was c: 69.6 ±8.2 (Ns/m, mean±1SD), k: 39.5 ±7.6 (x10^3, N/m) and m: 200.8 ±12.8 (g) in male and c: 55.1 ±5.7 (Ns/m), k: 23.3 ±6.3 (x10^3, N/m) and m: 143.5 ±15.4 (g) in female. Significant differences were found for viscoelastic parameters of the TMJ region between sexes ($p<0.01$). The normal range was determined as mean ±2SD in each parameter.

Measurement in Patients with Temporomandibular Disorders

During the first visit, the viscoelastic parameters fell outside the range for the normal subjects. Two patterns were observed in patients compared with normal ranges. The viscoelastic parameters in patients #1, #3, #4, #5, #6, #7, and #8 were larger than the normal subjects. On the other hand, the viscoelastic properties in patients #9 and #10 were smaller than those in the normal subjects *(Figure 5)*.

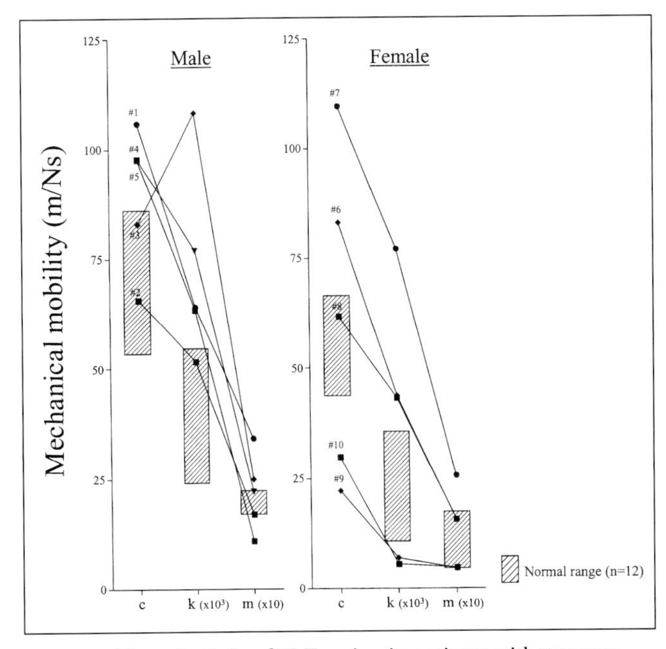

Figure 5. Viscoelasticity of TMJ region in patients with temporomandibular disorders.

Change with Treatment in Patients with Temporomandibular Disorders

With treatment utilizing a stabilization occlusal appliance, the values for viscoelastic parameters for patients began to fall within the range for normals and fell within the norms following treatment. *Figures 6 and 7* represented the treatment variation with appliance therapy for patients with temporomandibular disorders. We presented two patients who were selected from the patients list shown in *Table 1 (Patient #1 and #6)*. Their parameters were outside the scope of normal ranges at pre-treatment. As the treatment for temporomandibular disorders with appliance therapy proceeded, the viscoelastic parameters became more normal in both patients. Patient status improved with treatment.

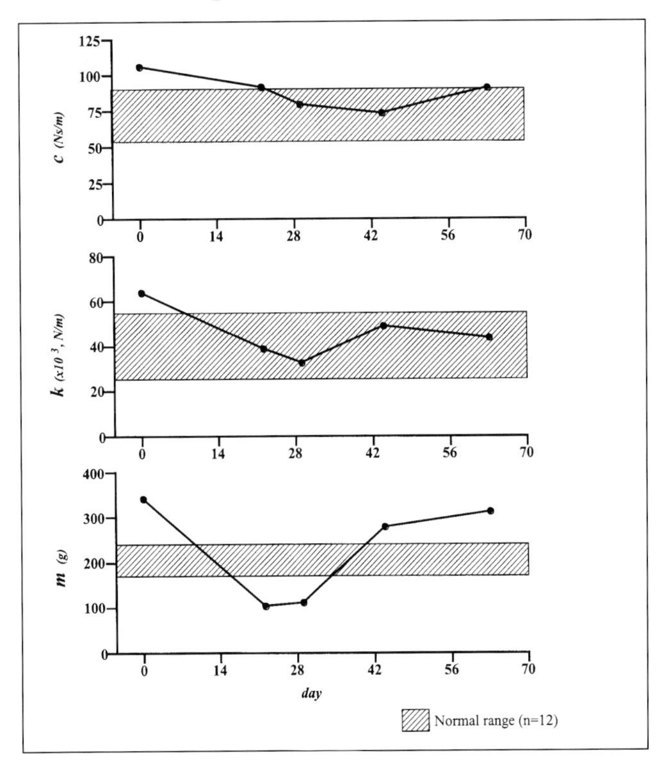

Figure 6. Treatment variation of viscoelasticity of the TMJ region with appliance therapy for patients with temporomandibular disorders (patient #1, male).

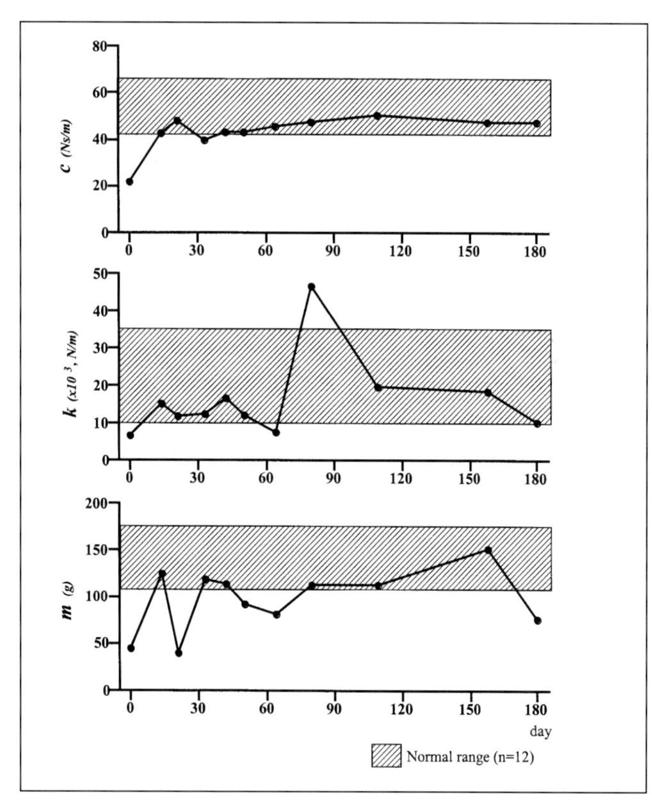

Figure 7. Treatment variation of viscoelasticity of the TMJ region with appliance therapy for patients with temporomandibular disorders (patient #6, female).

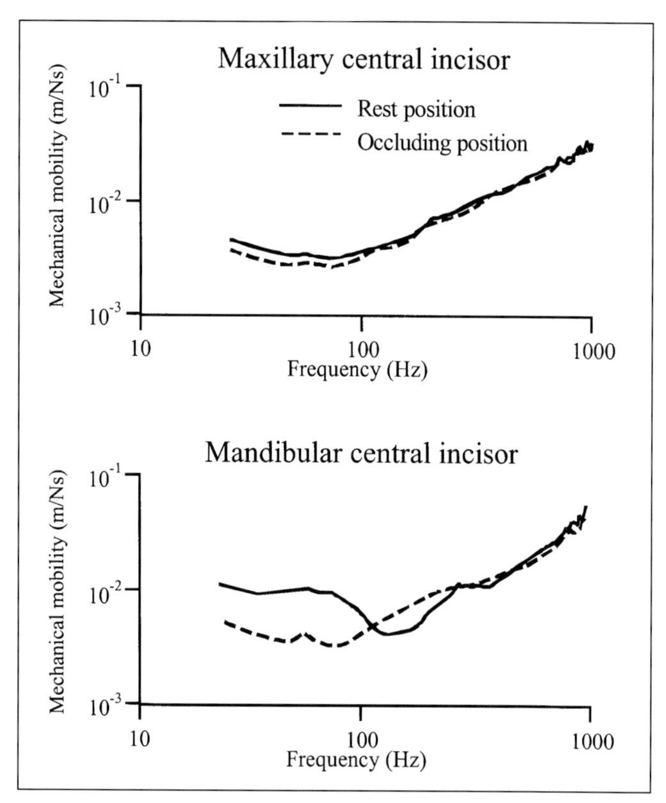

Figure 8. Changes in the mobility spectra for maxillary and mandibular incisors.

Discussion

TMJ Viscoelasticity Analyzer

The TMJ Viscoelasticity Analyzer was developed to determine tooth mobility.[6,7] *Figure 8* shows the mobility spectra for the maxillary and mandibular central incisors, which were measured using this system. The mobility spectra shown by the solid lines, which were measured with the mandible in the rest position, were different for the maxillary and mandibular central incisors. The mobility spectra shown by the broken lines were determined with the volunteers occluding on resin blocks in the molar region. Little difference was observed in the mobility spectra for the maxillary incisors when observed at rest position and at an occluded position. However, there was a significant difference between the two positions for the mandibular incisors, resulting from mobility of the mandible.

A measurement device and computer assisted program was developed to measure differences in biomechanical properties in the temporomandibular joint region.[8] However, no measurements could be made in the absence of mandibular central incisors. By changing the measurement point from the mandibular central incisor to the chin, it became possible to determine parameters for all patients. We named this new system the TMJ Viscoelasticity Analyzer. The actual measurements take about 30 seconds, and the computations another 90 seconds.

Biomechanical Model of TMJ Region

In order to assess the biomechanical properties of the TMJ region, we constructed a dynamic mechanical model of the TMJ region with a computer assisted spectral program *(Figure 3)*. Because it is difficult to understand viscoelastic information from only the mobility spectra, we decided to analyze mechanical parameters. The mobility spectrum in *Figure 3* shows the method for determining the viscoelastic parameters c, k, and m. Each parameter is based on the theoretical viscoelastic response at various frequencies *(Figure 9)*.

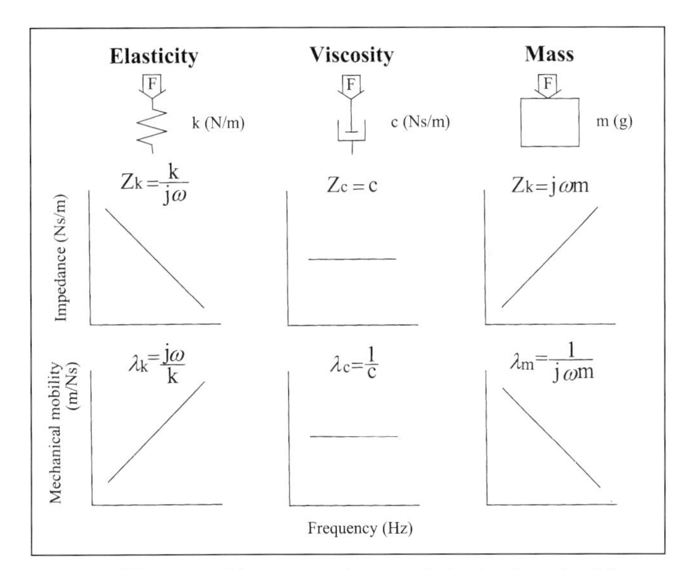

Figure 9. Theoretical frequency characteristics in viscoelasticity.

A mechanical model of the TMJ region was constructed for quantitative assessment.[9] Our mechanical model is superior to Noyes's model, where the mechanical mobility of the TMJ region was viewed based on oscillations. Moreover, because we applied curve fitting to the mobility spectra, it was possible to objectively assess biomechanical conditions in the TMJ region.

Viscoelasticity in Normal Volunteers and Patients

The TMJ Viscoelasticity Analyzer can estimate TMJ viscoelasticity non-invasively. The recording time takes about two seconds, and the analysis time for each measurement takes approximately five minutes. Our measurements were carried out between 2 PM and 6 PM, which was at least two hours after eating, to prevent any effect that mastication may have on the viscoelasticity of the TMJ region.

Viscoelastic parameters from normal volunteers were applied to viscoelastic values for patients with temporomandibular disorders. The viscoelasticity of the TMJ region is affected by many factors, including uncoordinated muscle movment, occlusal contacts, and stress, since the TMJ is a fulcrum or a mandibular lever.

Many epidemiological reports[10,11] indicate a patient ratio for TMD varying from 3:1 to 8:1, females to males. In normal volunteers, it was observed that females had significantly smaller viscoelastic parameters than those in males. The results of this study indicated that women have more soft and/or movable soft tissues of the TMJ region than males. It is inferred that viscoelastic differences between sexes may influence the number of patients with temporomandibular disorders.

In TMD patients, the viscoelastic parameters fell outside of the normal range when compared to normal subjects at the first visit. Observed were two patterns of high and low values compared with the normal ranges. However, it was found that with treatment these variations in viscoelastic parameters for patients ultimately fell within the ranges established for the normal subject. With treatment, no significant differences could be shown when comparing viscoelastic values for normal subjects and patients. It will be necessary to confirm what factors influence these parameters in the future.

Intra-articular soft tissues consist of the disc, retrodiscal tissue, synovium, synovial fluid, capsule, and associated ligamentous structures. In patients with temporomandibular disorders, these soft tissues may be traumatized and blood flow may be compromised. Appliance therapy has been developed for repositioning the mandible, possibly the disc, and influencing the investing and associated musculature. As the treatment proceeds, the condyle may move into a suitable position. It provides an environment which enables soft tissue to heal and normalization of the TMJ. Further, this environment allows viscoelastic parameters to normalize in the patient population.

These results indicate that the TMJ Viscoelasticity Analyzer can determine viscoelastic changes for the temporomandibular joint.

Conclusion

We may conclude the following:

1) The viscoelastic parameters of the TMJ region in normal individuals were significantly different between sexes.

2) The viscoelastic parameters of the TMJ region in patients with temporomandibular disorders were outside the scope of normal ranges.

3) In patients, the viscoelastic parameters fell within normal ranges following appliance therapy and occlusal adjustment.

References

1. Noyes DH, Clark JW, Watson CE: Mechanical input impedance of human teeth in vivo. *Med & Biol Engng* 1968;6:487-492.
2. Saratani K, Tatsuta M, Mizui M, Tanaka M, Kawazoe T: Quantitative assessment of laxity of the temporomandibular joint. *J Dent Res* 1994;73:262.
3. Bates RE, Stewart CM, Atkinson WB: The relationship between internal derangements of the temporomandibular joint and systemic joint laxity. *J Am Dent Assoc* 1984;109:446-447.
4. Westling L: Craniomandibular disorders and general joint mobility. *Acta Odontol Scand* 1989;47:293-299.

5. Tatsuta M, Saratani K, Furuichi E, Oka H, Kawazoe T: Development and validation of TMJ viscoelasticity analyzer. *J Osaka Dent Univ* 1996;30:7-14.

6. Oka H, Yamamoto T, Saratani K, Kawazoe T: Automatic diagnosis system of tooth mobility for clinical use. *Med Prog Technol* 1990;16:117-124.

7. Tatsuta M, Saratani K, Kawazoe T, Nakanishi T, Kuno Y, Matsumoto S: Normal range of viscoelastic properties of periodontium using automatic diagnostic system for tooth mobility. *J Jpn Prosthodont Soc* 1994;38:1265-1272.

8. Nabeshima F: Determination of the biomechanical properties of the temporomandibular joint region by mechanical mobility. *J Jpn Prosthodont Soc* 1992;36:299-313.

9. Noyes DH, Solt CW: Elastic response of temporomandibular joint to very small force. *J Periodontol* 1997;48:98-100.

10. Helkimo M: Epidemiological surveys of dysfunction of the masticatory system. In: Zarb GA, Carlsson GE, eds. *Temporomandibular joint function and dysfunction.* St. Louis, Missouri: CV Mosby Co.; 1979;175-192.

11. Rieder CE, Martinoff JT, Wilcox SA: The prevalence of mandibular dysfunction, Part 1: Sex and age distribution of related signs and symptoms. *J Prosthet Dent* 1983;50:81-88.

Utilization of Electromyographic Spectral Analysis in the Diagnosis and Treatment of Craniomandibular Dysfunction

Norman R. Thomas

Craniomandibular disorder is a chronic condition characterized by pain and dysfunction and dependent upon interaction between segmental and suprasegmental including righting or postural reflexes.[1] As a basis for understanding, it is helpful to revisit the Sherrington model of neuromuscular differentiation and integration.

Sherrington Model of Interrelationships Between Craniocervical and Axial Reflexes

The reflex figures that result from interaction of nociceptor and uprighting reflexes in the decerebrate state have been well described in the Nobel Laureate findings of Sherrington including interaction with jaw reflexes.[2] When a noxious stimulus is applied to the organism, the stimulated part is withdrawn from the point of stimulation. Ipsilateral flexor motoneurones are facilitated by noxious afferents, while ipsilateral extensor motoneurones are reciprocally inhibited.

A crossed extensor reflex simultaneously evokes contralateral extensor motoneurone facilitation and flexor inhibition. These reflexes serve to maintain posture of the animal while protecting it from further injury. Thus, there is muscle action in the nociceptor specific or relevant muscles and in the postural or nociceptor irrelevant muscle groups. Through feedback from muscle, joint, and tendon proprioceptors, as well as labyrinthine receptors in the semicircular canals of the inner ear, there is concomitant suprasegmental facilitation and inhibition of extensor and flexor motoneurones resulting in a cascade of righting reflexes so as to maintain body equilibrium in the presence of the nociceptor reflex.[3] With reference to the craniocervical system, the reflexes give rise to reflex figures exhibiting ascending and descending patterns (dependent upon whether the noxious stimulus is outside or within the craniocervical system respectively). The craniocervical system has been referred to as the fifth limb, with head and neck withdrawal occurring in all three planes: sagittal, coronal, and horizontal with respect to the site of nociception. For simplicity we will consider here responses in the frontal plane only.

Sherrington Model Applied to Acute Nociception in the Craniomandibular System

The mandible is an appendage of the craniocervical system. While the jaw elevators and depressors act homologously with postural extensors and flexors respectively, they also function reciprocally as flexors or extensors in nociceptor reflexes. Acute noxious stimulation of the trigeminal nerve afferents results in reflex withdrawal of the mandible, as well as the cranium, away from the site of stimulation essentially by cervical muscles but assisted by the jaw musculature. Thus, on the ipsilateral side, for example, the supra/infrahyoids and lateral pterygoid are facilitated while the vertical fibres of temporalis and masseter muscles are inhibited (jaw opening reflex). On the contralateral side to which the skull, neck, and mandible are deflected there is a crossed extensor facilitation involving the masseter and temporalis muscles accompanied by reciprocal inhibition of the lateral pterygoid and supra/infrahyoid musculature. Thus, the ipsilateral temporomandibular joint condyle is subluxed and the contralateral condyle is compressed with resulting premature contact of the contralateral teeth and disclusion of the ipsilateral teeth.

Chronic and Acute Pain Model

Acute nociceptor reflexes are normally evoked for short periods of time, but chronic pain dysfunction results from continuous, constant nociceptor stimulation and associated postural reflexes. The latter leads to a hypersensitive state thought to be due to increased neuropeptide concentration both at the receptor site and also centrally at the second and higher order neurones.[4-13] Calcitonin gene related peptide (CGRP) substance P, kinins, phospholipids, prostaglandins, and leukotrienes, etc. accumulate at the receptor sites with increasing pain and inflammation extending the original receptor field. Noxious afferent bombardment (particularly by C fibres) of the central nervous system produces hypersensitivity at synaptic terminals by what is believed to involve N methyl D aspartate receptor activation by centrally released neuropeptides at the pre-synaptic site. Central nervous system sensitivity has been analogized to hypersensitivity states in which C fos induction of Intermediate Early Gene Expression (IEGE) at ascending levels of the nervous system results in "wind-up" sensitization of central neural components of cortical and subcortical centres. The latter include limbic, basal ganglia, reticular activating (RAS), pyramidal and extra pyramidal systems. Alpha and gamma motoneurone hyperactivity is evoked by RAS, extrapyramidal and pyramidal system stimulation of lower motoneurones. Thus, in the chronic condition there is continuous concomitant activation of nociceptor and postural receptor sites. Co-contraction of antagonist muscles results. For example, chronic noxious stimulation of ipsilateral masseter, temporalis, temporomandibular joints, or periodontal nociceptors evoke ipsilateral and contralateral masseter and temporalis muscle hyperactivity which now become further sources of pain as do the involved cervical structures.

The overall effect is increased pain perception, central nervous system excitation/depression, and muscle co-contraction with muscle stiffness in which both extensors and flexors are simultaneously bilaterally hyperactivated with consequently increased trauma to the involved components. A cascade of inflammatory processes occurring within the continuously compressed or tensed joints, tendons, periodontia, and muscles produce destructive and dysfunctional changes in the tissues. The final chronic pain state corresponds somewhat to decerebrate rigidity in which range of movements of the body components are slow (bradykinetic), stiff, and tremorous (dyskinetic), characterized by co-contraction of normally opposing muscle groups.

Characteristics of the Chronic Craniomandibular Patient

In the chronic craniomandibular patient, due to the interaction of segmental, suprasegmental reflexes, muscle co-contraction, and central nervous system sensitivity, diagnosis becomes a complex process due to the added complication of central nervous system fatigue/clinical depression, as well as peripheral neuromuscular fatigue.

Descending Craniomandibular Dysfunction

In the CMD patient, the initial acute postural changes consisting of altered head, neck, and body posture, seen in the Sherrington model, continue to be expressed in the chronic state. The pattern of responses initially depends on whether the primary pain stimulus arises in the craniomandibular system (descending CMD) or elsewhere (ascending CMD). It must also be cautioned that, in the case of multiple injuries, regions with more extensive afferent feedback will take precedence over regions with less extensive afferent feedback. Thus, in a combination of jaw and hip injury, for example, the ascending pattern may be preferentially evoked rather than the descending pattern when involvement of hip afferents predominates.

In the descending pattern of craniomandibular dysfunction, when the noxious stimulus is applied to craniomandibular structures, the head is tilted away from the site of trauma by lateral flexion and rotation respectively at the atlantal-occipital and atlanto-axial joints of the upper cervical spine *(Figure 1)*. Righting reflexes horizontally correct the tilted aural, visual, and occlusal planes by compensatory contractions of ipsilateral lower neck, shoulder, and contralateral upper back and ipsilateral lower back muscles, as well as those of the pelvis and leg muscles. In this way, there develops on the ipsilateral side a raised shoulder, raised pelvis, and shortened leg. It should be understood that although the pelvic rim is raised the hip is actually depressed along with the shortened leg. Thus the body tilts in the direction of the shortened leg.

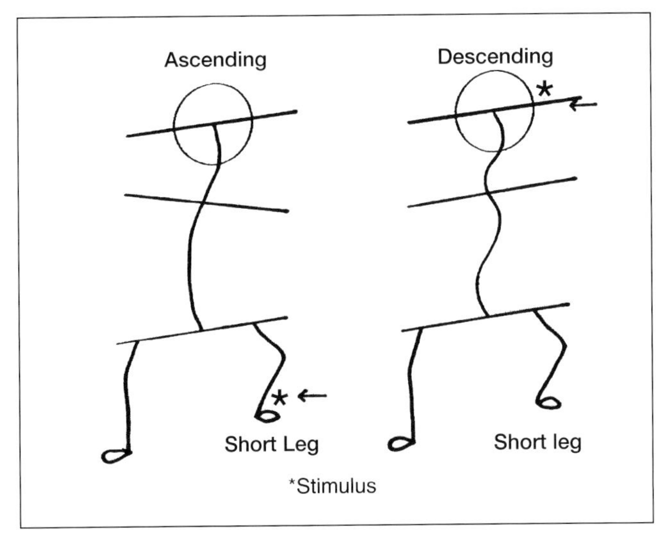

Figure 1.

In summary, in the descending pattern arising from stomatognathic or craniomandibular nociception, there is an observed parallelism between the occlusal, pectoral, and pelvic planes with tendency toward a double scoliosis of the cervical and thoraco-lumbar spines. Concomitant compression and subluxation of the affected vertebral, zygohypophyseal, and temporomandibular joints result with attendant pain.[14,15] It has been demonstrated that maintenance of the diameter of the oropharyngeal airway at the level of the hyoid bone is reflexly controlled by hyo-mandibular neuromuscular or portal reflexes.[16] Head changes in cranial posture must then necessarily result in jaw joint compression and/or subluxation at resting posture of the mandible so as to maintain the airway's diameter. Chronic co-contraction of the correcting postural muscle groups increases generalized pain, stiffness, and dysfunction.

Ascending Craniomandibular Dysfunction

In the ascending pattern, the tilt of the axial skeleton follows the nociceptively flexed "shortened" leg on the ipsilateral compensating contractions of the contralateral shoulder and neck which will attempt to horizontally correct the visual, aural, and hence the occlusal planes. The corrective or compensating tilt of the craniocervical structures is evoked by labyrinthine, cervical tonic and other righting reflexes to normalize the aural, visual, and occlusal planes relative to the horizon. Thus chronic flexion of the cranium and mandible to the contralateral leads to an opposite or rhomboidal orientation that characterizes the ascending reflex pattern. The compression of the jaw joint and occlusal prematurity on the contralateral side are accompanied by subluxation of the ipsilateral joint and disclusion of the dentition. Single cervical scoliosis will develop with associated joint compression, subluxation, and attendant pain. What we therefore see in chronic pain is a progressive painful postural stiffening and resultant abnormal postural pattern.

Chronic CMD and Hypersensitivity

Hu et al.[11] also demonstrated that mustard oil, which induces chronic pain supersensitivity, resulted in two phases of increased excitability and hyperactivity of the ipsilateral masseter and suprahyoid musculature when introduced into the temporomandibular joint. The demonstration of a second phase response by endorphin antagonist nalorphine was taken as evidence that both peripheral and central sensitization occur in chronic pain conditions and that endorphin production may mask the effect of chronic pain. In short, the effect of central pain sensitization in chronic CMD, especially in situations where endorphin production is low, will promote harmful muscle hyperactivity and progressive fatigue effects so as to exacerbate the results of trauma. The sustained muscle hyperactivity, by leading to altered central and muscle fatigue, may be accompanied by conflicting electromyographic (EMG) levels.

Importance of Electromyography and Computer Scan in the Diagnosis of Craniomandibular Dysfunction

From the above account it is seen that repositioning of the structural components of the craniomandibular complex in response to chronic noxious insult is accompanied by a complex interactive pattern of motoneurone recruitment and progressively fatiguing muscles with resulting limited range of joint movement and accompanying myofascial strain. Thus, palpation alone may lead to incorrect diagnosis since primary pain cannot be distinguished from secondary pain in compensating muscles. Indeed, it has been demonstrated that a false diagnosis may be derived in more than 50% of cases utilizing palpation alone.[17] Muscle tension and fatigue effects cannot be readily differentiated from joint compression/subluxation, fascial/ligamentous tension, or other traumatized soft tissues. MRI of the temporomandibular joints also often fails to provide a correct joint diagnosis because it is undertaken on the supine patient which alters gravitational effects and compromises the reflex figure. Nor does MRI differentiate specific inflammatory changes in the joints such as synovitis, exudation of tissue fluid, disc adhesions, or perforations.[18] While corrected tomography and transcranial plain radiography of the lateral third may indicate jaw joint space anomalies indicative of head, jaw, and body tilt, neither radiological assessment provides a reliable direct measurement of the compressive or tensional forces across the soft tissues of the joint. Similarly, when the patient is asked to clench the teeth together, any occlusal imbalance is masked or compensated by appropriate jaw elevator muscle contraction. Thus, the key to diagnosis is assessment of joint compression as indicated by electromyographic activity in the associated muscles including evaluation of the degree of muscle fatigue. Computerized mandibular scan incorporating pre- and post-transcutaneous electrical neural stimulation (TENS), electromyography, and sonography has thus been shown to be superior to other aids in diagnosis.[18]

Physiology and Biochemistry of Fatigue

Muscle fatigue is a physiological and biochemical process that is defined as the failure point in time when a muscle is unable to maintain constant force. Two effects have been demonstrated of diagnostic significance, one associated with local conditions and the other with central motor control.[19] These effects are: (1) a reduction in mean or median power frequency of the power density spectrum; and (2) an increase in IEMG (integrated electromyogram) power of the signal which reflects a change in central drive or recruitment to the motoneurones, i.e., motor neurone recruitment.[20-22] In profound fatigue, IEMG activity ultimately decreases as force declines to the failure point. Thus, assessment of IEMG alone may not indicate the presence or absence of fatigue.

Biochemistry of Muscle Fatigue

The biochemical mechanism of masticatory muscle fatigue is unclear. One longstanding hypothesis has been that fatigue occurs as a result of a rise in intracellular $[H^+]$ in consequence of sustained muscle contraction under anaerobic conditions.[23,24] But investigators have also noted that a decreased force of clenching is accompanied by a transient rise in pH early in muscle exercise. This is due to creatine phosphate/ADP/H^+ interaction as follows: $CrP + ADP + H^+ \rightarrow Cr + ATP$. Recent studies on adult skeletal and masticatory muscle[25,26] implicated monobasic phosphate $[H_2PO_4^-]$ as well as inorganic phosphate ions (Pi) as a primary factor in fatigue. Thus H^+ ions are indirectly related to fatigue through interaction with phosphate which is more directly associated with muscle fatigue. These studies utilized high time resolution p^{31} magnetic resonance spectroscopy during fatiguing exercise at maximum voluntary contraction. $[H^+]$ concentration is measured using chemical shift of Pi from PCr.[27] When comparing rest PNMR spectra with post 20 second clench spectra, the increase in inorganic phosphate (Pi) correlates with decrease in creatinine phosphate (CrP) while ATP remains unchanged and comparison is made of the time course of CrP, MVC, and $[H^+]$.[25] MPF is directly linked to pH and indirectly linked to $[H_2PO_4^-]$. The decline in pH both reduces the velocity of EMG action potential propagation and inhibits actin myosin interaction by moving the equilibrium, i.e., $HPO_4 + H^+ \rightarrow H_2PO_4^-$. The $[H_2PO_4]$, $[PO_3]$, $[HPO_4]$ ions are believed to complex with Ca^{++} to promote muscle contracture. This is because $[Ca^{++}]$ is essential for disclosing troponin sites for actin-myosin bridge interaction. During early contraction $[H^+]$ ions are consumed by inorganic phosphate, HPO_4, H_2PO_4, and CrP reactions. In summary, it appears that free H^+ ions are responsible for pain production and reduction in MPF in muscle fatigue but are not primarily responsible for muscle fatigue per se.

Electromyography

Many studies confirming the existence of a positive straight line or proportional relationship between muscle force and integrated EMG under healthy isometric conditions have demonstrated that such a relationship also exists for the masticatory muscles.[28-34] But in the fatigued state this relationship breaks down. Not surprisingly, there is lack of agreement in the literature that muscle hyperactivity is consistently present in CMD patients.[35] This is due to failure of the researchers to understand that surface EMG must be correlated with the primary source of noxious insult, as well as to its duration and particularly as these are expressed by muscle fatigue or motoneurone recruitment levels. Peripheral and central sensitization may at first be confined to the primary source of nociception but will progressively involve other areas as secondary sources of nociception develop. Thus, reporting only raw electromyographic data without assessing degree of fatigue of motoneurone recruitment has led to contradictory findings. Rasmussen et al.[36] also demonstrated that blood flow to the elevator muscles was reduced even with mild clenching. The blood flow varied from total circulatory arrest to normal at EMG levels less than 25% of maximal clenching. Blood flow was, in fact, obstructed even at 10 percent of maximal clenching levels. Restricted blood flow under such conditions of mild chronic muscle contraction clearly leads to fatigue. ATP, necessary for muscle contraction, is produced both by anaerobic and aerobic metabolism. An adequate blood supply is therefore essential for both processes as a replenishing source of glucose and oxygen. Inability to generate ATP also results in failure of muscles to relax. Under such conditions, the muscle remains in the contractured form, which characterizes the stiff craniomandibular dysfunctional state.

Lund et al.[37] demonstrated that passive stretching of an acutely painful muscle did result in increased muscle activity. Presumably then, gravitational effects on the mandible in the freely moving individual, particularly in the chronic posturally compromised situation, would certainly result in homologous muscle hyperactivity and fatigue. But Paesani et al.[35] showed that in chronic symptomatic female CMD subjects, EMG findings were generally more variable than those of asymptomatic subjects and were not reproducible from session to session. They rightly suggested that rest EMGs taken over a treatment period would not be reliable to evaluate the effects of treatment on chronic CMD patients.

It is therefore extremely important to assess the degree of fatigue accompanying the muscle activity. In fatigue, the force of muscle contraction may decrease even though EMG activity increases. Central fatigue will also lead to progressive decreased EMG activity. It was shown by Thomas[38] that EMG spectral analysis, unlike EMG activity, remains constant for a healthy subject over sessions separated by several weeks. It was also demonstrated that the EMG mean power frequency of masticatory muscles in maximally clenching subjects was shifted to lower frequencies in 71% while 29% actually increased in MPF at the point of fatigue. It was further demonstrated that pre-auricular TENS of the motor supply to masticatory musculature, whether hyperactive or fatigued, will result in normalization of the MPF of EMG signals to physiological levels, whereas in CMD rest alone does not.[38]

Spectral Analysis in the Pre- and Post-TENS Condition

Muscle pain is a common symptom of functional disturbances of the masticatory system known under variable diagnostic terms as temporomandibular joint dysfunction, temporomandibular disorder, craniomandibular disorder, musculo-skeletal dysfunction, or myofascial pain dysfunction. Experimentally induced hyperactivity of the masticatory musculature produces similar symptoms to TMJ dysfunction,[39,40] supporting the hypothesis that muscle pain is produced by muscle fatigue.[41-46]

Integrated electromyography (IEMG) has commonly been used as a quantitative measure of activity required to maintain a certain level of muscle tension, as well as to differentiate between muscle relaxation and fatigue, since it has been shown that relaxation is accompanied by minimal IEMG and fatigue by increasing IEMG as the time of fatiguing contraction progresses.[47] Many studies have confirmed the existence of a straight line (or proportional) relationship between muscle force and integrated EMG.[28-32]

Ahlgren[33] and Moller[34] have demonstrated that such a relationship also exists for the masticatory musculature. Furthermore, Kawazoe et al.[48] showed that the steepness of the straight line relationship increased on the non-preferred side of chewing and for fatigued muscles. Kawazoe et al.[49] provided evidence that the slopes of the fatigued muscle voltage tension curves decreased to a greater degree with percutaneous stimulation than by rest alone. But the effect of changing mandibular position was not assessed in this study nor was the effect on TMJ subjects investigated.

Indeed, it has been demonstrated by McKenna and Turker[50] that the IEMG will reduce as the jaw opens for a fixed muscle tension or constant load.[51] So a decrease in EMG activity is not necessarily a true indicator of elevator muscle relaxation if the jaw is simultaneously opened. Nor is the increase in jaw opening necessarily an indicator of muscle relaxation since this may also occur in muscle fatigue. It has been repeatedly demonstrated that TENS reduces IEMG activity in jaw musculature.[41,52] But without satisfactory evidence to the contrary, it may be argued that transcutaneous electrical neural stimulation, rather than producing relaxation, fatigues the masticatory musculature so that, as the load of the mandible opens the jaw, there is a reduction in EMG activity as a result of lengthening of the fatigued muscle.

Fortunately, there is a simple procedure that can be used to directly test the effect of TENS on fatigued masticatory musculature.

In 1912, Piper[53] observed that the peak frequency of the myoelectric signal decreases during fatiguing muscular contractions. Since that time, it has been repeatedly shown that fatigued muscle is accompanied by a decrease in the frequency of its EMG activity, causing the peak power frequency spectrum to shift to lower frequencies.[54,55,47] Indeed, Palla and Ash[45] and Lindstrom and Hellsing[46] demonstrated a similar shift in peak frequency for fatigued masticatory musculature.

The frequency shift is believed to be due to a reduction in the velocity of the muscle unit action potential and thus an increase in the duration of the motor unit action potential (MUAP).[23,56-61] Furthermore, the duration of the MUAP is indirectly related to the shape of the EMG power spectrum.[62,63,-65] Viitasalo et al.[47] and Kadefors et al.[65] have provided evidence that increasing muscle force or motor neurone recruitment shifts the spectral peak to higher frequencies whereas fatigue does the reverse, possibly indicating that the shift that occurs in fatigue is due to elimination of the more powerful fast twitch/fatigue sensitive phasic fibres and increased activation of the slow twitch/fatigue resistant tonic fibres.

It has also been shown by Vrendenbregt and Rau[66] that a shift in the spectral peak of EMG frequencies during fatigue is only minimally affected by electrode orientation or muscle elongation. The hypothesis that TENS does produce muscle relaxation and not muscle fatigue was led by Thomas[67,38] utilizing spectral analysis of elevator EMG on normal and TMJ patients pre- and post-TENS of the motor point of the masticatory elevator muscles.

Bipolar surface recording electrodes were applied to the skin overlying the masseter and temporalis muscles of 52 normal and 25 TMJ subjects. An indifferent electrode was attached to the skin over the 7th cervical vertebra. All subjects exhibited internal derangement of both temporomandibular joints, with clicking and crepitation. Palpable masseter muscle tenderness was also present in all subjects, and the patients complained of pre-auricular pain and constant headache. The myoelectrical potentials were amplified 1,000 times and filtered below 10 Hz and above 1 K.Hz, utilizing a 60 dB Grass preamplifier (p158). The raw EMG data were displayed on a 5113 dual beam textronix CRT and stored on magnetic tape for fast Fourier transformation using a 5L4 N textronix spectrum analyzer. The EMG recordings were rectified and integrated (40 msec time constant) for correlation with the patient's expression of fatigue and relaxation (IEMG).

Subjects were seated in a dental chair with the Frankfurt plane kept horizontal. Threshold transcutaneous electroneural stimulation was applied with a pulse duration of 500 msec at 1½ second intervals to the pre-auricular region overlying the masseteric notch.

EMG recordings were made prior to TENS stimulation while the subject was at rest for 20 minutes with a measurable freeway space varying between 2.2 and 3.1 mm. The subject was then required to maximally clench (MVC) for 10 seconds while EMG magnetic tape recordings were taken, using a Sony Tape Recorder (T.C.Fx600). Finally, the subject was asked to maximally clench until fatigue developed. A further ten second tape recording was taken. The subject was then provided with 20 minutes of TENS as described above. This procedure was repeated a second time with the exception that 20 minutes rest replaced the TENS treatment.

Results

Normal Subjects

The IEMG was seen to increase with the patient's expression of increasing fatigue. As fatigue developed, the spectral peak density gradually shifted to lower frequencies mean ~75 Hz. Twenty minutes of TENS, like rest, restored the spectral peak to the pre-TENS level of control subjects mean ~125 Hz.

TMJ Subjects

For TMJ subjects, it was observed that for both the pre and post fatigued conditions, the frequency spectrum peaked at low frequency levels of 75 Hz. No amount of rest or wearing of a Lucia jig splint between the incisor teeth could restore the peak to normal relaxed levels. TENS, however, succeeded in relaxing the musculature of the TMJ subjects' masticatory system shifting the spectral peak from ~75 Hz to ~125 Hz in all the subjects tested in this study.

Discussion

It was clear from this study that the masticatory musculature of TMJ subjects, as opposed to non-TMJ subjects, exhibited fatigue as objectively indicated by spectral analysis. Rest alone did not resolve the masticatory muscular fatigue. It was also found that rest with a Lucia jig also fails to eliminate the muscle fatigue.

TENS resolved the fatigue of both normal and TMJ subjects. The failure of rest to restore normal muscle activity in the TMJ subjects suggests that the masticatory muscular fatigue evident in these cases is more recalcitrant to rest than normal fatigued muscle. This indicates that other factors are involved, e.g., a metabolic deficiency such as relative ischemia and [H+] ion increase which cannot be resolved by rest alone.[69-72] The presence of internal joint derangement and joint tenderness were also factors. TENS may act by improving muscle function, through removing muscle metabolites and/or reversing muscular ischemia. Unloading of the temporomandibular joints, altered sensory feedback, and alleviation of pain are speculated as other possible effects of TENS.

Thomas[31] and Buxbaum et al.[72] demonstrated that band width and masseter EMG power spectrum of the myoelectropotential is stable and reliable over extended periods of time in jaw resting, chewing, and clenching activities, the power spectrum being particularly sensitive. These and other studies led to the development of Scan 18 in the electromyography series of tests that can be undertaken in conjunction with the computerized mandibular scan.[73] Scan 18 is the item of the computer that refers to the recording of the electromyographic activity (EMG) of the jaw and neck musculature utilizing multiple channels of specific activity in the variable modes of rest *(Figure 2, Box 1)*; initial maximal clench *(Box 2)*; following 10 seconds of clenching *(Box 3);* and post clench *(Box 4)*. In the healthy control subject, the temporalis and masseter activities are balanced. When there is postural imbalance of the head and neck, the temporalis activity including their frequencies are increased over masseter elevator activity. When the dysfunction is of occlusal origin, the masseter activity is increased over the temporalis activity including amplitude and frequencies. When there is combined occlusal and postural dysfunction, then the muscle imbalance will reflect both postural and occlusal abnormalities. If only the occlusal anomaly is corrected following TENS to the jaw elevators alone, then failure to correct the postural anomaly will be followed by continuing postural muscle imbalance. In short, TENS should be applied to both the elevator and postural muscles in those cases of combined occlusal and postural dysfunction. The following calculations will assist in the differentiation between physiological muscle activity and muscle fatigue. It is well established in the scientific literature that the myoelectric potential (IEMG) and frequency of motor unit potential (MPF) is directly related to muscle force under non-fatiguing conditions.

Therefore the quotient MPF/IEMG is subject and mode specific under physiological conditions of chewing, clenching, and rest. This, by comparison of MPF/IEMGs contralaterally and pre- and post-TENS, will differentiate between fatigued musculature in CMD.

When a muscle is maximally contracted, it develops maximal myoelectric potential (IEMG max) and maximal mean power frequency (MPF max).

In practice, utilizing Scan 18 as illustrated, MPF/EMG recordings are made at rest *(Figure 2, Box 1)*, immediate maximal clench *(Box 2)*, after 10 seconds clench *(Box 3)*, and during post clench relaxation *(Box 4)*. The MPF/IEMG ratios of Boxes 1, 3, 4 to Box 2 will provide a ready assessment of the degree of fatigue under the varying conditions and will be reduced vis à vis the control or non-fatigued state.

In *Table I*, the relative levels of MPF, IEMG, and MPF/IEMG are summarized for the rest, recruited, fatigued, and aerobic levels of muscle contraction. The effect of TENS on MPF/EMG is also tabled. It will be seen that TENS not only promotes blood flow and oxygen supply but also relieves pain effects by closing the pain gate and by stimulation of endorphin production. *Figure 3* demonstrates the effect of TENS on IEMG (decrease) and MPF (increase) in a CMD patient. It should be noted that not all jaw muscles in CMD are equally fatigued.

Table I
Ratio of MPF/EMG

	MPF	EMG	MPF/EMG	TENS MPF/ENG
Recruited	Hi	Raised	Hi	Mild Increase
Fatigued	Lo	Raised	Lo	Great Increase
Rest (non-recruited)	Lo	Lo	Intermed.	Mod. Increase
Aerobic Status	V. Hi	Lo	V. Hi	No change

Summary
Craniomandibular disorder is a chronic pathological condition of the masticatory system and is characterized by pain and dysfunction at segmental and suprasegmental levels. Neurophysiological studies have established that noxious stimulation results in local and general responses including postural and autonomic effects. Unresolved postural and anatomic responses to noxious irritation also become a further source of pain and dysfunction. Thus, with respect to the craniocervical system, the pain dysfunction processes may be classified into descending and ascending according to whether the site of pain origin is primarily in the masticatory system or outside of it. Studies on the neurological components of the chronic pain condition have revealed that release of neurotransmitters at the presynaptic site of the lower order neurone results in RNA-neuropeptide template induction of the neurone receptor genome to produce neural hypersensitivity of the higher order neurone in the pain pathway and consequently supersensitivity of the motor and autonomic systems. Hyperactivity may therefore be observed in the effector components. The latter can be objectively assessed by devices that measure such physiological parameters as electromyography, jaw posture and tracking, jaw joint sounds, and blood flow changes by computerized mandibular scan and infra-red emission. The latter modalities are superior to morphological studies such as MRI, radiography, and arthrography since the latter are either too gross or physiologically invasive in that they cannot be undertaken without interfering with the function of the masticatory system through altered gravitational effects and the like. Hyperactivity in the pain and final common pathway leads to

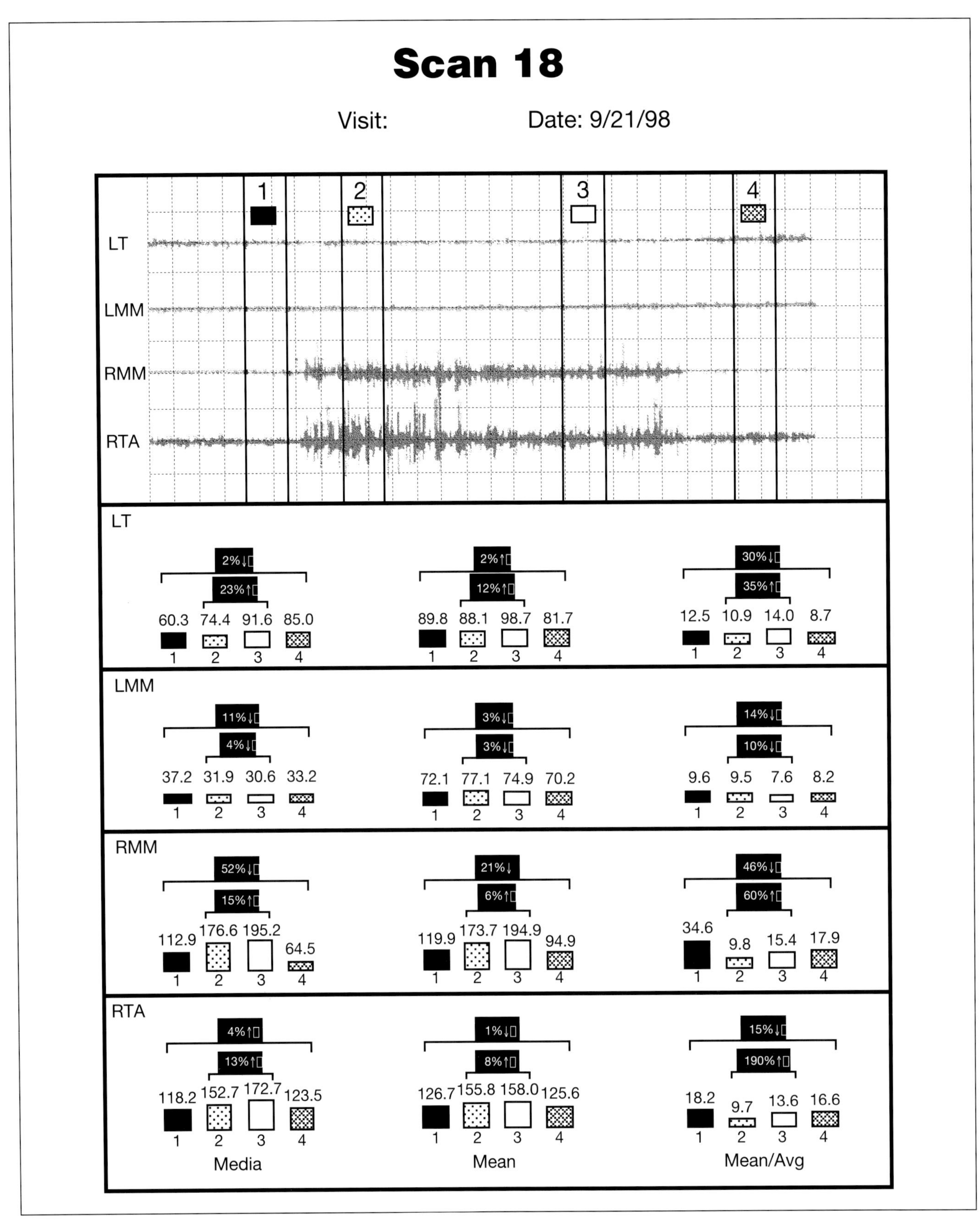

Figure 2. Scan 18.

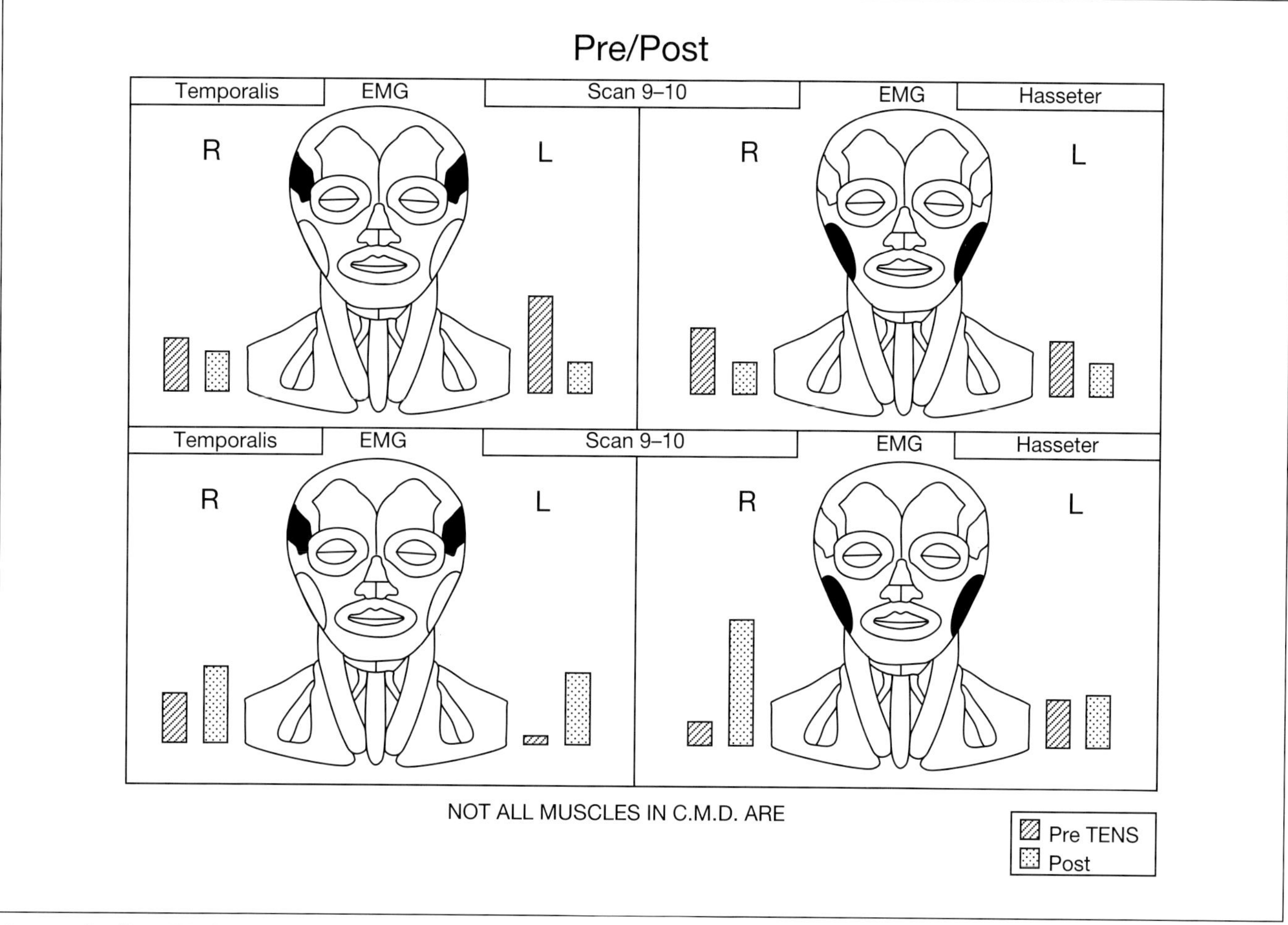

Figure 3. Pre/Post TENS.

fatigue, either constantly or peripherally. By utilizing surface electromyography, the presence or absence of fatigue is readily disclosed. In this context, it has been well established in the scientific literature that the force of muscle contraction under physiological conditions is directly proportional to the integrated electromyopotential (IEMG) and the frequency of motor unit firing (MPF). Thus the quotient MPF/IEMG is patient and mode specific, i.e., for clenching, chewing, and resting conditions.

Bibliography

1. Ormeno G, Miralles R, Sanbander H, Casassus R, Ferrer P, Palazzi C, Moya H: Body position effects on sternocleidomastoid and masseter EMG pattern activity in patients undergoing occlusal splint therapy. *J Craniomandib Pract* 1997;15:300-309.
2. Sherrington CS: *Integrative action of the Nervous System.* London: Archibald Constable, 1906.
3. Best and Taylor: *Physiological Basis of Medical Practice. Tenth Edition.* Brobeck JR, ed. Baltimore/London: Williams and Wilkins, 1981.
4. Meyer RA, Campbell JN, Raja SN: Peripheral neural mechanisms of cutaneous hyperalgesia. *Adv Pain Res Thera* 1985;9:53-57.
5. La Motte RH, Shain CN, Simone DA, Tsai EFP: Neurogenic hyperalgesia psychophysical studies of underlying mechanisms. *J Neurophysiol* 1991; 66:190-211.
6. Willis WD: Hyperalgesia and allodynia. In: Willis WD, ed. *Overview 1-11.* New York: Raven Press, 1992.
7. Neugebauer V, Schaible HG: Evidence for a central component in the sensitization of spinal neurones with joint input during development of acute arthritis in cat's knee. *J Neurophysiol* 1990; 64:299-311.
8. Woolf CJ: Excitability changes in central neurones following peripheral damage: role of central sensitization in the pathogenesis of pain. In: Willis WD, ed. *Hyperalgesia and Allodynia.* New York: Raven Press; 1992;221-243.

9. Cervero F, Laird JMA, Pozo MA: Selective changes of receptive field properties of spinal nociceptive neurones induced by visceral noxious stimulation in the cat. *Pain* 1992;51:335-342.

10. Willis WD: Mechanical Allodynia: a role for sensitized nociceptive tract cells with convergent input from mechanoreceptors and nociceptors. *A P S J* 1993;2:23-33.

11. Hu JW, Yu X-M, Sunakawa M, Chiang CY, Haas DA, Kwan CL, Tsai C-M, Vernon H, Sessle BJ: EMG and trigeminal brainstem neuronal changes associated with inflammatory irritation of superficial and deep craniofacial tissues in rats. In: Gebhart GF, Hammond DL, Jensen TS, eds. *Proc. 7th World Congress on Pain Prog. Pain Res. and Mgmt.* Seattle: IASP Press; 1994;2:325-334.

12. Woolf CJ, Wall PD: Relative effectiveness of C primary afferent fibres of different origins in evoking a prolonged facilitation of the flexor reflex in the rat. *J Neurosci* 1986;6:1433-1442.

13. Woolf CJ, Thompson SWN: The induction and maintenance of central sensitization is dependent on N-methyl-D-aspartic receptor activation; implications for the treatment of post-injury pain hypersensitivity states. *Pain* 1991;44:293-299.

14. Barnsley L, Lord SM, Walles BJ, Bogduk N: The prevalence of chronic zygohypophysial joint pain after whiplash. *Spine* 1995;20:20-26.

15. Bogduk N, Aprill C, Denby R: Discography. In: White AH, ed. *Spine Care, Diagnosis and Conservative Treatment Vol. I.* St. Louis: Mosby; 1974;219-238.

16. Bibby RE, Preston CB: The Hyoid Triangle. *Am J Orthod* 1981;80(1):92-97.

17. Paesani D, Westesson P-L, Hatala MP, Tallents RH, Brooks SL: Accuracy of clinical diagnosis for TMJ internal derangement and arthrosis. *Oral Surg Oral Med Oral Pathol* 1992;73:360-363.

18. Thomas NR, Thomas MR, Thomas NR: *The Fallibility of MRI Assessment as a Gold Standard in the Diagnosis of Craniomandibular Dysfunction Arising from Macrotrauma.* Toulouse, France: ICCMO Proceedings, 1995.

19. Maton B, Rendell M, Gentil M, Gay T: Masticatory muscle fatigue: endurance times and spectral changes in the electromyogram during the production of sustained bite forces. *Arch Oral Biol* 1992;37:521-529.

20. Bigland-Ritchie B, Cafarelli E, Vollestad NK: Fatigue of submaximal static contractions. *Acta Physiol Scan* (suppl 556) 1986;137-148.

21. Maton B: Human motor unit activity during muscle fatigue in submaximal isometric isotonic contractions. *Eur J Appl Physiol* 1981;46:271-281.

22. Maton B, Garret D: The fatiguability of two antagonist muscles in human isometric voluntary submaximal contraction, an EMG study II. *Eur J Appl Physiol* 1989;58:369-374.

23. Lindstrom LR, Magnussen R, Petersen I: Muscular fatigue and action potential conduction velocity changes studied with frequency analysis of EMG signals. *Electromyography* 1970;10:341-386.

24. Lindstrom L, Petersen I: Power Spectrum analysis of EMG signals and its applications in computer aided electromyography. *Progr Clin Neurophysiol* 1983. In: Desmedt JE, ed. Karger Basel 10:1-47.

25. Laurent D, Portero P, Goubel F, Rossi A: EMG Spectrum changes during sustained contraction related to proton and diprotonded inorganic phosphate accumulation: a P31 nuclear magnetic resonance study on human calf muscles. *Eur J Appl Physiol* 1993; 66(3):263-268.

26. Lam EWN, Hannam AG: Regional P31 magnetic resonance spectroscopy of exercising human masseter muscle. *Arch Oral Biol* 1992;37:49-56.

27. Moon R, Richards J: Determination of intracellular pH by P31 NMR. *J Biol Chem* 1973;248:7276-7278.

28. Inman VT, Ralson HJ, Saunders JB, Feinstein B: Relationship between muscle force and surface electromyogram. *EEG EEG Clin Neurophysiol* 1952;4:187-194.

29. Lippold OCJ: The relation between integrated action potentials in a human muscle and its isometric tension. *J Physiol* 1952;117:492-499.

30. Edwards RG, Lippold OCJ: The relation between force and integrated electrical activity in fatigued muscle. *J Physiol* (Lond) 1956;132:677-681.

31. Bigland B, Lippold OCJ: The relation between force, velocity and integrated electrical activity in human muscles. *J Physiol* (Lond) 1954;123:214-224.

32. Milner-Brown HS, Stein RB: The relation between the surface electromyogram and muscular force. *J Physiol* (Lond) 1975;246:549-569.

33. Ahlgren J: Mechanism of Mastication. A quantitative cinematographic and electromyographic study of masticatory movements in children with special reference to occlusion of the teeth. *Acta Odont Scand* 1966;24(Supp 44):1-109.

34. Moller E: The Chewing Apparatus. An electromyographic study of the action of the muscles of mastication and its correlation to facial morphology. *Acta Physiol Scand* 1966;280:1-129.

35. Paesani DA, Tallents RH, Murphy WC, Hatala MP, Proskin HM: Evaluation of the reproducibility of rest activity of the anterior temporal and masseter muscles in asymptomatic and symptomatic temporomandibular subjects. *J Orofacial Pain* 1994;8:402-406.

36. Rasmussen OC, Bonde-Petersen F, Christensen LV, Moller E: Blood flow in human mandibular elevation at rest and during controlled biting. *Arch Oral Biol* 1977;22:539-543.

37. Lund JP, Donga R, Widmer C, Stohler CS: The pain adaptation model: A discussion of the relationship between chronic musculoskeletal pain and motor activity. *Can J Physio Pharmacol* 1991;69:683-694.

38. Thomas NR: The effect of fatigue and TENS on the EMG mean power frequency. In: Bergamini M, ed. Pathophysiology of Head and Neck Musculoskeletal Disorders. *Front Oral Physiol* Basel: Karger; 1990;162-170.

39. Christenson LV: Facial pain from experimental tooth clenching. *Tandloe gebladet* 1970;74: 175-182.

40. Scott DS, Lundeen TF: Pain production in masticatory muscles in response to clenching. *Pain* 1980;8:207-215.

41. Jankelson B: Functional position of occlusion. *J Prosthet Dent* 1973; 30(4):559-564.

42. Jankelson B, Swain CW, Crane PF, Radke JC: Kinesometric Instrumentation: a new technology. *J Am Dent Assoc* 1975;90:834-840.

43. Lasken DM: Etiology of the pain dysfunction syndrome. *J Am Dent Assoc* 1969;79:147-151.

44. Derijk WK, Jones GL, Keith KD: Myographic characteristics and patient reported pain in patients with TMJ dysfunction. *J Dent Res* 1977;56:193.

45. Palla S, Ash MM: Effect of bite force on the power spectrum of the surface electromyogram of human jaw muscles. *Arch Oral Biol* 1981; 26:287-295.

46. Lindstrom I, Hellsing G: Masseter muscle fatigue in man objectively quantified by analysis of myoelectric signals. *Arch Oral Biol* 1983;28:297-301.

47. Viitasalo JHT, Komi PV: Interrelationships of EMG signal characteristics at different levels of muscle tension and during fatigue. *Electromyogy Clin Neurophysiol* 1978;18:167-178

48. Kawazoe Y, Kotani H, Hamada T: IEMG and bite force on non preferred biting side and fatigued muscles. *J Dent Res* 1978;58:1440-1441.

49. Kawazoe Y, Kotani H, Maetani T, Yatani H, Hamada T: Integrated EMG activity and biting force of fatigued masseter. *Arch Oral Biol* 1981; 26:795-801.

50. McKenna BR, Turker KS: Masseter integrated electromyography inter-relationship with mouth opening. *Arch Oral Biol* 1978;23:917-920.

51. Nordstrom S, Yemm R: Integrated electromyography of rat masticatory muscles: effect of jaw opening. *Arch Oral Biol* 1974;19:353-359.

52. Jankelson B: The Myomonitor: its use and abuse (I & II). *Quint Int* 1978; 9:21.

53. Piper H: *Electrophysiologie menschlicher.* Muskeln, Berlin; Springer; 1912;126.

54. Chaffin DB: Surface electromyography frequency analysis as a diagnostic tool. *J Occup Med* 1969;11:109-115.

55. Kwatny E, Klissouras V, Milsum JH: Electrical and metabolic activities and fatigue in human isometric contraction. *J Appl Physiol* 1970;29:358-367.

56. Cobb S, Forbes A: Velocity of muscle unit action potential in muscle fatigue. *Am J Physiol* 1923;65:234-251.

57. Scheiren J, Bourguignon: The motor unit action potential. *Am J Physiol Med* 1959;38:170-180.

58. Lippold OCJ, Redfearn JWT, Vuco J: The EMG of fatigue. *Ergonomics* 1960;3:121-131.

59. Viitasalo JT, Komi PV: Effect of fatigue on the motor unit action potential. *Eur J Appl Physiol* 1977;37:111-121.

60. Bigland-Ritchie B, Jones DA, Woods JJ: Conduction velocity and EMG power spectrum changes in fatigue. *Expl Neurol* 1979;64:414-427.

61. Gydikov L, Kosarov P, Dimitrov R: Fatigue effects on velocity of motor unit action potential. *Electromyogr Clin Neurophysiol* 1979;19:229-248.

62. Cencovich R, Gersten P: Duration of motor unit action potential and its relation to the EMG power spectrum. *Am J Phys Med* 1963;42:192-204.

63. Kaiser E, Peterson IL; Dynamic spectrum analysis and muscle fatigue. *Electromyogr* 1963;3:5-7.

64. Kaiser E, Peterson I; Frequency analysis of muscle fatigue. *Acta Neurol Scand* 1965;41(Suppl 13):213-236.

65. Kadefors R, Peterson I, Browman H: *New Developments in Electromyography and Clinical Neurophysiology Vol, I.* 1973;628-637.

66. Vrendenbregt J, Rau G: The stability and reliability of frequency analysis. In: Desmedt JE, ed. *New Developments in Electromyography and Clinical Neurophysiology Vol. I.* New York: Basal; 1973; 607-622.

67. Thomas NR: Spectral Analysis of the EMG in Pre and Post TENS Condition. ICCMO 5th Int Meeting October 1986.

68. Mortimer JT, Magnusson R, Petersen I: Conduction velocity in ischemic muscle effect on EMG frequency spectrum. *Am J Physiol* 1970;219: 1324-1329.

69. Kovacs R: *Electrotherapy and Light Therapy, 4th Ed.* Philadelphia: Lea and Febiger; 1984;185-187.

70. Stephens JA, Taylor A: Pain and muscle ischemia. *J Physiol (Lond)* 1972;220:1-18.

71. Merton PA: Muscle ischemia effects. *J Physiol (Lond)* 1954;123:553-564.

72. Frucht S, Jonas I, Kappert HF: Muscle relaxation by transcutaneous electric nerve stimulation (TENS) in bruxism [An electromyographic study]. *Fortschr Kiefirorthop* 1995;56(5):245-253.

73. Buxbaum N, Mylinski N, Parente FR: Surface EMG reliability using spectral analysis. *J Oral Rehab* 1996;23:771-775.

POLITICS AND PHILOSOPHY

Politics, Philosophy, and "TMD"

Allen J. Moses

The issues facing graduating dentists in the late '60s seemed clear. Few new graduates doubted their ability to make the diagnoses, "decay or not decay," "periodontitis or not periodontitis," "abscessed or not abscessed," "pathological lesion or normal tissue." Yes, there *was* subjectivity. Dentists could disagree whether or not to fill a small lesion, but the disease "dental caries" had definable criteria, and decisions such as whether to treat or not were based on clinical judgment.

As dentistry entered the '80s and the '90s, the enigmatic problem of "TMD" erupted into controversy. Clinical dentists were gaining more and more knowledge and success at treating temporomandibular disorders when a well-known academic clique declared that this clinical experience was unscientific.[1,2] "It works" they said was not scientific evidence but anecdotal theory. They did however declare pain as "The Gold Standard."[3,4]

As we approach the millennium, TMD remains a hot issue. Most of the disagreements however have reduced to political and philosophical rather than scientific issues. Is TMD a structural or psychological problem? Is it a disease or an illness? Can pain possibly be a valid gold standard? Does one most properly diagnose and treat to the specific etiologic conditions or the generalized non-specific symptoms? Is epidemiology a more appropriate methodology than ethology for the scientific study of TMD? Is subjective clinical judgment a better guide in diagnosis and treatment than objective measurement? Is there a causal relationship between TMD and malocclusion?

At the very core of the political arguments is the issue of money. Insurance companies seem to be under the assumption that TMD is a condition unrelated to human beings. They have isolated it from the rest of the body in singularly trying to deny coverage for anything related to pain and dysfunction associated with the temporomandibular joints. These insurance companies have approached as their allies and consultants the academic clique of research dentists who, for political and monetary considerations, attempt to hold the clinician/patient faction at bay by rejecting claims.

The academic faction has its agenda: (1) perpetuating their research grants; (2) gaining specialty status for orofacial pain; and (3) defending a very weak scientific position, by politically positioning themselves to dictate what is the "appropriate standard of care."

This political warfare also puts the clinician in a very bad light. The politics of TMD is such that clinicians too often feel obligated to list as diagnosis "whatever it takes" to get insurance reimbursement for their patients. They will call this disease/disorder virtually anything, such that their patients get insurance coverage for the proper treatment. Too often this "game" has no relationship to scientific diagnosis. Thus the academics report that clinicians want to do treatment that is experimental or unrelated to the diagnosis. They deny payment, and accuse clinicians of employing unscientific and unwarranted treatment, and an inconsistent standard of care. This chapter is an attempt to elucidate the opposing positions and facilitate clearer understanding of the issues.

From the time of Hippocrates to the present, the concept of both disease and diagnosis has undergone evolutionary change. In the era of Hippocrates, identification of disease was an act of observation, i.e., fever, consumption, or rash. Etiology was based on conjecture, such as deranged humors or angry gods. Sydenham in the seventeenth century originated the discipline of nosology, which proposed that each disease had a specific pathogenic cause. With the advent of the microscope, nineteenth century medical science searched for the histopathology of the diseased part.

Syndromes have been created to describe a concordance of multiple entities. In the 1930s, Costen reported successfully treating a group of patients with a mandibular overlay appliance which separated the teeth 2–4 mm.[5] The syndrome designated with his name manifested the following symptoms: hearing loss, aural fullness, tinnitus, preauricular pain, dizziness, eustachian tube fullness, headaches, and burning in the throat. Later renamed "TMD," the clustering station has been identified as the temporomandibular joint, but the etiology can be trauma, derangement, histopathology, or dysfunction, with the origin in either the masticatory system or a remote location.

TMDs pose many intellectual challenges for diagnosing and treating doctors. Identification of the pathology may be an effect rather than the diagnosis or etiology. Shared neurology of the head and neck often makes etiological identification difficult to ascertain. The location of the pain may not be the site of the pathological lesion. The quality and intensity of the pain may not relate to the extent or severity of the disease process.

Dentistry's predicament is that reproducible identification is necessary for scientific diagnosis of any disease. Definitive measurable, reproducible, objective disease criteria must be elaborated for identification of TMD or each disease or disorder categorized as a TMD. No such disease criteria for the entity called TMD have ever been suggested. Indeed the emerging consensus in dentistry seems to be that TMD is a collective term embracing a number of clinical problems involving masticatory dysfunction, the temporomandibular joints and associated structures.

When doctors discuss a disease, there is usually an unspoken mutual assumption that they share a common understanding of the medical model, conception of the disease process, definition of the disease itself, and that they are discussing the same level of disease. Often this is not the case, and confusion and disagreement ensue.

There are many levels at which doctors discuss disease. As noted, the evolution of a disease usually starts with a description of the symptoms, and this becomes the syndrome level. As the syndrome is studied, often the disorder or disease is localized to the specific system affected such as skeletal, muscular, vascular, neurologic, connective tissue, organic, etc. Further study of the problem by clinicians and researchers often reveals histopathological changes next, and the problem then reduces to the cellular level. When these cellular changes are further studied, often the genes responsible for the change can be isolated on the chromosomes. When the chemical changes resulting from and causing the problem are eventually isolated, the problem is reduced to the molecular level.

Satisfactory treatment for the disorder or disease can often be found at different levels. Analgesics are effective for controlling pain, which is a symptom, but they do not treat the cause (or etiology). Conventional medical wisdom is to treat diseases at the most basic etiologic level possible and reasonable. But what if doctors cannot even agree on whether or not the problem is a disease? What if they do not even agree on the definition of disease?

The term "TMD" has been used by some to characterize the generalized *nonspecific* symptom complex of headache, neck ache, ear pain, face pain, tenderness of muscles to palpation, sensation of bite change, difficulty chewing and/or swallowing, gross joint sounds, and limited range of jaw motion.

Hans Selye, in his classic book *The Stress of Life*,[6] relates how early on in his medical training he noticed a certain *nonspecific* symptom complex common to all infectious diseases. Each patient felt and looked ill, had a coated tongue, complained of more or less diffuse aches and pains in the joints, intestinal problems, loss of appetite, fever, enlarged tonsils, and skin rash. Each infectious disease had a few *specific* signs by which a differential diagnosis could be made and to which a specific remedy could then be directed.

The *nonspecific* reaction of the body common to all infectious diseases, the "syndrome of just being sick," Selye initially identified as the *General Adaptation Syndrome (GAS)*. He spent most of his career studying the *nonspecific* symptom complex, which relates to what we know as *stress*.

Selye defined *stress* as the state manifested by a specific syndrome which consists of all the *nonspecifically* induced changes within a biologic system. Briefly he summarized: "Stress is the *nonspecific* response of the body to any demand." He admits that the concept of stress is an abstraction. The study of stress is exploration and measurement of its tangible effects. Reduction and dissection of such an abstract concept has caused problems relative to temporomandibular disorders and orofacial pain.

Nonspecificity

In 1993, at an NIDR conference, Dworkin defined disease as an "objective biologic event involving disruption of specific body structures or organ systems caused by pathologic, anatomic or physiologic changes." He defined illness as "a subjective experience or self-attribution that a disease is present, yielding physical discomfort, emotional stress, behavioral limitations and psychosocial disruption." He claims progressive pathologic changes cannot be reliably diagnosed in TMDs and concluded that "TMD is more usefully considered to be an illness."[7] Dworkin thus created his psychosocial model of TMD.

This approach is fraught with problems and has pernicious implications for many clinical dentists. Relative to the generally accepted Selye Stress Model, Dworkin's **psychosocial model fractionates TMD to the *nonspecific* symptom complex only,** and, of necessity, limits all treatment to the nonspecific components, because his ***definitive* position** states that progressive pathophysiological changes cannot be reliably diagnosed in TMDs. Certainly stress reduction therapies can be appropriately directed at TMDs, but isn't this just symptomatic treatment, aimed at reestablishing homeostasis, and not addressing the specific etiologic factor?

Specificity

The problem simply stated is this: Can the clinician get beyond the *nonspecific* components common to all temporomandibular disorders to diagnose *specifically*, and direct more effective treatment at the specific etiological component of each disorder? Each of the 25 or so individual temporomandibular disorders discussed in the literature has specific definitive diagnostic criteria that differentiate or define them. These unique identifiers also suggest treatment that is disease-specific, which is different than the nonspecific treatment suggested for TMD in the Dworkin Model.

If dental clinicians perceive of themselves as diagnosticians and treaters of orofacial pain, on any given patient they must make a differential diagnosis from approximately 145 possibilities. Weldon Bell has taught that, "An accurate diagnosis is the first step in the treatment of any TMD and the process cannot be abridged." He believed that a diagnosis should do the following: properly identify and classify the disorder, establish the mechanism of dysfunction and the source of pain, determine the etiology, if possible, and provide a basis for prognosis in the light of effective therapy. He, of course, advocated that the treatment should specifically and appropriately relate to the diagnosis.[8] It seems self-evident then, that no knowledgeable, self-respecting clinician would treat muscle trismus secondary to infectious disease the same as MPD, or treat disc displacement without reduction the same as rheumatoid arthritis. Thus it would seem that in temporomandibular disorders dentists must concern themselves with the "specific diagnosis."

Gould's Medical Dictionary defines disease as "a response to injury, sickness or illness; a failure of the adaptive mechanism of an organism to counteract adequately the stimuli or stresses to which it is subjected, resulting in disturbance in function or structure of any part."[9] Diagnosis involves analysis of the scientific evidence of what is wrong with a patient, and why, and applying a tentative name to the disease. This approach to masticatory problems is based on "disease," not "illness."

When a patient presents to a health professional and asks, "Doc, have I got TMJ?" it is imperative that the doctor consider all the possibilities in making a differential diagnosis. A patient obviously feels some pain and/or dysfunction in the head, face, or joint area as the basis for their office visit. It would certainly be beneath a reasonable standard of care, and might even result in a malpractice case, should the doctor treat a patient for TMD and miss a diagnosis of infectious disease or cancer whereby the patient dies or ultimately loses half their face to radical surgery. It could cost the doctor his or her livelihood, life savings, and sanity, and the patient could lose their life or any semblance of a quality life and endure constant pain and suffering.

There are about 145 diseases and disorders manifesting orofacial pain. In studying textbooks[10-15] on the differential diagnosis of these 145 possibilities, it was found that the expert authors consider about 18 categories of factors or rubrics in arriving at a diagnosis. *(The Rubric Sheet, Figure 1)*. Each of these rubrics has between 5 and 27 possible responses, most of which are not mutually exclusive. This means that, while a disease cannot be both painful and not painful at the same time, symptomatology can simultaneously be sharp, continuous, throbbing, unilateral, preauricular, infraorbital, and severe. Actually, the number of permutations and combinations one might possibly consider in making such a differential diagnosis approximates 1.5×10^{55}. If a supercomputer could sequentially consider 1 billion possibilities per second and started on its first such diagnosis at the "big bang" (origin of the earth), it would not have completed its first diagnosis by the year 2000 A.D.

Psychological studies have shown that the human mind can consider only a few variables (in the range of 4–7) in making complex decisions.[16] Thus, a clinician is faced with a difficult task in diagnosing diseases and disorders manifesting complaint of pain in the area of the head, face, and jaws.

Certainly, not all of the approximately 145 diseases and disorders with the symptom of orofacial pain are temporomandibular disorders. In fact, only about 25 of these involve the masticatory apparatus, and a significantly smaller amount involve the temporomandibular joint itself. Yet there seems to be little disagreement in the dental literature that myogenous problems with **no TMJ pathology** be included in the category "temporomandibular disorders," soon to be retitled "masticatory diseases and disorders."

TMDs, or temporomandibular disorders, certainly have posed many philosophical and conceptual problems to dentists and other health professionals. The panel statement at a 1996 NIH/NIDR Technology Assessment Conference on Management of Temporomandibular Disorders[17] determined the following:

- *The term "TMD" has been used to characterize conditions as diversely presented as pain in the face or jaw joint area, headaches, earaches, dizziness, masticatory musculature hypertrophy, limited opening, closed or open lock of the TMJ, abnormal occlusal wear, clicking or popping sounds in the jaw joint, and other complaints.*
- *Temporomandibular disorders have no common etiology or biological explanation and comprise a heterogeneous group of health problems whose signs and symptoms are overlapping but not necessarily identical.*
- *The name "TMD" is not universally endorsed. Generally accepted, scientifically based guidelines for diagnosis and management of TMD are unavailable.*
- *There are significant problems with present diagnostic classifications of TMD in that these classifications appear to be based on signs and symptoms rather than on etiology.*
- *Validated diagnostic methods for identification and classification of TMD patients are needed.*
- *A classification system based on measurable criteria should be developed as the first step in a rational approach developing diagnostic protocols and appropriate methodologies. This should lead to a labeling of subtypes that could permit the elimination of the term "TMD" which has become emotionally laden and contentious.*

Summarizing so far, there seems to be no agreement as to what constitutes TMD. There are no universally accepted diagnostic criteria for TMD. What constitutes normal has never been definitively established. We have no means of scientifically determining what constitutes diseased or disease-free relative to TMD, thus making it impossible to conduct an epidemiological controlled study. And we need a new, less contentious name for TMD.

Perhaps a new paradigm is in order. Logic dictates that the variables that must be dealt with in arriving at the differential diagnosis for orofacial pain patients must be crunched and organized into categories and subcategories in a manner in which they can be reasonably contemplated by human minds. It is suggested that clinicians consider themselves diagnosticians of orofacial pain. A methodological algorithm is suggested *(The Orofacial Pain Diagnostic Hierarchy, Figure 2)*. It is a result of a search of the medical/dental literature for all diseases and disorders having orofacial pain as a symptom in which there is not an observable pathological lesion. Thus diseases such as pemphigus, herpes, and aphthous ulcers are not on the list. The term "Temporomandibular Disorder" has been eliminated.

It should be generally agreed that the area of treatment expertise for most dentists is the "masticatory" category in which all diseases and disorders share the characteristic of dysfunctional movement of the masticatory apparatus, and the odontogenic category which may result in dysfunctional movement, but not as a primary identifying characteristic.

A diagnosis of "TMD" or "TMJ Syndrome" is no longer appropriate. The acquisition of the signs, symptoms, and patient characteristics that constitute clinical data is sine qua non for arriving at a correct diagnosis. Doctors must readjust their thinking to be more specific. The recommended treatment must be appropriate for the *specific* condition or conditions diagnosed.

Most importantly, doctors are largely dealing with physiologic problems. All conditions on the Orofacial Pain Diagnostic Hierarchy except those few under the category Psychogenic have a physiologic basis. They are characterized by pathophysiologic findings as diagnostic criteria. They are diseases not illnesses. They can be stress-related, but psychological stress is not the primary etiology.

Pain as Gold Standard

Illness, defined as subjective self-attribution of pain experience or pain as "gold standard," must be examined further. Horal's study[18] showed that the only difference between controls and subjects in a stress disorder is that the patient group is complainant. Thus it has been said that TMD patients are self-selected. But TMD has no definitive diagnostic criteria. Horal's study simply demonstrates the inappropriateness of epidemiology as a methodology for the study of TMD because one cannot distinguish normals or controls from the subject group and that pain as gold standard is unreliable.

Most clinicians have had the experience of dealing with the patient who presents complaining of toothache in the upper, only to have the correct diagnosis be abscessed tooth in the ipsilateral lower arch. This is an example of poorly localized pain. Many have had patients who present with complaint of pain over the TMJ, where local anesthetic injection does not relieve the pain, but on closer examination find trigger points in a remote location such as SCM or trapezius where local anesthetic injection of the trigger point relieves the pain over the TMJ. This is referred pain. Often, when asked if palpation hurts, a patient will reply, "not really." This does not say yes or no and affirms that pain is often vague and quantification difficult. If palpation of a muscle on the right side evokes pain on the left side, it is an example of psychosomatic pain. There is no known neurological circuitry to account for this response. It is well-known that patients can lie about pain for financial gain, such as insurance fraud. So how scientific can pain be as gold standard if it is untestable, unreliable, referred, poorly localized, poorly quantified, imagined, vague, and lied about?

Referring to the Diagnostic Hierarchy for Orofacial Pain *(Figure 2)*, each condition has distinct diagnostic criteria. Pain without the criteria necessary for any diagnosis may be psychogenic. Pain in the presence of the appropriate diagnostic criteria constitutes a pathophysiological condition. This pathophysiologic condition in the absence of pain may or may not necessitate treatment. That decision is based on the clinical judgment of the doctor and the willingness and understanding of the patient to undergo treatment. Often this is based on risk/reward considerations and frequently on financial considerations. Decisions are often based on political factors rather than need, but the diagnosis does not change and should be based on scientific criteria.

Ethology

The process of scientific discovery often begins with an unexpected observation that forces researchers and/or clinicians to reconsider [their thinking relative to] existing theory and formulate new hypotheses that better explain their findings. Koch's Postulates, Harvey's work on blood flow, Darwin's evolution, Fleming's penicillin are examples of ethological discoveries. Facts that can be well-established from observation, and hypotheses supported by evidence, become specific explanations. Accurate observations of human behaviors have proven invaluable in sound scientific research and diagnosis of disease.

It is a major point of this chapter that reliable methods such as clinical ethological study, using non-invasive objective measurement, may represent a far better investment of research funds than controlled epidemiological studies. Astute clinical observation aided and corroborated by objective measurement and new imaging methods offers significant promise for identifying the causes of masticatory diseases and disorders and susceptibility characteristics of patients.

For dentistry to advance in the management of masticatory disorders from an art to a science, a systematic approach to gathering and interpreting clinical evidence must be refined. Its elements must be consistent with those of basic sciences such as morphology, physiology, and biochemistry. This body of knowledge must be fed by relevant clinical research and, as a result, generate better strategies for identifying and solving problems in diagnosis and management of masticatory diseases and disorders.

Clinical Ethology

By coming to a dentist a patient asks to participate in the reproduced experiment that is dental care. They are asking, "Doctor, can you repeat your most successful results of past therapy on me?" Treatment of human beings demands a methodology capable of identifying and reproducing the conditions of past

THE RUBRIC SHEET

Patient Version

Patient Name ______________________ Age ________
Address ______________________
City, State, Zip ______________________
Tel ______________________ E-Mail ________
Dr (Name) ______________________
Address ______________________
City, State, Zip ______________________
Tel ______________________ E-Mail ________

Intensity of pain no pain mild moderate severe excruciating/unbearable variable
other ______________________

Quality of pain throbbing pulsating paroxysmal/sudden stabbing bright deep dull
pressure tight/vice-like twitching superficial radiating aching stabbing
distinct itching pricking tingling burning sharp
other ______________________

Common site/locations of pain maxilla temporal parietal occipital orbital
peri-orbital retro-orbital intra oral throat ear neck nose sinus tongue
forehead top of head mandibular shoulder localized spot pre-auricular
other ______________________

Pattern/flow of pain unilateral bilateral referred site specific
building/crescendo no pattern crosses midline diffuse
other ______________________

Length of time illness has been present days weeks months years
other ______________________

Duration of pain episodes seconds minutes hours days constant
variable ______________________

Frequency of pain steady/constant intermittent/recurrent/occasional infrequent
daily weekly monthly hours minutes increasing decreasing
other ______________________

Origin/source of pain infection inflammation/swelling myogenic osteogenic
muscle contraction vascular vasodilation odontogenic trauma neurogenic ligamentous
other ______________________

Onset Initiation (of pain) spontaneous triggered aura gradual
other ______________________

Figure 1. The Rubric Sheet.

Precipitating factors auto injury dental procedure medical procedure
none trauma systemic disease other ______________________________

Aggravating factors (of pain) face movement jaw movement tongue movement
malocclusion tension fatigue provocation time of day swallowing
head position body position activities foods chewing poor posture sleep disorder bowel movement
parafunctional habits yawning endocrine/hormonal systemic disorder psychological stress
other ______________________________

Mitigating factors (which alleviate pain) analgesic anesthetic injection
avoidance of function medication relaxation electrical modalities thermal modalities manual modalities
nothing works orthotic other ______________________________

Age of patient at onset child youth adolescent young adult middle age old age

Patient characteristics psychological stress family history male female
smoker alcoholic substance abuse overweight underweight eating disorder weight change intense
history of trauma history of surgery other ______________________________

Characteristic symptoms pain swelling dry mouth
nausea vomiting no pathosis ringing in ears restricted jaw movement
restricted neck movement numbness swallowing difficulty chewing difficulty dizziness loss of balance
burning tongue sensation of bite change other sensory changes stuffy ears
clenching/grinding and oral habits anxiety depression insomnia subjective hearing loss light sensitivity
muscle weakness muscle tightness clicking jaw other jaw sounds grating sounds in jaw
other ______________________________

Characteristic signs pain referred from trigger points hypermobility fever
autonomic dysfunction joint sounds neurological deficit diminished head motion diminished neck motion
diminished vertical jaw motion diminished lateral jaw motion deviation on jaw opening/closing
uncoordinated jaw motion motor deficit abnormal/excessive wear patterns on teeth skeletal assymetry
craniofacial assymetry muscle pain from palpation abnormal blood chemistry joint clicks crepitus
abnormal radiograph findings radiopaque radiolucent occlusal factors diminished protrusive movement
hypomobility positive intrameatal palpation
other ______________________________

Previous diagnostic tests/Treatment with positive results/Findings
biopsy local anesthetic injection electromyograph radiograph blood chemistry ☐ N/A
electrokinetic tracking sonograph CT scan MRI tomographs endoscopy
range of movement auscultation
other ______________________________

Previous diagnostic tests/Treatment with negative results/Findings: conservative
antibiotic orthotic thermal modalities manual modalities ☐ N/A
electrical modalities analgesic diet modification exercise other medication remove causative factor
trigger injection rest/relaxation other ______________________________

Figure 2
Diagnostic Hierarchy for Chronic Headache and Orofacial Pain

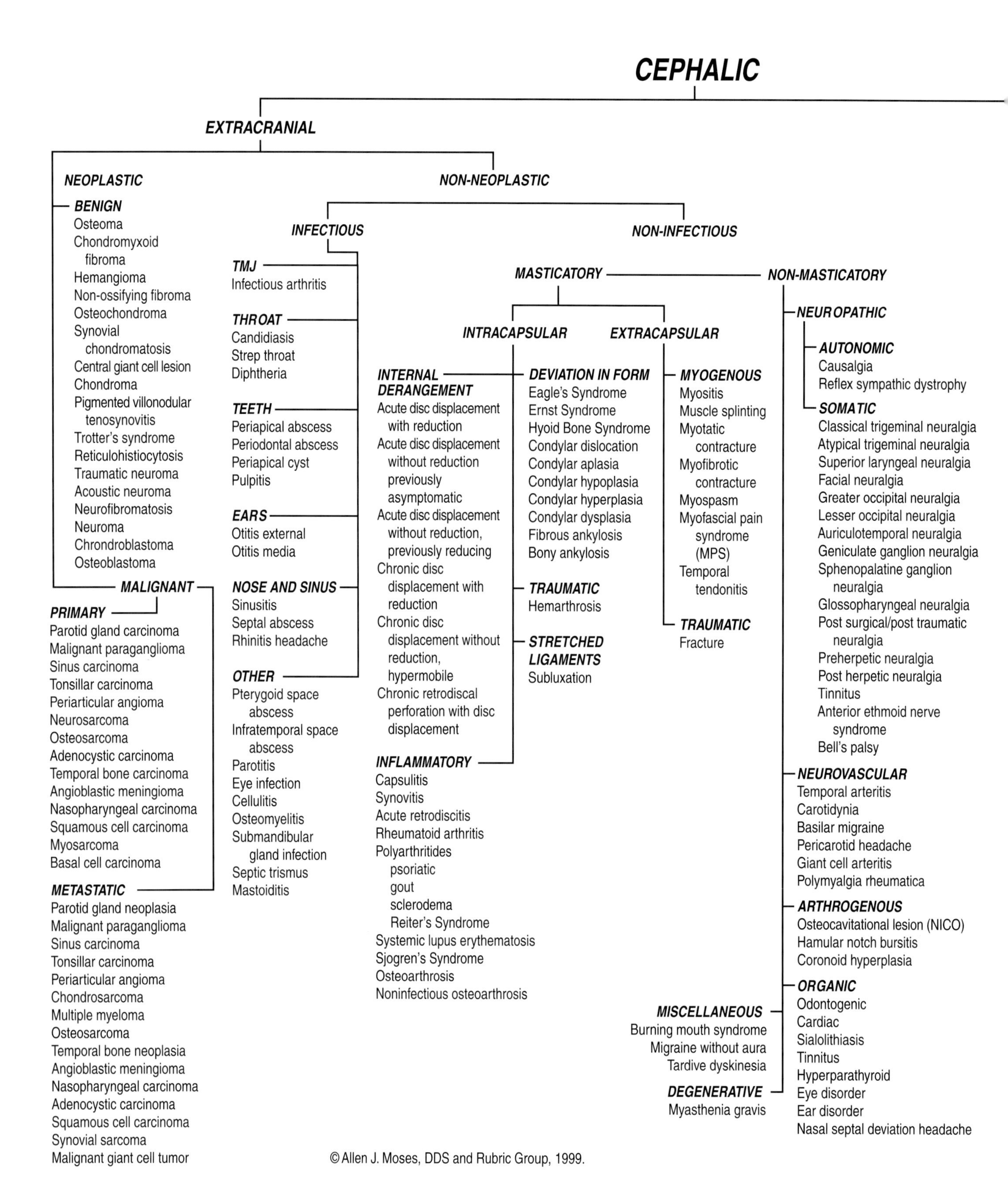

© Allen J. Moses, DDS and Rubric Group, 1999.

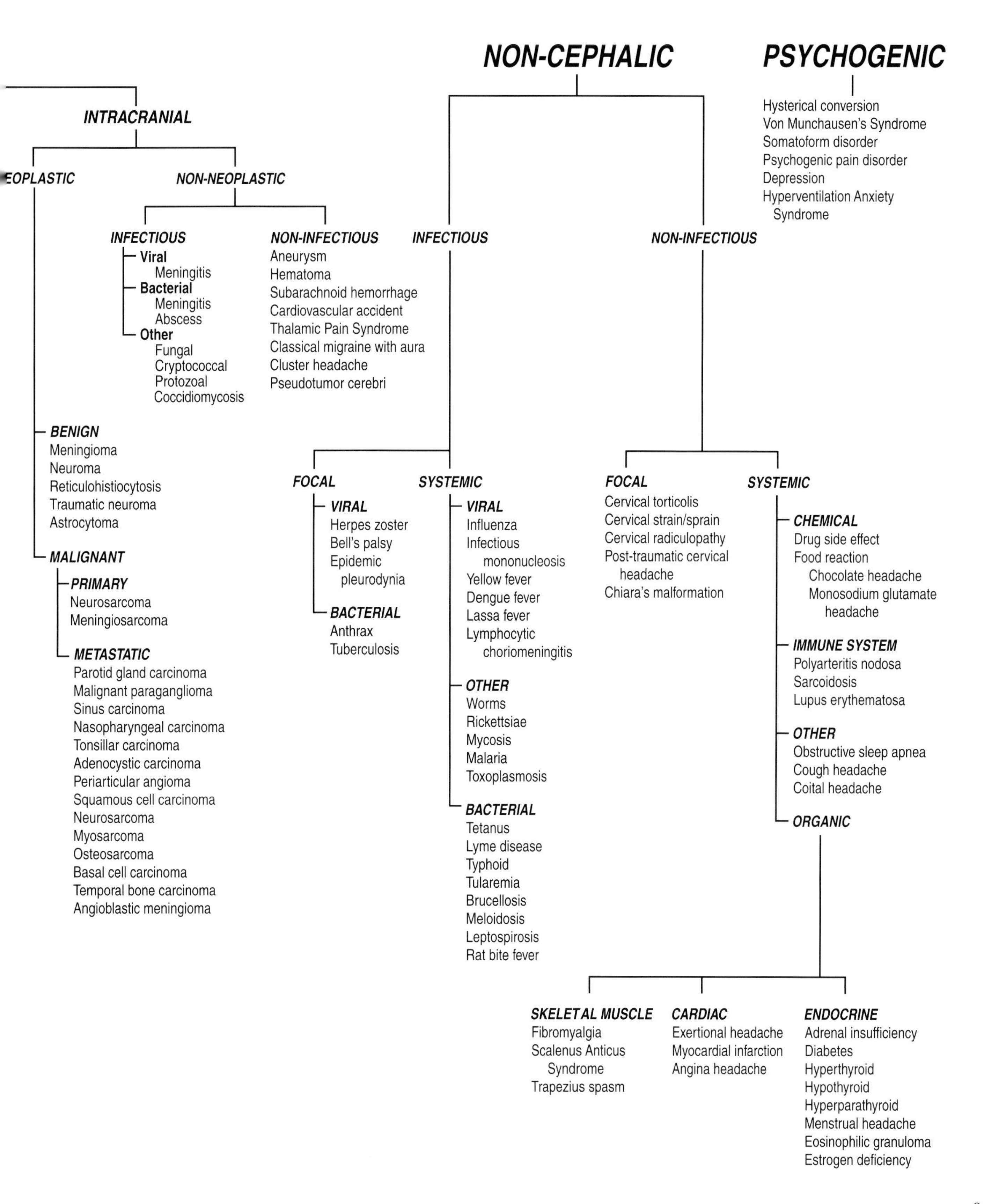
NON-CEPHALIC
PSYCHOGENIC
Hysterical conversion
Von Munchausen's Syndrome
Somatoform disorder
Psychogenic pain disorder
Depression
Hyperventilation Anxiety Syndrome
INTRACRANIAL
EOPLASTIC
NON-NEOPLASTIC
INFECTIOUS
Viral
Meningitis
Bacterial
Meningitis
Abscess
Other
Fungal
Cryptococcal
Protozoal
Coccidiomycosis
NON-INFECTIOUS
Aneurysm
Hematoma
Subarachnoid hemorrhage
Cardiovascular accident
Thalamic Pain Syndrome
Classical migraine with aura
Cluster headache
Pseudotumor cerebri
INFECTIOUS
NON-INFECTIOUS
BENIGN
Meningioma
Neuroma
Reticulohistiocytosis
Traumatic neuroma
Astrocytoma
MALIGNANT
PRIMARY
Neurosarcoma
Meningiosarcoma
METASTATIC
Parotid gland carcinoma
Malignant paraganglioma
Sinus carcinoma
Nasopharyngeal carcinoma
Tonsillar carcinoma
Adenocystic carcinoma
Periarticular angioma
Squamous cell carcinoma
Neurosarcoma
Myosarcoma
Osteosarcoma
Basal cell carcinoma
Temporal bone carcinoma
Angioblastic meningioma
FOCAL
VIRAL
Herpes zoster
Bell's palsy
Epidemic pleurodynia
BACTERIAL
Anthrax
Tuberculosis
SYSTEMIC
VIRAL
Influenza
Infectious mononucleosis
Yellow fever
Dengue fever
Lassa fever
Lymphocytic choriomeningitis
OTHER
Worms
Rickettsiae
Mycosis
Malaria
Toxoplasmosis
BACTERIAL
Tetanus
Lyme disease
Typhoid
Tularemia
Brucellosis
Meloidosis
Leptospirosis
Rat bite fever
FOCAL
Cervical torticolis
Cervical strain/sprain
Cervical radiculopathy
Post-traumatic cervical headache
Chiara's malformation
SYSTEMIC
CHEMICAL
Drug side effect
Food reaction
Chocolate headache
Monosodium glutamate headache
IMMUNE SYSTEM
Polyarteritis nodosa
Sarcoidosis
Lupus erythematosa
OTHER
Obstructive sleep apnea
Cough headache
Coital headache
ORGANIC
SKELETAL MUSCLE
Fibromyalgia
Scalenus Anticus Syndrome
Trapezius spasm
CARDIAC
Exertional headache
Myocardial infarction
Angina headache
ENDOCRINE
Adrenal insufficiency
Diabetes
Hyperthyroid
Hypothyroid
Hyperparathyroid
Menstrual headache
Eosinophilic granuloma
Estrogen deficiency

successes. Every act of treatment is an experimental attempt to reproduce successful results of the past.

The clinician must contemplate previous patients with the same disease and whose characteristics resemble the patient being considered. This process is called "clinical experience." Understanding of that experience is "clinical judgment." A good clinician must evaluate the conditions associated with success or failure to decide how to improve future performance. Such method of investigation is called "retrospective study." The data for such study is patient records. This is the clinical use of ethologic methodology. It is scientific.

Clinicians are capable of correlating the knowledge gained from such retrospective studies with proper non-invasive measurement tools to find solutions to problems previously thought to be unsolvable and thus provide better care for sick people. A good clinician can benefit from any inanimate objective measuring device which improves his or her sensory acuity. It should be self-evident that scientific precision in making accurate diagnoses can be increased by improving the detail, accuracy, objectivity, and consistency of protocol in obtaining clinical data from patients.

Evidence-based Care

Information obtained from electromyography, electrosonography, and electrokinetic tracings analyzed properly in retrospective studies aid in assessing what a specific masticatory disease does to a patient and the effect treatment has on that disorder. This is scientific. It is the essence of evidence-based care.

A clinician whose sole measure of success is relief of pain does not know what was done to the patient to get that result. This is not scientific. It does not constitute evidence.

Human beings often have a strong desire to identify trends and infer causes which cannot be intellectually sustained. People often confuse correlation with causality. They often correctly identify certain parameters of a trend but wrongly assume something else happening simultaneously to be cause. It is important, therefore, to differentiate experiential learning from intellectual learning.

Intellectual learning is independent of emotion and is dominated by language, books, instruction, logic, and analysis. Science is the human intellectual effort to make sense out of nature. Science represents a medium for logical analytical resolution of conflicts between experiential learning, which is subjective and coincidental, and intellectual learning, which is meaningful and objective.

In our search for understanding of the diseases and disorders manifesting orofacial pain, this differentiation between intellectual learning and experiential learning is crucial. The U.S. Congress has established Federal Rules of Evidence[19] for use in the courts. Rule 702 states that the word "knowledge connotes more than just subjective belief or unsupported speculation." The ultimate test of scientific knowledge is whether it can be tested. Scientific methodology is based on generating hypotheses and testing them to see if they can be falsified. The criterion of refutability, testability, or falsibility is what distinguishes science from pseudoscience.

Evidence vs. Inference

Evidence has been defined variously as the means by which a fact is established; a body of facts on which a proof is based; and facts that tend to clarify, support, or prove a point in question. Inference is a probable conclusion, not based on deduction, but loose usage, experience, or statistical correlation. Inference does not absolutely establish a premise but constitutes a demonstration of probability.

"Circumstantial evidence" is events and occurrences which establish reasonable grounds by which a fact is substantiated. Circumstantial *evidence* is an example of inference. It is considered soft rather than hard evidence.

Epidemiology is another example of inference. Epidemiology is concerned with the incidence of a disease in populations. It addresses whether an agent can cause a disease, not whether it did cause any one patient's disease. Specific causation is beyond the domain of the science of epidemiology. It is a soft science based on manipulation of statistics.

There is often confusion between correlation and causality based on subjective experience. The vast majority of correlated sequences cannot be causally related. The study of TMD is overladen with experiential subjective beliefs.

There are those such as Greene,[20] Mohl,[4] and LeResche[3] who advocate pain as a gold standard for the diagnosis of TMD. Pain is a presumption, however, which is untestable, unfalsifiable, unmeasurable, and unreliable, and therefore must be considered unscientific as criterion for research. Inferential use of such statistics must be regarded as weak and very soft science. Epidemiologic studies of TMD based on statistical manipulation of pain complaint is really pushing the limits of scientific reasonableness.

We are often led to believe that natural systems conform to a Bell Curve. "Normal" has been defined by Gaussian distribution or the Bell Curve as we know it. Researchers leave out two standard deviations at each end of the Bell and define normal as the 95% in the middle of the curve. This usage begs the question, "What value can there be in definition of normal relative to TMDs in which extremes of good health are as abnormal as extremes of bad health?" If the occurrence of any such disease were greater than 5%, normal controls in epidemiological studies could be both symptomatic and complainant. Such a definition of normal is also contrary to a defined purpose of epidemiology, which is to discover the distribution of diseases in populations, not define it. In reality, few biological problems conform to a Bell Curve, and TMD is one that does not. Basing evaluation of treatment efficacy for any patient on reliance of statistics and results of double-blind controlled studies from the dental literature defines "inference" not "evidence." The United States Federal Judicial Center recently published *The Reference Manual on Scientific Evidence.*[21] It establishes that epidemiologic double-blind studies cannot prove causation. Based *not* on individual case study, but on representative samplings, such studies cannot ascertain very small effects. They address whether an agent can cause a disease or a treatment might work, not whether it did cause a disease or will work for treatment. There is no logically rigorous definition of what a statement of probability means with reference to an individual instance. Interpretation and manipulation of epidemiologic statistics does not constitute scientific evidence or explanation; it is *inference.*

Epidemiology and double-blind controlled studies on TMD are being challenged. Normal has never been unequivocally defined, and there are not two well-delineated states such as diseased and disease-free relative to masticatory diseases and disorders. TMD is not one disease entity but a grouping of many different conditions (now known as masticatory diseases and disorders). In virtually all epidemiological research, TMD has been studied as a group entity, so the results are meaningless. Pain as a gold standard is unscientific. It is irrefutable, having no testable, observable, or measurable phenomenology. Psychometric testing based on the patient's self-report of pain has never been proven to be more appropriate than objective physiologic measurement of the study of TMD phenomenology. No double-blind study based on pain can possibly be considered hard scientific *evidence.*

Fortunately, hard scientific evidence is available to aid in documenting the physiologic status of our patients, advancing our understanding of temporomandibular disorders and guiding doctors toward better patient care. Intellectual learning is alive and well in the diagnosis and treatment of orofacial pain.

Evidence-based care is being practiced by many clinicians. Using non-invasive, objective, electronic measurement such as electromyography, electrosonography, and electrokinetic range of motion tracings[22,23], doctors are now able to confirm the status of the musculoskeletal facial pain patient before, during, and after treatment. Thus one can accurately evaluate what was done to the patient to get the result. This is *evidence.* The validity construct and ethological methodology for clinical study are well established in the scientific literature.[24-30]

Relative to making a differential diagnosis in masticatory diseases and disorders, objective electronic measurement can aid in:

- judging the severity of the disorder
- strengthening the diagnostic hypothesis
- predicting the prognosis
- estimating the responsiveness to alternative therapies in the future
- determining the response to present therapy

These instruments are FDA-approved for safety and have earned the ADA seal for accuracy of their measurement. When non-invasive instrumentation is used:

- There is no variation in the senses of the examiner
- There is no tendency to record inference
- There is never entrapment by prior expectations

Is There a Causal Relationship Between Malocclusion and TMD?

The proper approach to this disagreement should now be obvious. With TMD no longer considered an appropriate diagnosis, then the question properly rephrased becomes "Could there be or is there a causal relationship between malocclusion and any of the 24 specific masticatory diseases and disorders?" Any respectable scientist would study the *evidence* presented on each of the 24 problems, listed on the Hierarchy *(Figure 2),* on an individual basis to answer the question appropriately. Broken down to this level of specificity, a causal relationship can be demonstrated such that successful occlusal management of certain myogenous problems results in repeatable improvement of relevant measurable parameters and symptoms.[31-42]

References

1. Stohler CS: Epidemiology and Natural Progression of Muscular Temporomandibular Disorder Conditions. NIH Technology Assessment Conference on Management of Temporomandibular Disorders. Bethesda, MD: April 29–May 1, 1996;37-39.

2. Marbach, JJ, Raphael KG: Future Directions for Advancing Treatment of Chronic Musculoskeletal Facial Pain, NIH Technology Assessment Conference on Management of Temporomandibular Disorders. Bethesda, MD: April 29–May 1, 1996; 117-120.

3. LeResche, L: Assessing Physical and Behavioral Outcomes of Treatment, NIH Technology Assessment Conference on Management of Temporomandibular Disorders. Bethesda, MD: April 29–May 1, 1996;41-45.

4. Mohl ND, Dixon CD: Current status of diagnostic procedures for temporomandibular disorders. *J Am Dent Assoc* 1994;125(1):56-54.

5. Costen JB: Syndrome of ear and sinus symptoms dependent on disturbed function of the temporomandibular joint. *Am J Otol Rhinol Laryngol* 1934 43:1-5.

6. Selye H: *The Stress of Life.* New York: McGraw-Hill, 1955.

7. Dworkin SF: Perspectives on the interaction of biological, psychological and social factors in TMD. *J Am Dent Assoc* 1994;125:856-863.

8. Bell WE: *Temporomandibular Disorders. 3rd Ed.* Chicago: Yearbook Medical Publishers, 1990.

9. *Gould's Medical Dictionary. 4th Ed.* New York: Grove Hill Pub; 1979;399.

10. Okeson JP: *Orofacial Pain: Guidelines for Assessment, Diagnosis, and Management.* Chicago: Quintessence Publishing Co., Inc., 1996.

11. Pertes RA, Gross SG: *Clinical Management of Temporomandibular Disorders and Orofacial Pain.* Chicago: Quintessence Publishing Co., Inc., 1995.

12. Friction JR, Kroening RJ, Hathaway KM: *TMJ and Craniofacial Pain: Diagnosis and Management. 1st Ed.* St. Louis: Ishiyaku EuroAmerica, Inc., 1989.

13. Bell WE: *Orofacial Pain: Differential Diagnosis. 2nd Ed.* Chicago: Yearbook Medical Publishers, Inc., 1979.

14. Kaplan AS, Issael LA: *Temporomandibular Disorders: Diagnosis and Treatment.* Philadelphia: W.B. Saunders Co., 1991.

15. Shankland WE: Craniofacial pain syndrome that mimic temporomandibular disorders. *Ann Acad Medicine.* Singapore 1995;24(1):82-112.

16. Faust D: *The Limits of Scientific Reasoning.* Minneapolis: University of Minnesota Press, 1984.

17. *National Institute of Health Technology Assessment Conference Statement on Management of Temporomandibular Disorders.* Bethesda, MD: Draft of May 2, 1996.

18. Horal J: The clinical appearance of low back disorders in the city of Gothenberg, Sweden—Comparisons of incapacitated probands with matched controls. *Acta Orthop Scand* 1969;18(1):109.

19. *Federal Rules of Evidence,* United States Congress.

20. Greene CS, Marbach JJ: Epidemiologic studies of mandibular dysfunction: A critical review. *J Prosthet Dent* 1982;48(2):184-190.

21. *Federal Judicial Center: Reference Manual on Scientific Evidence.* St. Paul, MN: West Publishing Co., 1994.

22. Myotronics—Noromed, Inc. 15425 53rd Ave., South Tukwila, WA 98188

23. Bio Research, Inc. 4113 Port Washington Rd. Milwaukee, WI 53212

24. Moses AJ: *Controversy in Temporomandibular Disorders: Clinicians' Guide to Critical Thinking.* Chicago: Futa Book Publishers, 1997.

25. Moses AJ: Scientific methodology in temporomandibular disorders. Part II Ethology. *J Craniomandib Pract* 1994;12:190-193.

26. Tinbergen N: Ethology and stress diseases. *Sciences* 1974;185:20-27.

27. Feinstein AR: Scientific methodology in clinical medicine, I. Introduction, principles and concepts. *Ann Int Med* 1964;61(3):564-569.

28. Feinstein AR: Scientific methodology in clinical medicine, II. Classification of human disease by clinical behavior. *Ann Clin Med* 1964;61(4):757-781.

29. Feinstein AR: Scientific methodology in clinical medicine, III. Evaluation of therapeutic response. *Ann Clin Med* 1964:61(5):944-65.

30. Feinstein AR: Scientific methodology in clinical medicine, IV. Acquisition of clinical data. *Ann Clin Med* 1964;61(5):1162-1194.

31. Cooper BC: The role of bioelectric instrumentation in the documentation and management of temporomandibular disorders. *Oral Surg Oral Med Oral Path Oral Rad Endod* 1997;83:91-100.

32. Sheikholeslam A, Moller E, Lous I: Postural and maximal activity in the elevators of the mandible before and after treatment of functional disorders. *Scand J Dent Res* 1982;90:37-46.

33. Chong-San S, Hui-Yun W: Postural and maximum activity in elevators during mandible pre- and post-occlusal splint treatment of temporomandibular joint disturbance syndrome. *J Oral Rehab* 1989;16:155-161.

34. Helkimo E, Carlsson GE, Carmeli Y: Bite force in patients with functional disturbances of the masticatory system. *J Oral Rehab* 1975;2:397-406.

35. Crain JR, Klemons IM: EMG: comparisons in craniofacial muscles following therapy for head and neck pain. *Med Electr* 1988;106-110.

36. Gervais RO, Fitzsimmons GW, Thomas NR: Masseter and temporalis electromyographic activity in asymptomatic, subclinical, and temporomandibular joint dysfunction patients. *J Craniomandib Pract* 1989;7(1):52-57.

37. Riise C, Sheikholeslam A: The influence of experimental interfering occlusal contacts on the activity of the anterior temporal and masseter muscles during mastication. *J Oral Rehab* 1984;11:325-333.

38. Riise C, Sheikholeslam A: The influence of experimental occlusal contacts on the postural activity of the anterior temporal and masseter muscles in young adults. *J Oral Rehab* 1982;9:419-425.

39. Sheikholeslam A, and Riise C: Influence of experimental interfering occlusal contacts on the activity of the anterior temporal and masseter muscles during submaximal and maximal bite in the intercuspal position. *J Oral Rehab* 1983;10:207-214.

40. Humsi ANK, Naeije M, Hippe JA, Hansson TL: The immediate effects of a stabilization splint on the muscular symmetry in the masseter and anterior temporal muscles of patients with craniomandibular disorder. *J Prosthet Dent* 1989;62:339-343.

41. Ingervall B, Carlsson GE: Masticatory muscle activity before and after elimination of balancing side occlusal interference. *J Oral Rehab* 1982;9: 183-192.

42. Sheikholeslam A, Holmgren K, Riise C: A clinical and electromyographic study of the long-term effects of an occlusal splint on the temporal and masseter muscles in patients with functional disorders and nocturnal bruxism. *J Oral Rehab* 1986;13:137-145.